BE THE BEST YOU CAN BE IN SPORT

A BOOK FOR IRISH YOUTH

By Paul Kilgannon.
With insights from many of Ireland's
top coaches and sportstars

Published by Book Hub Publishing with Offices in Galway and Limerick.

First Edition 2020

Book Design and Layout:
Declan Durcan, Cloontubrid, Ross, Castlebar, County Mayo.
+353 (0)86 2658038 decdurcan@gmail.com

Cover Illustrator: David Sweeney
ISBN: 9 781838 169138

www.bookhubpublishing.com

(091) 846953   (087) 2246885
Twitter: @bookhubpublish
Instagram: bookhub_publishing
For further information re international distribution contact
info@bookhubpublishing.com

Paul Kilgannon may be booked to speak or present on the themes of the book
by contacting Paul Kilgannon at
www.CarverCoachingFramework.com
or (086) 3304062.

Contents

Thanks

To the multiple contributors for saying 'Yes', sharing their story, and giving of their time and energy. I hope you are proud of your contribution and I am very grateful to you for coming with me on this book journey.

For helping with contributors - some of whom came off, some of whom didn't: Kieran Shannon, Philip Murphy, Kieran McDermott, Ciarán Mollahan, Rob Dolan, Mícháel Fahy, David Matthews, Pascal Kellaghan, Phillip Lanigan, Sylvia Gee, Derry McVeigh, Damien Joyce, Sharon O'Connor, Jack Coyne, Ruadhán Cooke, Paul Kelly, David McHugh.

For feedback, input and opinion: Mark Finlay, Fran Keenan, Alan Moran, Ciara O'Flynn, Shane Keegan, Michael Hannon Jr., Conor Walsh, Keith Duggan, Ava Sheehan, Joe Canney, Christy O'Connor, Anthony Watson, Fiona Morley and Stephen Behan.

To Barry Smith for the incredible level of detailed feedback and direction he gave me.

To Brendan Egan for helping me to pull some of the pieces of this book together.

To David Sweeney for the top class illustrations. Thanks for being so diligent and a pleasure to work with.

To Éanna Shalvey and Dhani McGuire for their great work on the videos that accompany this book. Also to Sean O'Flynn, Aoibhe O'Flynn and Dáithí Mac Ginley for their help here too.

To the lads in Grafton Digital for their help with various bits and pieces.

To Paul Burns for saying, "I'll help you in any way I can" and following through on it.

To Irish Examiner Archive for contributing the beautiful image of George O'Connor free of charge.

To Sportfile for many of the photographs throughout the book.

To Niall and Susan in Book Hub Publishing for doing their thing and making this book happen.

To my comrades in Carnmore Hurling Club. Viva La Reds Forever!

To my family and friends for forgiving me for often not being there…even when I'm there.

To my mother, Joan Kilgannon, for supporting me and enabling me to work hard when I need to.

To my dear Lauren for helping me in this. For reading through it, correcting my many typos and mistakes, and for being there when I was struggling. My sincere hope is that someday I can return the favour for you. Go do it Loz! Love P x

Dedication

This book is dedicated to the memory of the late Enda Flaherty.
Enda was a man who cared for others and lived a life of truth, courage and conviction. He was a sportsman, a gentleman, a teacher, a coach and so much more. He embodied all that is good about sport, and life.
His advice to you would be to find joy through sport.

Rest in Peace 'Fla'. Your memory will live on.

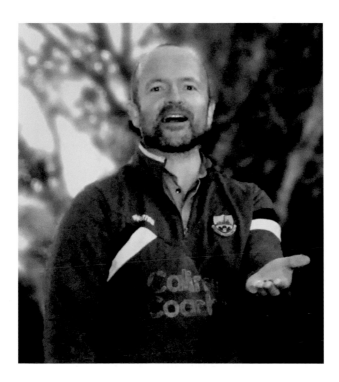

JIGSAW
Young people's
health in mind

A percentage of the proceeds raised from this book
is being donated to Jigsaw.

Our Vision

We are Jigsaw and our vision is an Ireland where young people's mental health is valued and supported.

We work towards achieving this vision in three ways:

1. We Influence Change

   We use our experience and knowledge to create a more supportive environment for young people. By working together with our partners, we want to secure changes to awareness levels, policies and funding to advance our vision for the mental health of Ireland's young people.

2. We Strengthen Communities

   We believe in a community-based, holistic approach. We cannot achieve our vision without the active involvement of communities across Ireland. To make essential change happen, we want to inform, support, and educate everyone across Ireland about young people's mental health.

3. We Deliver Services

   We continue to grow and develop our youth mental health services and supports. We want to ensure that we are there for all young people when they need us most. We offer a listening ear, and give expert mental health advice and support, to young people. We give families, teachers, and those who support young people, ways to cope and skills to be there for young people.

To see how Jigsaw can support you visit www.jigsaw.ie

Introduction

My name is Paul Kilgannon. I have spent a large portion of my adult life practicing, learning and studying coaching in sport. It has been a challenging endeavour. As a coach, you try to help those in your care. Often, you feel inadequate and inept. Human performance is a vast and complex subject. Trying to connect with every individual athlete at a human level, and working with them, in order to help them get the best out of themselves. The prudent coach's dream athlete is always the one that is in constant endeavour to become the best version of themselves.

Sports can be divided into collective (team) and individual categories, and my hope is that this book will be of use to teenagers across all sporting disciplines. Many similar fundamentals and principles apply across all sports. This is a book about principle based learning and improvement. Excellence is excellence, no matter the domain. High performers across domains are defined more by their similarities than their differences.

Whether coaching collective or individual sport, the true nature of coaching lies in coaching the individual. If we can get the best out of the individual in collective sport, the team will take care of itself. In coaching, rather than focusing on building teams, it is more prudent to build people and understand that these people will go on to build the team. The biggest challenge in coaching collective sport can often be delivering valid and meaningful feedback to the individual. Often we end up giving generic, collective feedback. We can struggle to get to the core needs of the individual.

I spent a large part of the last few years of my life writing a coaching book. As I was nearing its end, the outline of this new book began to appear in my mind. I wanted to create a book full of information, insights and inspiration for Irish youths to practice self-improvement and self-coaching in sport and beyond. It is my hope that the principles of this book transcend sport.

We live in the age of easily accessible information. With an abundance of information, comes an abundance of misinformation. The challenge is always: what information can I trust and what is the right information for me, at this point in my sporting journey? I hope this book will provide you with a worthwhile and practical tool. Sport, and indeed life, is a journey. We are all at different stages in the journey, but I hope there is much in this book to help you find your way.

As human beings, our lives, sporting and otherwise, are hugely influenced by the environment which surrounds us. By this I mean factors such as: our family, our school, our peer group, our sporting clubs and coaches. In negative undertones, you could say we can be a victim to our geography or our environment and the supports that surround us. In a sporting context, you may be very lucky and be part of a progressive club with a host of good people, expert coaches and professionals. As most of Ireland's sports clubs are run by very well meaning volunteers, it is unrealistic to expect this.

To optimally support a young athlete in reaching their sporting potential requires multiple professional inputs. There is a call for the input of expert professionals across athletic development, skill acquisition, sports psychology, sport nutrition and beyond. These inputs can allow you to become more efficient and intelligent in your approach. Again, it can be said it is unreasonable to expect such infrastructures to be in place country-wide. As with everything in life, circumstances offer us all different hands.

In this book I will try to provide a solution to this. I have enlisted the help of a number of learned and trusted academics and professionals, as well as some of Ireland's most respected athletes and coaches across a wide variety of sports. These contributors have great information, insights and advice to offer you, and interesting and inspiring stories to tell.

I want this book to be simple, yet comprehensive, thought provoking and useful. It is designed as an aid for continuous learning and personal development in sport. I am fully aware that this is a book that will challenge you in many ways. Some of you will struggle with it, but that is ok; after all - the struggle is the pathway. I see it as a book you might read, and then reread various parts again and again. You will need to reread many pieces, and each time you do so, you will get a deeper appreciation of the content.

For you, it is not about maximising every area in the book. It is about prioritising what you feel can work well for you. It is about maximising certain qualities in order to optimise learning, development and ultimately performance. If you have little interest in a particular subject area, or find it beyond you at this point, simply move on and you can return to it in time.

I have broken the book into 3 distinct parts and it could be said that it is 3 books in 1:

- Part 1 focuses primarily on performance related topics.
- Part 2 focuses on sports science type content.
- Part 3 focuses on lifestyle and pastoral orientated content with an emphasis on balance, holism and wellbeing.

Rather than aiming to take all the information on board, you can use the content as a menu to aid continuous improvement and self-discovery. This is a book that aims to both challenge and serve you for the duration of what I hope will be a long and fulfilling sporting career. There is a lifetime of learning in this book.

One thing I certainly don't want this book to be is a jumped up 'you can do anything you set your mind to' type book. It cannot be denied that elite level sport requires a baseline level of talent. For every individual that 'makes it' in sport, there are thousands of the hard luck stories. However, we all have dreams and it's certainly not my job to tell you to be 'realistic'. Instead, my purpose is to offer you the skills and tools that can help you chase that dream, if you so wish. It simply cannot be denied that as a human race we would accomplish much more, if we did not think things to be impossible.

This is a book for you in sport. This is your book. This is not a book about comparison. Comparing yourself to others very often leads to unhappiness. The only great person and athlete you can be is the greatest version of yourself. You are enough.

This book is my attempt at pulling together a guide that I believe can serve every young person in sport in Ireland, and beyond. It is an Irish book, by Irish coaches, for young Irish sportspeople. I believe it is a book worth writing, and I hope you deem it a book worth reading and using.

Be the best you can be,
Paul Kilgannon.

Note:

- For the purpose of consistency and clarity what we would traditionally call 'players' in many sports (not all sports are 'played') will frequently be referred to as 'athletes'.
- This is a book for youths from approximately 13 years and upwards. There is no 'correct' age for readers; when the athlete is ready, this book will be there. A certain level of maturity is required of the reader. Similarly, you will never be too old for this book.
- This book can be read alone, or in conjunction with teammates, in order to stimulate discussion and further learning. A useful idea would be for a team to read it in unison, over the course of a season, and hold structured discussions weekly, on a chapter-by-chapter basis.
- For the purpose of differentiation and acknowledgement, all contributions other than those of the book's author, Paul Kilgannon, will be written in Italics.

PART 1

This section of the book is designed to educate you in a number of areas that will allow you apply yourself in sport, focus on improvement and learn how to perform to the best of your ability.

Paul Kilgannon.

CHAPTER 1 : THE VIRTUES OF SPORT

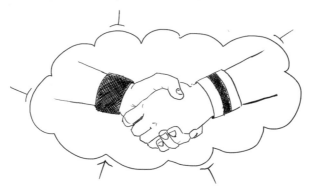

First Things First

If you haven't read the 'Introduction' of the book please take five minutes to do so. It includes information, and context, that is important for you to appreciate when reading what is to follow. If you have already done so…Read on!

The Ancient Greeks introduced formal sport to the world with the first Olympic Games, in Olympia in 776 BC. The Games remained the sporting, social and cultural highlight of the Ancient Greek calendar for almost 12 centuries. From its very inception, sport played a central and positive role in people's lives. Interestingly, from an Irish perspective, modern Irish folklore challenges the originality of the Greek Games and claims that the Tailteann Games started in Ireland around 1600 BC.

The majority of the sports we know and love today, only developed into their current form in the 19th and 20th centuries. For example, on 1st November 1884, a group of Irishmen gathered in Hayes' Hotel in Thurles and founded The Gaelic Athletic Association. In 1823, William Webb Ellis was the first man to pick up the oval ball and run with it, thus beginning the modern version of rugby; up until this point, the ball had been kicked forward as opposed to being carried. 1892 saw the first formal rules of basketball being drawn up, with the previous year, 1891, seeing the introduction of the penalty kick in football (soccer).

In historic times, many sporting endeavours revolved around the preparation for war, or training as a hunter. It involved the throwing of spears and rocks, as well as one-on-one wrestling and sparring. However, the modern iterations of sport were formulated for more peaceful, moral and pastoral reasons.

Any search for a definition of sport will uncover words such as 'physical exertion, skill, pleasure and play'. Sport, at its most morally praiseworthy, is a place of human endeavour. It is a place where learning and development comes about through challenge. Sport is a place to explore the limits of human potential and to maximise what we have been given. It is a place to express identity. The power of the human spirit to compete and excel is most beautifully demonstrated in the sporting arena.

There is beauty in sport. At its most moving and noble, it doesn't have to involve cups and medals. It provides the opportunity to both exhibit and develop great moral courage, to find enjoyment and connection. Sport brings people together; it connects, it unites. It is a means of communication which transcends language, race, religion and nationality. It enhances society. It can support people, lift them and guide them.

Sport provides endless opportunity, and opportunity is the mother of all learning and development. For me, the primary role of sport is to teach young people lessons for life. Sport should be a vehicle to help people 'get better' at life.

Sport is a place for you to learn about yourself on a number of levels. It gives us all the opportunity to test ourselves mentally, physically and emotionally, in a way no other aspect of life can. Sport adds to the wellbeing and health of people in communities. It is an antidote to laziness and a comfortable life; a preserver of physical, social and emotional health and wellbeing. Your body is designed to be active and sport gives it the perfect opportunity to realise this.

Sport brings order to our lives, builds character, teaches winning and losing. It is a place where 'failure' is inevitable. It gives us the opportunity to develop mental and physical resilience, self-discipline, self-control, personal responsibility and self-reliance. It imbues loyalty and brotherhood/ sisterhood. It develops interpersonal and communication skills, teamwork skills, as well as leadership qualities. Sport is built on cooperation. It is a spiritual thing.

We must now begin to attune your perspective on sport, and the opportunity it offers you. I often say to the athletes I coach that, in choosing sport, they are choosing to go down a road of struggle and suffering. This may sound dramatic, almost negative, but in many ways it is true. Bernard Suits, in his book, 'The Grasshopper: Games, Life and

Utopia', defines the playing of a game as "the voluntary attempt to overcome unnecessary obstacles". Again, this may sound severe, but there is truth to it. I feel it is important to appreciate the road to true achievement will be difficult, but please don't allow that difficulty to deter you from making the effort.

In writing this book for Irish youth in sport, I am seeking (to paraphrase the name of Marlo Thomas' famed book) to provide you with 'the right words, at the right time'. I am hoping this book can help you to get the best out of yourself in sport, while getting the best out of sport. I am obviously hoping that a large number of youths across the country will read it so my challenge is to have something for everyone in it: from the elite to the recreational, from the performance orientated to the participation orientated, from the gifted to the not so gifted. Not all prospective readers are going to be exceptional sportsmen and women, but sport is, and must be, for everyone and, therefore, this book should be for everyone.

"You are never really playing an opponent. You are playing yourself,
your own highest standards, and when you reach your limits.
That is real joy".
Arthur Ashe

My challenge is: can I write a book for every youngster in Irish sport? However, in your choosing to read this book, I have to make a number of assumptions. I have to assume you are interested in maximising your potential in sport to some degree. I have to assume that, to some degree, you are ready to invest in your sporting self, and I have to presume you are leaning towards the more performance-orientated side of the spectrum.

We will begin with you and your relationship with sport and I will commence with a number of questions. This book is full of questions and exercises that will help you create your 'sporting world' and draw your attention to what you feel is important. Self-coaching begins with facing the truth and becoming self-aware. Some of the questions may be challenging, but in sport and indeed in life, it is critical to develop the ability to reflect, and ask yourself difficult questions. Questions open the mind and bring clarity. In order to sacrifice, you must believe in what you are doing; there must be purpose and passion.

No one can give you the answers to the questions in this book. They can certainly help with some information, guidance and inspiration, but you must create your own 'sporting world'. I urge you to get a pen and take the time to complete them as you read through the book. I understand the human condition wants you to skip ahead, and continue on reading to 'find the answers'. Perhaps this may happen on first reading, and that is ok, but my hope is you will never be finished with this book. I am confident if you take the time to answer the questions, you will surprise yourself with the level of your answers, and the clarity they bring you. There are no right or wrong answers, and indeed your answers will change over time as you grow and evolve as an athlete.

We will begin by establishing why you play? Never forget your greatest contribution to sport, and indeed humanity, is your own self-realisation. Your motives will anchor your strength and drive your passion. Understanding meaning and purpose is critical. Clarity of purpose is key.

Note: while there may be spaces for you to write in this book, may I suggest you acquire your own journal and add your learnings and insights to it as you go- see Chapter 2. An exercise like this may be best suited to the front or back of your journal. This will allow you access them easily and take a moment daily, or maybe weekly, to read and review them.

WHY ARE YOU INVOLVED IN SPORT?

_____

_____

WHAT DOES SPORT MEAN TO YOU?

_____

_____

WHAT DOES YOUR INVOLVEMENT IN SPORT MEAN TO THOSE AROUND YOU?

_____

_____

OUT OF 10, HOW INTERESTED ARE YOU IN ACHIEVING YOUR POTENTIAL IN SPORT? _____

WHAT DO YOU WANT FROM SPORT? (Note, here I am not looking for medals and prizes as the answers. I am more looking at it from if you couldn't win the plaudits or succeed in the conventional sense; what would you want to gain from your involvement in sport?)

_____

_____

CHAPTER 1

Liam Moggan

Liam Moggan has been involved with coaching and coach development for over 40 years. He is affectionately known in Irish sport as 'The Coaches' Coach'. Liam has served in the background with numerous Irish teams and individual sporting successes across a diverse range of sports. He is recently retired from his role as Coach Educator in Coaching Ireland where he served with distinction. He has both an educated and truly unique insight into the value of sport and what it can offer you. I feel this insight is something that can be of great benefit to you. My advice is to read and reread this fabulous piece of writing. Enjoy!

A group of Kenyan athletes stayed in my home a few years ago. After their first meal, their young leader stood up and thanked my wife for making them "fed up!" It was a good meal and I've stretched my wife's patience by repeating that story many times! Words carry weight, they have meaning. And yet, we all carry a vocabulary of what I call 'words when we've nothing else to say 'words'. Those words stretch meaning. They lose context. They lose punch. Words can be dangerous.

Sport is one of those words. It covers a multitude and can be wrapped around so much it eventually means little. What is it? I've been involved in sporting activities all my life. I was an athlete. I played basketball. For years I worked as a Physical Education teacher. In another life I delivered Tutor Development courses for people educating coaches. I, too, am a coach. I walk. I cycle. Much of what I do falls under the umbrella of that ubiquitous term 'sport'. The most common description of sport is broad. It covers competitive and recreational activities. It includes traditional games as well as exercises aimed at improving physical fitness, health and well-being. It all sounds good; a word when we've nothing else to say 'word'.

Those wide descriptions miss what I believe is the very essence of sport. Let's be honest it is difficult to explain. I got involved in sport and stayed involved because of the experience, the feeling, the joy, the challenge, the company and the craic. How can a single word encompass all of that? Passion describes it best for me. Above all else, sport is about passion.

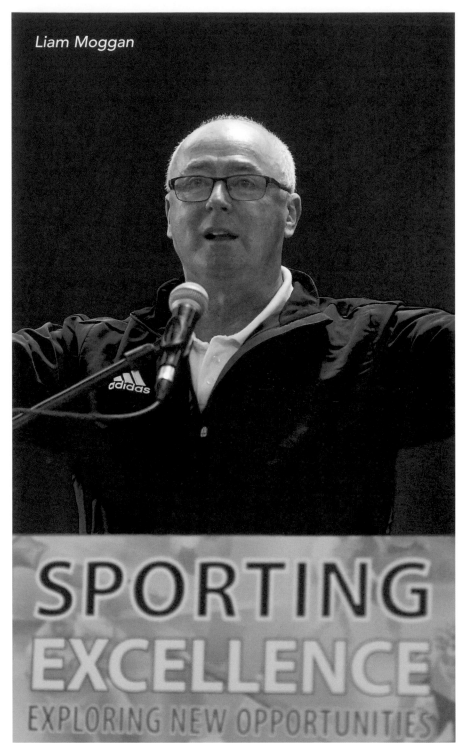

Liam Moggan

SPORTING EXCELLENCE
EXPLORING NEW OPPORTUNITIES

For me that passion started a long time ago. The Mossy Bank is a bowl cut out of the earth with soft grass for a carpet. It was at the bottom of McGrath's field. Behind it lay the railway line and the spires of Tuam's two Cathedrals guarded its side. We rarely walked to the Mossy Bank. It was a place to rush to.

If it was to be Croke Park the goals of the double ESB poles defined the Hill 16 end. For the Ryder Cup, bucket size holes were permanent fixtures near the edges. Olympic sprint finals were contested along the straight stretch near Farragher's field. A show jumping course of stonewall fences and leafy branches was a temporary fixture. Trains to the Sugar Factory provided perfect props for Cowboys and Indians.

The Mossy Bank was my first gym. We ran there. We strolled home. In between we jumped, tumbled, wrestled, rolled, sprinted, threw things and kicked footballs. We rested and chatted within its soft slopes. We had accidents. We fell and got hurt. Sometimes we had fights. Far enough from town and adults our imaginations ran free. It was anywhere or anything we wanted it to be. We were anyone we wanted to be. It was the best sports facility I've ever known. I loved the Mossy Bank.

I am one of the lucky ones. More formal competitive settings came along when I started to race and play basketball. I was passionate about those too. I developed an appreciation for new challenges and satisfaction in the mastery of new skills. There were friends again, sometimes fights again, sometimes accidents. It didn't always bring out the best in me. But imperceptibly, bit by bit there was improvement. Improvement in self-belief, movement skills and social skills. Mind, body and soul.

The sense of what I am today is shaped by those activities. The people I met and the places I visited contributed to make me who I am. I'm immensely grateful. The commitment, effort and dedication embedded then has stood to me all my life. Change is inevitable, improvement is earned by the sweat of one's brow. The sporting activities and good people I met helped me improve over time. There's no shortcut to improvement. Good things can happen and bad things can happen along the way, but improvement only comes about with hard work. True success is to labour.

Time spent acquiring skills that have absolutely no application outside of sport might seem to some like time wasted. Being able to run fast or dunk a basketball or kick a football has limited social value. Even if they have, time will diminish it. The best athletes slow down eventually.

Playtime can have added value when participants learn vital life skills and are encouraged to grow into fully-rounded, caring, human beings. Sport has potential to offer that.

Dedicated, committed adults played a significant part along the way. I was lucky to have supportive parents. I was blessed to meet Bro. Willie Morgan in secondary school who guided, nurtured and taught with patience and expertise. He helped create a climate where I was allowed to express myself, to extend myself and evolve my own style, my own personality. Sport shaped what I've become. Sport was and still is my passion. After all what's engraved in youth is engraved in stone.

Pat Duffy, a friend and colleague who was Director of the National Coaching Training Centre in Limerick and who sadly passed away a few years ago, led many innovative and effective programmes around the development of sport worldwide. Pat believed that sport had the potential to offer an experience such as mine to everyone. He was passionate that sport is not just for the talented, the champions, the big children and early developers. Pat saw sport as an enormous resource for good. He saw sport as a vibrant part of any decent society. Pat believed that there is an appropriate sporting activity for everyone. He had the foresight too to understand that in order to bring about improved participation levels we first must find the right way and a better way to explain and promote sport.

If others are to benefit as much as I have we must search for and find a right way and a better way. We need to encourage people to do something they enjoy rather than be better doing something than someone else. We need a climate that promotes learning rather than structures that make participants dependent; less about what coaches do and more about how people, particularly children and teenagers, learn.

All God's creatures have a place in the choir. We need to accommodate and encourage those who sing high and those who sing lower. Variety is key. Sport is for everyone. It is not just for those who conform to some predetermined body type or shape or age. If people want to participate they will. If they don't, they won't. It's all about the passion. We need to promote a love of movement, not sport. We should emphasise feel good factors, like self-belief, confidence, commitment and control, not just competition.
Sport is not always about sport. It can be about commerce and money

and sponsorship. Much of how it's promoted is about winning. National Governing Bodies have well-financed High Performance units that plan and prepare elite senior athletes for international competition. They have stolen the term 'high performance' as their own. It implies that what happens in clubs and gyms and fields and pitches and Mossy Banks all over the country every day is all well and good, but it's not high performance. It is too easy to discredit high performance everywhere by kidnapping words and labelling them to specific targeted areas. High performance sport can be experienced in many ways by many people and it starts in homes, clubs and communities.

In the Mossy Bank we played and in playing we became problem-solvers, risk-takers and innovators. We played. We designed rules and stuck to them. We included everyone. From those generations of active thinkers and active youngsters came an explosion of new ideas and innovation. From that environment grew a passion to stay active, a resilience to face the unknown, to face issues of right and wrong and to oftentimes extend ourselves beyond our comfort zone. From that environment grew many great sportspeople. Sport provided us with a background to trust our own initiative and to learn for ourselves.

Deep down we know that all kinds of sports are valuable. Banner events get attention. They catch the eye but there are examples everywhere. Let me share one. Near the end of a morning session of the Paralympic Games at the Olympic Stadium, London in 2012, a Men's 1500m heat took place. A runner who finished nearly 6 minutes behind the second to last competitor made an impression that will never leave me.

Houssein Omar Hassan from Djibouti was missing a right arm. At the start of the race he injured his right ankle. Yet he was determined to finish. Hassan never strayed from lane three, allowing faster runners the freedom of inside lanes. His progress was slow. As he moved around the track he was identified by name and as the only athlete from Djibouti competing at the Games. Gradually, each section of the 84,000 crowd stood in sequence to applaud and cheer. It was like a Mexican wave in slow motion. He finished in 11 mins. 23.50secs, the slowest 1500m I ever saw! It was not what we call high performance. Nor was it in tune with the Paralympic message of elite sportspeople competing on the world stage. Houssein Omar Hassan moved to a different beat. The spontaneous, spectacular outburst of applause was heartfelt. It was not patronising. So what was going on?

This impulsive expression of joy and admiration demonstrated that what was happening before us was something special, something genuine, something precious. We may not have been able to describe it, but we knew it was happening. 84,000 of us knew it! Such moments are not always palpable but when they happen, we know it. We sense it. This was one of those unforgettable moments. It felt wonderful. It was an honour to be there. Passion was abundant.

Somehow, someway, all the time, we must get those stories out there. Sport matters. Our country has a rich, proud tradition of sport. We need sporting heroes all the time. We need heroes that we can see and believe in and admire; heroes for the next generation to dream about and make-believe with down the Mossy Bank.

It is my dream that sport will reach beyond the formal and connect with a passion that exists in every person, home, club and community. Formal, top-down structures are petrified of passion and therein lies a real challenge. Sport is not meant to be about commerce and money and sponsorship. There must not be an institution of sport because sport by its nature cannot and should not be institutionalised. Localised is the way forward.

The prevalence of a 'winning' mentality has thrown an imbalanced spotlight on tangible assets. Leagues titles and championship medals have their place. I've been alongside winning teams and individuals and enjoyed being there. However, there is more to sport than records and results. Intangible assets like passion do not fit an institutional image because passion cannot be measured. Like sport, it's a feeling, an experience, a joy.
I love the Arts. They thrill me and contribute to my life every day. Sport does not have a monopoly on that kind of fix. However, our bodies are designed to move and within an active healthy body other joys are amplified.

The most common guidance offered down the Mossy Bank was to 'go in there and play any old how'. It was fierce liberating. It released me to be me, to do my best, to bring my own style, to make my own decisions, to enjoy myself. If future generations are to be liberated and to thank us for making them 'fed up' we need to up our game. We need to feed the passion of a new generation, feed their enthusiasm and integrate fun and enjoyment into the wonderful world of sport.

Miles to Run and Promises to Keep,
Liam Moggan.

SUMMARY POINTS - Chapter 1

- Sport is for everyone.
- There is more to sport than results and records.
- Sport can, and should, be an enormous resource for good.
- Sport can add much to your life.
- Understanding meaning and purpose is critical, in order for you to get the most out of sport.

CHAPTER 2: JOURNALING THE JOURNEY.

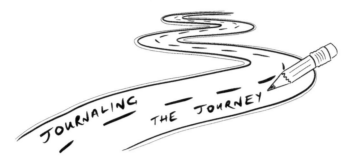

Before we go any further, I must address what I believe is a key learning and development tool namely: journaling. The practice of journaling has been around since humans first learned to write. Indeed, many of history's greatest minds including: Isaac Newton, Abraham Lincoln, Leonardo Da Vinci and Charles Darwin, all acknowledged and endorsed it as an essential habit. As a human race, we have long known about the benefits of writing about personal experiences, thoughts and feelings.

Athletes who espouse the value of journaling include Tennis player Serena Williams who has won, an Open era record, 23 Grand Slam singles titles.

"Writing down your feelings in a notebook or journal can help clear out negative thoughts and emotions that keep you feeling stuck".
Serena Williams

Others include, 28 time Olympic medallist Michael Phelps and renowned 'Free Solo' rock climber Alex Honnold who became the first person to scale the iconic 3,000-foot granite wall known as El Capitan, without using ropes or other safety gear. He is an obsessive note taker, who journals every workout and climb in great detail. Indeed, many of the athletes who have contributed to this book have reported journaling and note taking, as a key skill and habit.

For you, journaling can include comment and observation on any, or every, facet of your life, both sporting and otherwise. As we will see throughout this book, most of the various facets of your life are intertwined, and it is often the interaction between these different elements, that allow you to access your sporting ability at a higher level. To this end, your journal can be as sport, or life orientated as you please. Journaling improves and develops your most potent athletic asset, your mind. It can provide you with a place to: set goals, reflect on experiences, gain insight, celebrate successes, make sense of setbacks, as well as track and record important training information. Journaling improves your relationship with yourself, as it facilitates introspection and drives self-awareness. Journaling is an excellent self-development tool to help you 'keep the most important things, the most important things'.

The challenge of sport, and indeed life, is to get better at getting better, and journaling is one of the most effective means to allow you to consciously, and actively, reflect and learn as you go. Non-judgemental reflection is a process of self-discovery; as we discover ourselves we are creating ourselves. By non- judgemental reflection I mean being level-headed and fair in your self- critique and not being overly self-critical or harsh. Journaling can make you more conscious of your thoughts and more intentional with your actions. Throughout the chapters of this book you will see me advise you to, 'add this or that', to your journal, so I will briefly give an overview on journaling, and what it might entail for you.

What is Journaling?

Journals can come in many formats, shapes and sizes. Keeping a diary, or a training log, are similar concepts and come under the umbrella of journaling. Physically, they can take the shape of a hardback notebook, a 'page a day' type diary, or anything of that nature. I suggest you invest in a quality one, with a drawstring closing mechanism. Indeed, you can actually keep two; one for more diary type, day to day scheduling and planning (see Chapter 21), and one for journaling type reflection, learning practices, and introspection. I believe this to be the best format, but feel free to be creative and learn as you go.

One format of journaling is simply noting random observations about daily events, happenings or learnings. For a more life-focused style of journaling, simple questions, or journaling prompts, can also be used and completed at the end of each day. For example:

- What were the positive things that I am grateful for today?
- What did I do well today and why?
- What could I have done better today and how?
- What relationships did I strengthen/ weaken today and why?
- Did I take care of my priorities today?
- What did I learn or relearn today?
- What do I need to start / stop / continue doing?
- Did I work towards my goals today?
- Was I true to my personal values today and how?

Simple questions can be a powerful journaling and reflective tool, and we will see this throughout the book. Maybe pick three or four of your favourites from above. Vary and change your questions or prompts if, and when, a new stimulus is needed. Google journaling ideas and prompts for further ideas. Effective journaling can be very structured, quick and to the point, or it can be more free flowing and therapeutic. There is no 'wrong way' to journal. It is a relatively simple habit.

Journaling and note taking can be a great help when it comes to tracking goals, prioritising things, monitoring athletic progress, and measuring or tracking skill levels. It can also be a great confidence tool, as you can go back and relive previous accomplishments, written in your journal. Training and nutrition logs, can be included to help drive improvement. Honest and precise, post competition reflections can be incorporated to drive learning. Journaling can help unlock knowledge and energy.

How and Where to Begin
Start small. Don't make a huge commitment. Commit to journaling for 30 days. If you miss a day or two don't worry, simply get back to it. Spend five to 10 minutes a day reflecting. After the 30 days are up, go back and review what you've learned. You will see the progress you have made, leading to greater self-confidence, and improved development and performances.

It must be noted that journaling can be something people struggle to sustain over long periods. Rather ironically, the busier you are and the more you need it, the harder it can be to include it in your everyday practice. However I must double down here and urge you to focus on it as a critical learning and support tool for sport and indeed life. Aim for five to 10 minutes of uninterrupted time daily, ideally at the same time every day.

Journal the journey. Build your 'sporting world'. Consciously and actively learn and develop as you go.

(Note: Throughout this book, I advise certain content to be placed at the front or back of your journal, so you can access it with ease and review it frequently. This content may include: values and priorities, core principles, key habits, personal definitions and mantras and so on. If you prefer to journal digitally, OneNote or Evernote are good tools that can be accessed via phone or computer.)

See Appendix for sample journal.

Stuart Lancaster

Stuart Lancaster is the Senior Coach with Leinster Rugby. Prior to this he was England RFU's Head of Elite Player Development before being appointed England Head Coach where he served for four years. He is a respected leader in the fields of coaching, leadership and player development. Here he shares with you what he feels is the value of journaling and writing things down.

I will begin with a story to bring to life the point I wish to make. My family live in Leeds, and I work in Dublin coaching Leinster Rugby. For the last four years I've commuted backwards and forwards, driving my car from training, leaving it at the airport, flying to Leeds, getting a taxi home and then returning the following day. Many times I have arrived back into Dublin airport and found myself thinking...where did I park my car?!

What I do now to avoid this is when I have parked my car, I walk into the departures area at the airport and write down the bay where I have parked. This ensures I recall it twice in my mind, as well as writing it down. Now, every time I arrive back in Dublin, sometimes after a day or two off, I always remember.

The process of memory recall is critical in life, but also in sport.

There are many times I am delivering meetings at Leinster packed full with information. Some of it is logistical: where we need to be, why we need to be there, here is the plan for the future etc. Some of it is technical: here is the game plan, here is the review, here are the attacking sequences we want to use etc.

It amazed me how many players used to turn up to these meetings without a journal or a notebook. If you don't write anything down, you have nothing to refer back to, nothing to recall. I guarantee you players who make notes, write things down, constantly look ahead, reflect on experiences, ask themselves appropriate questions and intentionally plan their future development, make much more of their potential than players that don't. They are simply clearer in their thoughts and more focused on what's important.

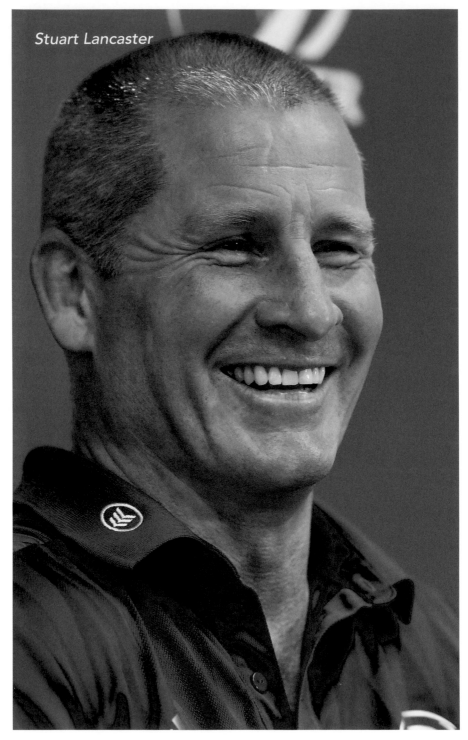

Stuart Lancaster

Journaling is key to success. It can take many forms and cover a wide variety of content: information, thoughts, reflections, learnings, planning and so on. I simply can't stress strongly enough its value as a learning and personal development practice.

Somebody once described that successful leaders have the ability to lead with a telescope and a microscope. So they have the ability to see and plan into the future, yet they have the ability to see the detail also, just like a great player should. There is simply no way I could lead and coach in a club like Leinster without my journal, and the many notes that I make.

The notes are the one thing that I constantly refer back to, and the journal is where I am constantly planning ahead. By having these notes, I have something to recall and it becomes hard wired in my mind so I don't forget really important information, just like where I have parked my car!

Best wishes,
Stuart Lancaster

SUMMARY POINTS - Chapter 2

- Journaling and notetaking help bring clarity and focus.
- Journaling can provide you with a place to: set goals, reflect on experiences, gain insight, celebrate successes, make sense of setbacks, track and record important training information, as well as plan, ponder and question.
- Journaling comes in many different forms and styles.
- Journals can come in many formats, shapes and sizes.
- Questions can be a powerful means to stimulate reflection and introspection.
- Commit to journaling as a daily habit.

CHAPTER 3 : VALUES & CHARACTER

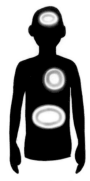

We will start with you, 'the person', before we come to you, 'the athlete'. Never forget, the world needs better people, more than it needs better athletes. When you are clear on who you are as a person, it can lift your performance to new levels in whatever domain you wish to excel in. Be assured, sports participation and performance are extremely important, but it does not define who you are. You are much more than this. If you develop an exclusive 'athletic identity' your entire sense of self, and self-worth, will come from being an athlete, and this is both unhealthy and self-limiting.

The question, 'Who am I?' is an extremely important question for us all to ask, and answer. At times we can lose sight of who we are because the outside world relentlessly attempts to tell us who, or what, we should, or should not be. The challenge is always to strive to live according to your values, as opposed to the circumstance or situation you find yourself in.

You did not invent the sport, you play it and experience it. It is only part of your life and self- identity. Your 'athletic identity' or who you are 'on the pitch' is only a part of who you are 'off the pitch'. Sport affords you an opportunity to express your identity.

I AM MORE THAN JUST A _____

(SPORT YOU PLAY, E.G. RUGBY PLAYER)

I PLAY _____ (SPORT E.G. RUGBY)

When you over-identify with something you do (sport), rather than who you are as a person, it can affect your perception of yourself in a negative manner. If you lose a game or underperform, you can use negative self-talk towards yourself, for example, 'I am useless'. If you perform poorly in your sport, it doesn't make you a useless person. It simply means you may have performed poorly at a given task, in a given moment.

Your personal wellbeing should not be reliant on your sporting performance. If you rely on your sporting performance in order to generate personal self-worth, the performance space can unnecessarily become an anxious and stressful place for you. Great performances do not equate you to being a great person, or even great at your sport. Alternatively, the same is true for bad performances, they do not equate you to being a bad person, or bad at your sport.

The challenge is to not allow your 'athletic identity' to limit or restrict you as a person, or affect your perception of what the world has to offer you, or indeed, what you have to offer the world. A narrow self-concept will severely restrict your development as a person. Sometimes you have to let go of the limiting stories you've told yourself about who you are, in order to live a fuller life.

Below is an exercise to highlight some of the identities, or groups we have in our lives. We mean different things to many different people.

Potential Group Identities

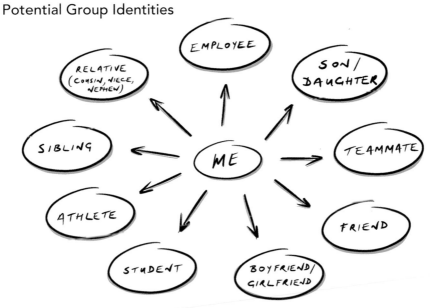

Create a similar graph and fill in the various groups/identities that you associate with. Then establish a level of importance you attach to each identity from 1 to 10: 1 being not at all, to 10 being you strongly associate with this identity and it is really important to you. Indeed, on reflection, you may score very high in all groups/identities and so appreciate further that sport is only part of your life.

(Note; an exercise like above, may be best suited to the front or back of your journal. This will allow you to access it easily and take a moment daily, or weekly, to read and review).

When you are underperforming in a certain part of your life, you have plenty of other areas you can gain a sense of achievement and fulfilment from. This can come from many different sources, activities and interactions with others, inside and outside of sport. We are all important human beings. We all have much to offer this world.

Character

'Character first' is a mantra of many great coaches. Character is the foundation of the athlete. By character I mean, what are the personal and performance qualities of the individual and I will explain these shortly. Like all qualities, these are not fixed and throughout the book we will see how you can develop them. Your youth is the perfect time for you to begin to actively and consciously develop your character. If you wish to be someone who excels in their chosen field, then you will be required to evaluate and look at new ways of thinking, feeling and behaving, at different stages on your journey.

Your character is the key to unlocking your talent and ability. It will be what sustains you. Coaching for character focuses on the athlete developing character strengths and using their sport as a source of, and opportunity for, personal growth. One of my favourite mantras in coach education is, 'we must coach character and self-awareness.' The absolute best part about this is that if you develop these areas, you will go on to be a much better athlete in the long term. Character qualities are what drive technical qualities.

Andy Friend

Andy Friend is the Connacht Rugby Head Coach. He is highly experienced having previously worked as Head Coach for the Australian Men's 7's Rugby, Suntory RFC and Canon RFC in Japan, The Brumbies RFC in Australia and Harlequins RFC in England. He believes in a holistic approach to athlete development, ensuring that players are nurtured and guided both on and off the field, with a strong focus on building character and leadership in a positive, sustainable culture. I have asked Andy to share with you what he believes is the importance of character in sport and indeed life.

It has been said that sport is a microcosm of life – a statement that I truly believe in. As coaches, we have a huge responsibility to educate our chargers, not only in the skills and attributes to play the specific sport that we teach, but more importantly, to guide them in developing the right character traits that will assist them in being the best versions of themselves, both on and off the sporting field.

So what are the ideal character traits that I believe are integral in both life and sport? Below I have listed my top SEVEN...

1. RESPECT
Treat people the way you wish to be treated. Sport offers you many opportunities where one can 'take advantage of' or disrespect another person. It is important for athletes to stay true to one of life's golden rules – 'do unto others what you would have them do unto you'.

2. HUMILITY
In nearly all sporting events, there are winners and there are losers, and most accept this as the likely outcome whenever competitors face off. Nothing is more disheartening than to see a winner who lacks humility. The competitor who can win on the scoreboard and remain humble in doing so, is the true champion of the contest.

3. ACCOUNTABILITY
Own your actions. Too often we see people use what I call the 'BCD' principles when something that they're involved in goes wrong. They either Blame, Complain or Defend the action that led to the error. The real champions in life take responsibility by holding themselves to account, regardless of the outcome that is delivered as a direct consequence.

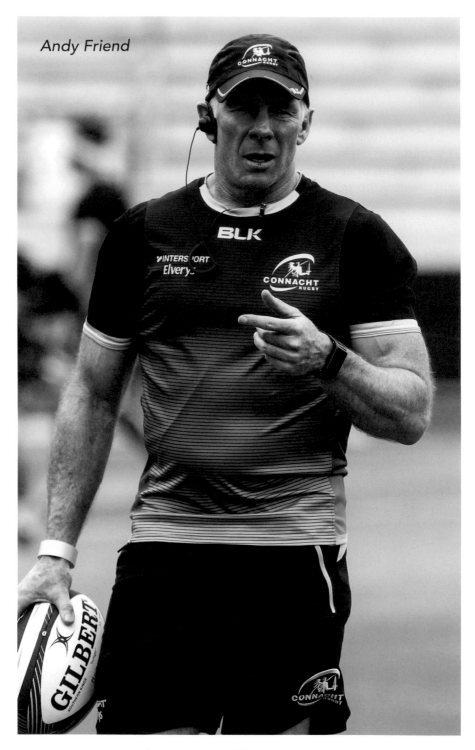

Andy Friend

4. HONESTY
It is important that we teach our athletes to earn their victories through being truthful and fair, and not through taking cheap wins through dishonest means. Rules will always be broken, and individuals will test them to their limits. But if a victory is offered that wasn't earned fairly, it's dishonourable to accept it.

5. DEPENDABILITY
One of the greatest attributes you can possess is that of dependability. If a teammate or coach says 'I know I can count on you', then you have truly earned the trust of that person. Whilst that sounds like a simple message to receive, it's only ever earned through a huge amount of self-discipline and hard work. The commitment you show at training, the diligence you display in the way that you prepare, the honesty with which you speak to your coach & peers, and your everyday focus and determination is what will earn you that highest of praises from your teammates and coaches.

6. COURAGE
Courage is the choice and willingness to confront agony, pain, danger, uncertainty or intimidation. Sometimes this is for the betterment of oneself, but more often than not it's for the betterment of the team or a teammate. Sport offers many an opportunity for someone to either display courage, or to shy away in the face of it. If you can learn to face your fears head on, then you're opportunity for growth is greatly enhanced.

7. COMPASSION
The capacity of an individual to identify and feel another person's suffering, and to then feel compelled to offer support in order to ease that suffering, is a character trait that is rare and special. Whether the suffering be physical, mental or a combination of both, the sporting arena lends itself to this type of situation on a regular basis. Those who can show the appropriate amount of compassion at the right time, are unique and special.

Those are the character traits that I believe are paramount to success both on and off the sporting field. I once read the following letter in a newspaper section titled 'Letters of Significance'. I believe it sums up exactly how sport and life are so uniquely intertwined.

The letter was titled:

'A Fathers Wish'…

"Dear Coach,

Tomorrow morning my son starts football. He's going to step out on the field and a great adventure that will probably include joys and disappointments begins. So I wish you would take him by his young hand and teach him the things that he will have to know.

- *Teach him to respect the Referee and that his judgement is final.*
- *Teach him not to hate his competitors, but to admire their skill.*
- *Teach him that it is just as important to be a team player and set up a try as it is to score one.*
- *Teach him to play as a team and never be selfish.*
- *Teach him never to blame his teammates if the team is losing.*
- *Teach him that winning isn't everything, but trying to win is.*
- *Teach him that it is far more honourable to lose than it is to cheat.*
- *Teach him to be a competitor.*
- *Teach him to close his ears to the howling mob and stand up for himself if he thinks he is right.*
- *Teach him gently but don't coddle him, because only the test of fire makes fine steel.*

This is a big order Coach, and I place my son in your hands. See what you can do for him. He's such a great little fellow.

His Dad"

I wish you well on your way,
Andy Friend

As Andy has so eloquently explained, how you carry yourself and how you compete is crucial. When you fail in these areas you commit what can be termed 'character errors' and character errors are the ones we are always aiming to avoid. These are the errors that, from a performance point of view, are unacceptable.

Your character is determined by what you value as a human being. In many ways it is influenced by your environment, your peer group and the leaders you have been exposed to. It is generally accepted that 30% of character is innate (what you are born with) and 70% is nurtured by environment. The premise of this book is that I am trying to influence you in multiple areas, no matter your circumstances, so it is necessary for you to accept a high level of personal responsibility. Again, self-coaching begins with facing the truth and being self-aware.

Values are the starting point, and the challenge for you is to then align your actions with your values. Values lived out become character qualities. Build what you do around clear values, however understand that actions bring values to life and these character qualities make a difference to you as a person and athlete, your team environment and indeed your community.

You can break character qualities into two categories: 'personal character qualities' and 'performance character qualities'. Personal character qualities are the ones we associate with 'off- field selves' for example: kindness, friendliness and integrity. Performance character qualities are the ones we associate with our 'on- field selves' such as doggedness, aggressiveness and bravery. As we will see shortly, there is a significant overlap in how the two categories relate to each other.

I strongly suggest, personal character qualities should be your first focus. For me, it must always be 'person first'. I feel it shouldn't necessarily be a case of being someone when doing your sport, and then being someone else outside of that. For sure you can develop what might be termed a 'game face' but I feel it should be all the same person, just a matter of understanding and tapping into different dimensions of yourself.

Sport is a place for you to express your identity. Gaining a clear understanding of who you are 'off the field' will enable you to widen your sense of self, gain clarity over your other strengths and allow you access the full spectrum of your human qualities.

Below is an exercise which challenges you to separate a jumbled list of 'personal character qualities' and 'performance character qualities' into a Venn diagram. The purpose of this exercise is to give you an appreciation of the overlapping relationship between the two categories of character qualities. Please don't get too bogged down in this activity. I am not so sure there is a right or wrong answer here. I am using this exercise to allow you explore the concept of values and character deeply.

Character Qualities:
Kindness, Dependability, Adaptability, Drive, Integrity, Loyalty, Humility, Doggedness, Friendliness, Honesty, Aggressiveness, Fun, Diligence, Open Mindedness, Sportsmanship, Self-Discipline, Gratitude, Accountability, Friendship, Joy, Compassion, Focus, Spirit, Commitment, Self–Awareness, Respectfulness, Work Ethic, Competitiveness, Courage, Resilience, Bravery, Relentlessness, Enthusiasm, Passion, Leadership, Positivity, Fairness, Generosity, Composure, Sincerity.

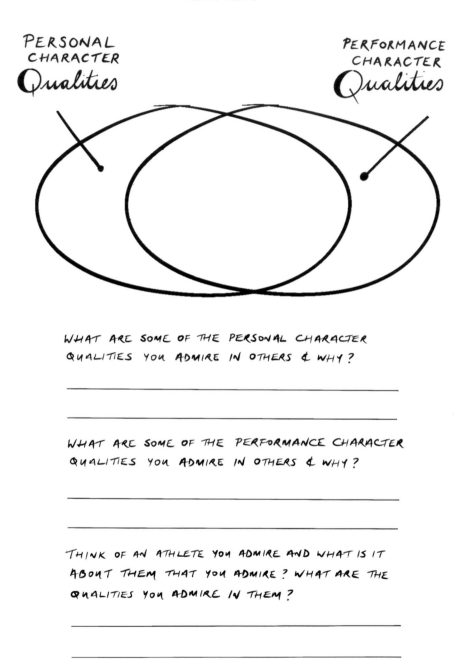

PERSONAL CHARACTER Qualities

PERFORMANCE CHARACTER Qualities

WHAT ARE SOME OF THE PERSONAL CHARACTER QUALITIES YOU ADMIRE IN OTHERS & WHY?

_____

_____

WHAT ARE SOME OF THE PERFORMANCE CHARACTER QUALITIES YOU ADMIRE IN OTHERS & WHY?

_____

_____

THINK OF AN ATHLETE YOU ADMIRE AND WHAT IS IT ABOUT THEM THAT YOU ADMIRE? WHAT ARE THE QUALITIES YOU ADMIRE IN THEM?

_____

_____

(Note, an exercise like the one that follows may be best suited to the front or back of your journal. This will allow you access it easily and take a moment daily, or weekly, to read and review).

LOOKING INWARD, WHAT ARE THE KEY VALUES OR 'PERSONAL CHARACTER QUALITIES' & 'PERFORMANCE CHARACTER QUALITIES' YOU WANT TO BE KNOWN FOR?

_____

_____

Now take each value or quality and assign standards of behaviour to them.

EXAMPLE VALUE: DILIGENCE

STANDARD OF BEHAVIOUR: I COMMIT 100% TO WHAT I AM DOING; NO SHORTCUTS IN MY PREPARATION. I LOOK AFTER THE SMALLER DETAILS OF EACH TASK & DAY AS I UNDERSTAND THIS IS WHAT LEADS TO THE BIG OUTCOMES. MY DAILY HABITS WILL REFLECT MY PERFORMANCES IN THE FUTURE.

_____

_____

Now put 3-5 key values or character qualities that you have identified into a coherent 'personal mission statement' that sums up who you are, and what you are about. It could look something like this:

"HONEST, KIND & DRIVEN IN LIFE & IN SPORT"

"I AM LOYAL, HARDWORKING & STRIVE FOR EXCELLENCE IN EVERYTHING I DO"

"A ROLE MODEL OF DILIGENCE, KINDNESS & HUMILITY IN MY TEAM ENVIRONMENT & COMMUNITY"

_____

_____

You can then ask yourself this simple question after practice or a game: Did I display the character qualities I am proud of, and wish to be associated with?

Alternatively, you can create something like a 'Character Weapons & Work-Ons Tool' where you could identify five character strengths i.e. 'weapons', that come naturally to you and five areas you feel you need to consciously develop i.e. 'work-ons'. I suggest you should have a balance between personal character qualities, and performance character qualities, although as we have just seen, many if not most, overlap.

You can use this tool as one of your journaling or reflection tools from time to time, where you can score yourself out of ten and use this feedback to feedforward as part of your 'personal improvement plan/goals'. When scoring each item you can reflect on times when the standard of behaviour or 'character quality' has been displayed or not (a 'character error'). Remember that character qualities will drive technical qualities. When character qualities are matched with technical qualities we get ultimate performance. Alternatively, 'character errors' rob us of the opportunity to utilise our talents.

SAMPLE CHARACTER WEAPONS & WORK-ON'S TOOL

WEAPON CHARACTER QUALITIES	SCORE	WORK-ON CHARACTER QUALITIES	SCORE
HONESTY	/10	POSITIVITY	/10
GRATITUDE	/10	FUN	/10
DOGGEDNESS	/10	SPORTSMANSHIP	/10
BRAVERY	/10	LEADERSHIP	/10
COMPETITIVENESS	/10	SELF-DISCIPLINE	/10
TOTAL		TOTAL	

WHERE, WHEN & WITH WHOM AM I DOING WELL?

_____

WHERE CAN I FOCUS ON IMPROVING?

_____

WHAT'S IMPORTANT NOW (WIN)?

_____

Successful people rarely make excuses. Never forget that your character is not something that is handed to you, it is something you must consciously develop over the course of your life. You are designed to be constantly improvable, and my hope is as you work your way through this book you will reflect, refine, and indeed redefine. A question you must honestly answer is- How do I want to show up in sport, and in life?

Your character will guide and drive your application, self- discipline and ambition. Strong character qualities will get you through the challenges, and allow you to learn and develop as you go. They will allow you explore the limits of your potential. Remember that all great failures are 'character failures'. A big part of character is the self-discipline needed to avoid complacency and resist temptation.

One of the simplest pieces of advice you can give a person is to:
"Do the right thing when no one is looking".

This is far easier said than done, and is the ultimate test of character. The challenge for every athlete, and indeed person, is to try to improve a little every day.

Remember, you are not your sport; you play it, you experience it. You are your character. You should be less concerned about what others may think of you; it is far more prudent to be concerned about what you think of yourself. Some days will go well, and others may not. It is important for your wellbeing that you identify more with yourself as a person, as opposed to 'the athlete'. You are much more valuable to your family, friends and your community than solely what you 'do'. Be clear on who you are as opposed to what you 'do', but know that over time, who you are, will show in what you do in sport and more importantly, in life.

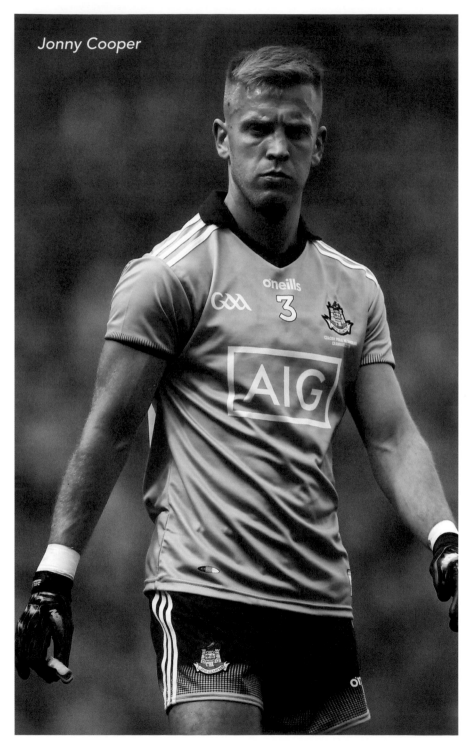

Jonny Cooper

Jonny Cooper

Jonny Cooper has been a key playing figure throughout the recent glory years of Dublin football which has seen him winning six All-Irelands, seven Leinster Titles and two All-Stars. In his youth, he was a dual-athlete playing both hurling and football at inter-county level. His Grandfather was a founding member of Na Fianna GAA Club which Jonny proudly plays with and serves today. Here he discusses the important role, character development has played in his life.

Your athletic identity can often precede your human identity. This can prove self-limiting. In my experience you need to always ensure that YOU are presented first. It is your background and experiences that add to your human self, being an athlete comes after.

I am from Glasnevin, Dublin, youngest of four with a great bond with each of my siblings. From a very young age, the four of us were working in our family business doing all sorts - lifting boxes, sweeping floors and taking orders. This 12-year summer job was where I honed behaviours that have stuck with me right through to this day. From an early age I worked in a team environment where the group output was appreciated more than the individual. I was given ownership of tasks that required me to think on my feet and, as we were involved in a competitive market, it required not only repeated excellence, but also an expectation to ignite growth and improvement when the opportunity arose.

My family values met those of my club, Na Fianna. From my younger days, into my teenage years, I received a unique opportunity to learn (and fail). For example, I learned to have a certain level of self-awareness to recognise my own skills and limitations, as well as those of my teammates. Self-awareness was critical in my development as an athlete. My ambition to learn, develop and grow allowed me to identify weaknesses and opportunities, and to ask for help from older and wiser heads. I have gone on to complete my BSc, MSc and a couple of diplomas to help me figure out a number of questions; all as a result of being self-aware enough to know I needed to learn continuously. I am unsure how many times I have asked for help with a problem or challenge, but it must be in the thousands. Na Fianna was the training ground for a large portion of my personal growth, particularly as a teenager.

I have had a fascination with high performance, both individual and team, from a very young age. I am intrigued as to how I can figure out myself, respect those around me and strive to maximise potential. I recall taking a General George S. Patton speech, adapting it before our Under 14 Féile, and dropping a copy in each of my teammates' bags. We didn't win the Féile, but I learned more about connecting with others that weekend, than any other training course I have completed. Some of my teammates missed the point, others had tears in their eyes and for some it was motivation, but as a whole, it connected me with them in a different way than was the norm.

Character is who you are when no one is looking. Sometimes it's your tone, other times it's your language, and most of the time it is your actions. Say hello, say thank you. Be the king of the simple things.

My biggest learning has been to be open-minded and curious – someone, somewhere has what you are looking for. Ask the right questions, and this helps craft the story you are trying to create. It is this curious mindset that allows you to break away from norms, and do something that has never been done before. If you find the right group environment, your influence can rub off on others – this is Leadership. The more you give the more you get. If you are willing to accept none of the credit, and I mean truly, accept none of the credit – you will be surprised how many opportunities will come your way.

Yours in Sport,
Jonny Cooper

CHAPTER 3

Rena Buckley

Rena Buckley is a recently retired Cork ladies football and camogie star. Between 2005 and 2017 she won 18 All-Ireland medals, making her one of the most decorated sportspeople in Gaelic games. She also has the unique honour of being an All-Ireland winning captain in both codes, and was named an All-Star on 11 occasions. She was named joint-winner of the 2015 Irish Times/Sport Ireland Sportswoman of the Year Award. Below Rena shares with you the important role, values and character play in her life inside, and outside of sport.

I come from a family of five- myself, my older brother Jerry, my twin sister Mary and my parents. My two siblings and I were always treated equally growing up, with each of us expected to contribute to the family as best we could. Discipline was strong in our house, which suited our personalities and we had a very happy childhood. Jerry introduced Mary and I to sport, and the three of us had hours of fun playing Gaelic games together. My parents had strong values of hard work, discipline and honesty. The Catholic faith was very influential in my upbringing, and Catholic values of love, giving, gratitude and forgiveness were very much to the fore.

Success in our house was understood as each of us doing our best in whatever we were doing-sport, education, relationships or work. There was an acceptance that each of us had gifts and talents, and each of us were equal. Any achievements or failures we experienced were not dwelled upon for too long. We looked forward to the next challenge.

From a young age it was clear what my passion in life was. I was driven to become the best I could be in sport. I showed personal leadership by leading a disciplined life in relation to training. I believed that through hard work and commitment I could achieve in sport. I was also very lucky to have a supportive family, who accepted me for who I was. During my teenage years, I made choices which aligned with my passion to achieve in sport, and my commitment to education. I was not the 'normal' teenage girl, but instead I was a very healthy, ambitious and determined young woman. On occasions, I skipped social events and gatherings with family and friends, and instead looked forward to every training session and match. I became completely immersed in the world

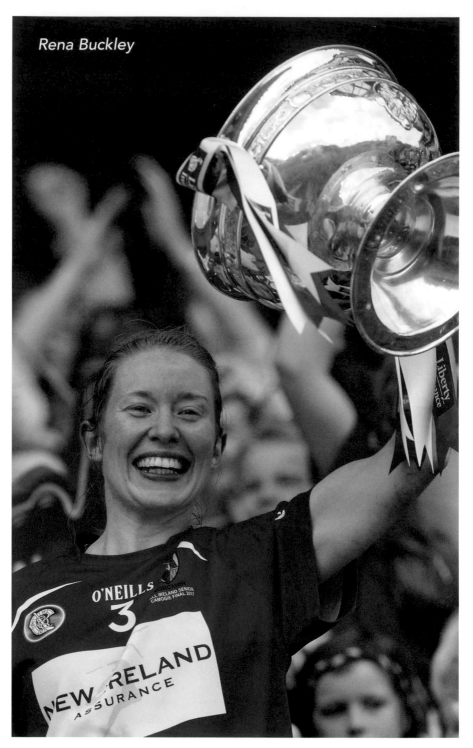

Rena Buckley

of sport. Did I miss out on some developmental aspects of my life? I did without question, but I gained in other areas. I was lucky enough to experience the joy, and the feeling of really being alive while playing sport.

While sport was taken seriously, we had brilliant fun at training and going to and from matches. My life was enriched with hugely positive people who helped me hone skills which are beneficial in sport and in life. I learned organisational skills, time management skills, interpersonal skills and teamwork. I was pushed by peers and coaches to be the best I could be.

My resilience was also developed and challenged. I learned that sometimes my best just wasn't good enough to gain victory on the scoreboard. This can be very hard to take, especially the bigger the effort you put into something. However, life is much bigger than sport. Sport is only one part of every person's life, and competition is just one part of sport. A poor performance, or a few mistakes, doesn't make you a poor player or less valuable as a person.

The most important lesson I have learned from sport is understanding that all that can be expected from anyone is their best-no more and no less. This applies to sport as well as all areas of life. I have been lucky enough to have had this understanding reinforced down through the years by teammates, coaches and family.

My journey of learning and developing is a journey which I am still on. I'm constantly learning more about myself as a person. My philosophy is that everyone should continue to develop throughout their lifetime, in an attempt to reach their potential. Our development can focus on the mental, physical, emotional or spiritual aspects of the person. Attending to each area is important and development is possible in all areas. I enjoy learning and improving, and find learning experiences hugely rewarding.

I can look back on my sporting journey so far with huge pride. Did I play poorly at times? Of course I did. Did I make mistakes? Plenty of them! But I feel I got the most out of myself and therefore I have very little regrets. My life has been blessed with friendships, fun and health and I am still enjoying my sporting journey. As I make my way through this phase of my life, my values are becoming clearer.

The values which are important to me are:
- *Love: love and understanding of self, of family, of community and of life itself*
- *Authenticity: being myself and being at peace with myself*
- *Joyfulness: enjoying life, being healthy, reaching my potential and helping others reach their potential*
- *Integrity: being honest, loyal, hard-working, disciplined and respectful.*

All the best,
Rena Buckley.

SUMMARY POINTS - Chapter 3

- The question, 'Who am I?' is an extremely important question for us all to ask, and answer.
- The challenge is always to strive to live according to your values.
- Your personal wellbeing should not be reliant on your sporting performance.
- We all have many group identities. We mean different things to many different people. Sport is only part of your life.
- Character is the foundation of the athlete.
- Character is made up of the personal and performance qualities of the individual. These qualities are not fixed and can be developed.
- Character qualities are what drive technical qualities.
- Character errors are the ones that, from a performance point of view, are unacceptable.
- Your character is determined by what you value as a human being.
- Values lived out become character qualities.
- Sport is a place to express your identity.

CHAPTER 4: MINDSET FOR LEARNING

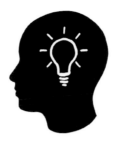

I have often heard it said that the best students are those who want to learn. The same can be said of athletes. The starting point of the learning process must be a willingness to learn. As life continually changes, so must our minds, beliefs and behaviours. Athletes who are unable to motivate themselves to learn must be content with relative mediocrity, no matter their talents. Learning is the product of the activity of the learner.

Race's 'Ripples' Model of Learning, developed by British educational and training developer Phil Race, places the internal motivation (motivation that comes from within you) that makes a person want to learn something, at the very centre of the learning process. In Race's opinion, four basic elements constitute successful learning:
- Needing/Wanting – motivation.
- Doing - practice, trial and error.
- Digesting - making sense of it, gaining ownership.
- Feedback - seeing the results, other people's reactions.

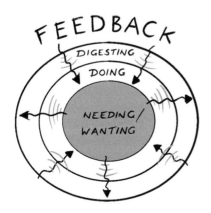

Again, 'needing / wanting' is the heart of the model, and it permeates or radiates through all the other elements. The 'doing' must be wanted, 'feedback' must be actively sought and welcomed, and opportunities for 'digesting' seized.

Adapted from Phil Race's 1993 Ripples Model of Learning.

The questions you must honestly ask yourself are:

OUT OF 10:

- HOW OPEN-MINDED ARE YOU ? _____

- HOW COACHABLE ARE YOU ? _____

- HOW WILLING TO LEARN ARE YOU ? _____

- HOW ABLE TO LEARN ARE YOU ? _____

I feel these are an extremely important questions to consider deeply, because often as humans we are programmed to self- persevere as opposed to self- improve. The first principle is that you must be honest and true to yourself.

Our mindsets can be our downfall. In any given moment you have two options: step forward into learning or backward into safety. Having a personal philosophy of 'continuous improvement' is priceless. Again, as with most things, your character is what drives this. It can be said that character is the golden thread that connects everything.

"My best skill was that I was coachable.
I was a sponge, and aggressive to learn".
Michael Jordan

Being 'coachable' means being humble and vulnerable enough to know you are not perfect. It means being open to honest and constructive feedback, even if it is tough to take. Being 'uncoachable' includes behaviours such as being arrogant, negative, judgemental, cynical or pessimistic, unable or unwilling to self-reflect or self-critique. Being unwilling to learn new things, or take on board constructive feedback, is a fatal barrier to development and improvement. You must work to develop the ability to listen, learn and reflect.

"Only fools despise wisdom and instruction".
Proverbs 1:7 NIV

In short, it is usually better to be curious than judgmental. The 'beginner's mindset' is critical. Spend time striving to learn from the thoughts, behaviours and experiences of learned others. Be curious-read books, watch documentaries, listen to podcasts, ask questions. Be a student of your game and its leading lights. Success leaves clues. I must reinforce the power of reading and study of principled-based excellence. Reading, and other mediums, broaden the mind by giving you an insight into the minds of others who can help you along the way.

Be a truth seeker. It is better to be a 'figure-outer' than a 'know it all'. Surround yourself with wisdom, seek opinion and inspiration. Keep a journal (see Chapter 2) and learn to reflect on experience. Learn from experience. Learn to analyse your performance (see Chapter 7). Learn how to face the truth, and how to learn from it. When we 'self-preserve', blame others, or deflect responsibility, our ego gets out safely but the underlying issues go unresolved.

It is too easy to 'believe what you believe', and it is hard to 'know what you don't know'. Welcome and invite feedback and learn how to use it and take it on board. Understand and appreciate, that the best never stop learning and striving to improve. Your growth depends on your willingness to get comfortable being uncomfortable.

In the 'beginner's mindset' everything is possible. To paraphrase Henry Ford, 'whether you think you can or whether you think you can't, usually you are right'. 'I can, I am, I will' is the language of learning. Your mindset is a way of thinking that determines your outlook, and therefore drives your actions and behaviours.

Mindset
Carol Dweck is the lead researcher in the area of mindset. Dweck's subject is motivation. She proposes two classes of goals that individuals carry in achievement situations, 'learning goals' and 'performance goals'. Individuals who strive to learn something new, or master a skill, are driven by 'learning goals', whereas those who are driven by 'performance goals' are preoccupied with their ability, and seek to cultivate favourable judgements or avoid negative ones. The 'learning goal' individuals are interested in increasing their competence. The 'performance goal' individuals are less likely to accept challenging tasks for fear of revealing inability, thereby denying themselves the opportunities to truly learn.

An individual who is driven by 'learning goals' will seek challenge and apply themselves to it. If their perceived ability is low, they will choose tasks that promote learning and improvement. If they have high-perceived ability, they will accept further challenges in order to improve more. They are less preoccupied with how they will be judged, more willing to display their inability, and are focused on the process of learning.

Dweck has championed the concepts of 'Fixed' and 'Growth Mindset'. It is a tangible and usable concept. Her book 'Mindset- How you can Fulfil your Potential' explains it in detail. Put simply, individuals with a 'growth mindset' have huge levels of 'coachability'. They are 'mastery orientated'. They think talent can be developed through strategy, effort, feedback, perseverance and hard work. They see challenge as an opportunity to learn; energising and invigorating. They read more, reflect more, practice more, ask more questions and so on. They surround themselves with knowledge, learning and wisdom.

Those with a 'fixed mindset' believe ability is a fixed trait. They avoid challenges, because challenge may result in mistakes and error, being more probable. Mistakes crack their self-confidence, leaving them fearful of challenges and unmotivated to strive valiantly, because they attribute failure and error to lack of ability. They find themselves in a downward spiral of rejecting growth opportunities and self-preservation. They render themselves unable to learn and become 'uncoachable'.

FIXED Mindset		Growth Mindset
SOMETHING YOU'RE BORN WITH	skills	COME FROM HARD WORK CAN ALWAYS BE IMPROVED
SOMETHING TO AVOID COULD REVEAL LACK OF SKILL TEND TO GIVE UP EASILY	challenges	TO BE EMBRACED AN OPPORTUNITY TO GROW PERSEVERE
UNNECESSARY SOMETHING YOU DO WHEN YOU ARE NOT GOOD ENOUGH	effort	IS ESSENTIAL THE PATHWAY TO IMPROVEMENT
GET DEFENSIVE TAKE IT PERSONAL	feedback	USEFUL SOMETHING TO LEARN FROM IDENTIFY AREAS TO IMPROVE
BLAME OTHERS GET DISCOURAGED	setbacks	PART OF LEARNING NECESSARY FOR GROWTH

IS MINDSET IMPORTANT TO YOU? IF SO, WHY?

_____

_____

You can, and absolutely must, develop a 'growth mindset' but be assured, the world isn't divided into those who have a 'growth mindset' and those with a 'fixed' one. As with all skills, mindset can be changed and developed. Most of us have different degrees of both, and this can vary from situation to situation or domain to domain. Focusing on process, not ability, is key to success in sport and in life. Many of the skills and principles shared in this book will help you develop a 'growth mindset' and lead you to being a better learner. Once again, sport and indeed life, is a journey of continuous learning, and learning is the most important skill.

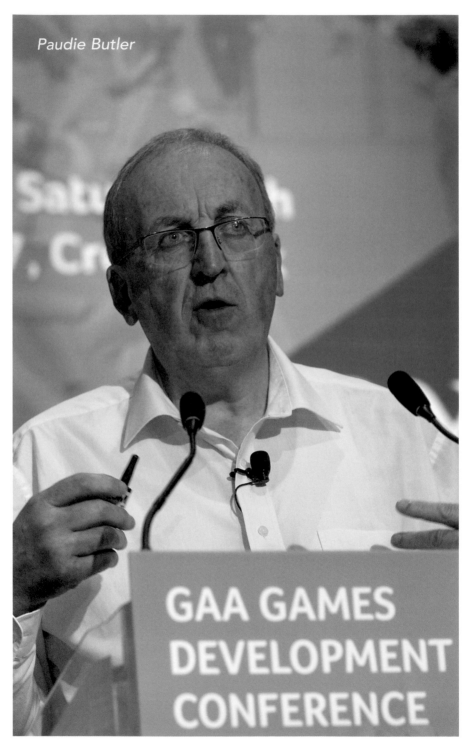

Paudie Butler

Paudie Butler

Paudie Butler is a renowned coach and coach developer. In his youth, he represented Tipperary in both senior hurling and football. He is a former National Director of Hurling and is revered by many for his lifelong service to the game of hurling and to coaching in Ireland. He has travelled the country spreading his word on the value of sport in the lives of Irish youths. Here he gives an insight into the importance of self-awareness and the role mindset plays in maximising your talents

Self-awareness is the key to growth. You have chosen an ambitious path that will be demanding of yourself and others. If you are to achieve your dreams you will need guidance and support from experienced people. Excellence is never easily achieved and talent will only take you so far. In sport, the challenges come thick and fast. Careers are short and learning opportunities must be recognised and taken to heart.

I have been coaching for fifty years. It has been a wondrous experience. I have been so lucky to come under the experience of so many great coaches and mentors. They have helped me see things in new ways that I would never manage on my own. I have coached thousands of teenage boys and girls. Their enthusiasm and hunger for knowledge always inspires me. I have also tutored thousands of coaches who now guide and coach teams all over the country.

I understand how ambitious you are, how you love this sporting life. You love to test yourself and let yourself be tested at the highest level. That demands great humility. One must accept the ups and downs of competitive sport. There's no such thing as failure, only opportunities for learning. Of course you worry sometimes that you might not be good enough or strong enough or fast enough or pretty enough or popular enough or whatever. These are the challenges every human being has to deal with. You are not your thoughts. You are yourself-precious and unique.

"If it's going to be it is up to me" is a sentence that helped me greatly along the way. It is from Declan Coyle's book The Green Platform. We take responsibility for our own actions and reactions. 60,000 thoughts run through your head every day. You choose your path and let all the other thoughts sail on past. Negative thoughts will destroy you if you

linger on them. They must be consigned to the trash bin.

Being self-aware means you are able to recognise how you react to feedback and instruction from coaches, parents, teachers and mentors. These are people who have your best interests at heart. Defensiveness indicates that you are coming from a place of fear and self-doubt, instead of love and confidence. Self-belief will enable you to seek out feedback and benefit from it.

We are all born into a definite time and place and get conditioned very early. Becoming self-aware means you can stand back and examine your beliefs and how you are thinking. In the pursuit of your dream you must set high standards for yourself and hold yourself accountable. Sport is a fierce tester of truth and courage. How you do one thing is how you do everything. We can't switch on and off. We must learn to live in the present moment. We get opportunities every day to fully participate in life or turn a blind eye. There's always lots to be done.

Victor Frankl wrote his highly influential book 'Man's Search for Meaning' after surviving the concentration camps of Germany and Poland during World War 2. He faced death every day. Thousands died in the gas chambers. Starvation, disease, prison guard brutality and despair claimed thousands more lives of utterly innocent men, women and children. He tells us how he used every trial as an opportunity to grow. "What is this situation teaching me now?" he would say to himself. He confided in a small group of positive people who spoke of what they wanted to achieve when they found freedom. He kept his dream in front of himself even when it looked hopeless. He was able to forget about himself and help others who were losing hope. We will never be in such a desperate situation. But the same question is relevant, 'What is this great opponent teaching me now?' 'What is my coach saying now that will enable me to thrive and meet my challenges?'

Games now are more complex than before. The pace is very high, new tactics are being used and analysis of opponents is normal. To meet these demands we need the support of older and wiser heads and we need to be active learners.

Many ambitious people keep a journal. It enables them to write out their objectives and map out their pathway step by step. Normalising excellence is the path of the great sportsperson. They recognise the power of habit. They replace old lazy ways with integrity and discipline.

Good habits make good character. Not only are you becoming a great player but you are becoming a leader also. Leaders choose their actions and they live up to their beliefs, they know how to fuel the body, they know how to practice their skills at match pace. They know that to operate at full capacity they must have a growth mindset and an even tempered disposition. Great players enjoy the feedback on their performance. They know they need the insights and the intelligence of others. They know they need to continuously learn and improve.

Pride and arrogance are the great enemies. It takes courage and humility to ask for help. The love of the game will help you keep your lofty goals in the forefront. Enjoy your game, your family and your friends. Seek out the honest opinion of trustworthy people. They will be the signposts you need to help you travel the road.

Slán,
Paudie

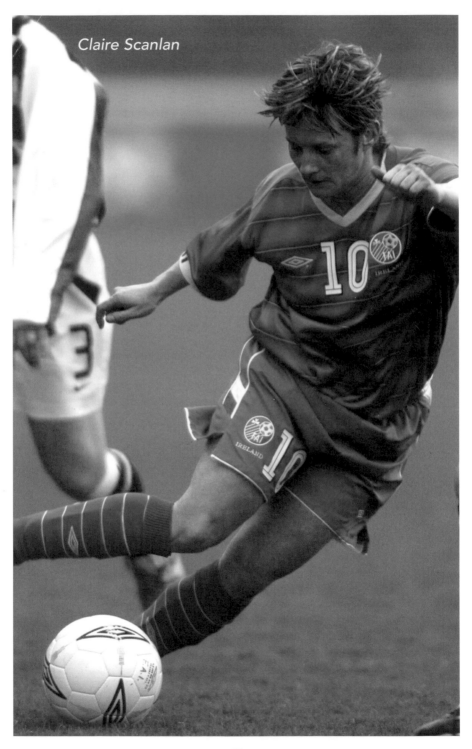

Claire Scanlan

Claire Scanlan

Claire Scanlan is a retired Irish International Footballer who has coached and played in numerous countries around the world, seeking growth and new challenges everywhere she has gone. Where there was no path, she forged her own. In 2009 she was presented with a Legend Award for services to Irish football. Her playing and coaching career is a story of seeking challenges, breaking new ground and learning at every opportunity.

Playing football on the green with my father and brother was the beginning of my soccer education. Soon after, playing with the local boys in Kenure Park and St. Maur's Park became a daily activity. Little did I know that competing and getting pushed around by the boys was all part of my football development. I was a girl that wanted to be a professional soccer player and I was very much in the minority!

At 11 years old, I played on my first female team, Rush Athletic Ladies. The sporting landscape of 1980's Ireland was not what it is today. There was no underage soccer structures for girls. If I wanted to play competitive female soccer I had to play with adult women and in hindsight this was the best possible start for me. I loved playing with my hometown club, my manager was the local bread man, Charlie Armstrong, and he took great care of me.

It was around this time I started writing to professional clubs in England. The hunger to learn, improve and seek new challenges was deep inside. I felt a need to be proactive. I had to go in search of what I wanted. I remember Man City getting back to me, saying I had to be 16 to play for their ladies team, I was 12 at the time. I was also a Man United supporter, so maybe that worked out for the best!

I knew that playing for Ireland would be the ultimate honour for me. My performance with Rush Athletic allowed me to get noticed by Irish management. Playing football on the green with the boys, had prepared me and now I had to forge my own path. On November 26th, 1988 I captained the Irish U18's and scored 2 goals on my debut in a friendly International. I was quickly thrust into the Senior Squad and got my first senior cap at age 17. This gave me the platform to receive a number of scholarship offers from American universities. I chose to accept a scholarship in Mercyhurst College in Erie, Pennsylvania. I knew little about either scholarships or America. I knew of only one other who had taken this route. All I knew was that I would be playing football every day! I wanted to test myself, I wanted to see how good I could be, I wanted to be a professional footballer and was willing to do whatever it would take. At the time there was nothing in Ireland that replicated this opportunity and so it was an easy decision for me to make.

I attended Mercyhurst College for four years and got a degree in Business. During my time there I enjoyed considerable success being a two-time All-American, a Conference Player of the Year and the NCAA Division II Player of the Year. Best of all my dream of playing professional football was still alive. With limited professional leagues worldwide, I began calling prominent coaches around the USA to see if there was an 'in'. Once again, I felt a need to be proactive. Eventually, I was invited to a trial in California to play professionally in Japan. Off I went, dreams in tow, and spent three days competing against other professional hopefuls. A day after returning home, I received a call offering me a one year contract with Oki FC Winds. I was a professional footballer and I was going to Japan!

I spent a full season in Japan with Oki and I immersed myself in the culture and attempted to learn the language. It was a real education especially with training sessions that were 4 hours in length. We trained on dirt pitches as grass was at a premium, but the game day stadiums were the best in the country. When my contract was up, I returned to Ireland to play with Shelbourne FC and resumed playing with the Irish team. In 1999, I was named the FAI Irish Women's Player of the Year.

I returned to America to get my Master's Degree in Education while still playing with the National Team. During that time I played my club football with Springfield Sirens where we became National Champion's and then with Memphis Mercury, where we were Conference Champions. Once I graduated, I signed for Leeds United to continue my football career and after four years there, I was offered a fulltime coaching and playing role at Bristol Rovers (soon to become Bristol Academy). It was at Bristol that I coached the Filton College Female Football Academy and played with the senior women's team. Filton had some very good young players and we won the English League and British Cup double. We also won the 2007 English FA Charter Standard Academy of the Year Award that was presented to me at Old Trafford by Trevor Brooking.

In 2008, I had an opportunity to return to America to coach in college soccer. I had always loved the college environment because of the resources available to develop players and as my playing career was coming to an end, I made the decision to move. At the same time I also accepted offers from then Irish manager Noel King to be involved in many Irish coaching set-ups. If I couldn't play for Ireland, I wanted to serve Ireland in any way possible. In 2010, Noel invited me to be a part of his backroom staff for the U17 Women's World Cup in Trinidad and Tobago. The team reached the quarterfinals after a heroic display in the tournament.

Over the past 12 years I have coached at four American Division One Universities and won two conference titles along the way. Through my experiences in coaching and from my study of the various elements of performance and development, I can see clearly why I had such a comprehensive and diverse playing career. As a player, I was driven to search for ways to enable myself to play football as a career. I believe I had a classic growth mindset long before the term became part of common vernacular. I was willing to leave the comforts of home and be adaptable to all countries, cultures and environments. I was coachable in each environment I was in. I was willing to accept challenge and setbacks and my mindset was one of growth and continuous improvement. I had a laser like focus on achieving my goals and was willing to make the sacrifices required. I was in love with the learning process.

Nowadays the very same qualities drive me in my coaching, a relentless pursuit of personal growth and challenge. The growth mindset is a quality I continually try to nurture in those I coach. I believe this is the key to maximizing your potential. Similar to my playing career, I have had to move to progress and develop as a coach, but I have had a career in football that has spanned 37 years, and for me, that is a decent result. Learning as I go and seeking new challenge has been my approach.

Best wishes,
Claire Scanlan

SKILLS FOR DRAWING
ON YOUR INNER STRENGTH
By Tony Óg Regan

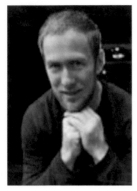

Tony Óg Regan is a performance psychologist who has worked with some of Ireland's highest performing athletes and teams including: All Ireland Champions Tipperary Senior Hurlers 2016, Limerick Senior Hurlers 2019 and Olympic and professional athletes with backgrounds in rugby, athletics, swimming & modern pentathlon. He has supported elite amateur athletes in sailing, show jumping, ultra-marathons, golf, soccer and horse riding. He competed as a player at the highest level with the Galway senior hurlers from 2003 to 2013. I have asked Tony to explain a number of mental skills that can be utilised in order to improve performance. These skills are numbered and scattered through the book for you to develop and use throughout your sporting career and beyond.

SKILL NO. 1- OPTIMISM

Why is it important?

Optimism is a lens through which you can see the world. Optimism is the fundamental belief that something good is about to happen. This is a mindset skill that you can train and improve. Optimism is the emotional skill that enables you to see opportunities, maintain a positive mood, and be resilient in the face of setbacks.

Building an Optimistic Mindset (Martin Seligman)

1. Permanence

Optimists tend to see negative experiences as temporary setbacks whereas people who give up easily believe the causes of bad experiences are permanent.

2. Pervasiveness

Optimists can compartmentalise the struggles they are having into a sports issue, a homework issue, a disagreement with a friend. They do not let this issue affect everything else in their lives. Pessimists let one issue dominate and affect all aspects of their life.

3. Personalisation

When optimists face misfortune or bad news, they tend not to take it personally. They see the influence of external factors in their issues.

Whereas pessimists will often attach the misfortune down to them and their lack of ability.

Reflection Exercise
Can you remember the last time you were optimistic about something and how did it impact your performance?

WRITE ABOUT THIS CHALLENGING SITUATION. WHAT WORKED WELL? WHAT IMPACT DID IT HAVE ON YOU? WHAT CAN YOU LEARN FROM IT FOR NEXT TIME? HOW CAN YOU PRACTICE & IMPROVE THE AREAS MENTIONED?

_____

_____

CAN YOU REMEMBER THE LAST TIME YOU WERE NOT OPTIMISTIC ABOUT SOMETHING & HOW DID IT IMPACT YOUR PERFORMANCE?
WRITE ABOUT THIS EVENT FOR 2 MINUTES, WHAT YOU WERE THINKING & FEELING BEFORE, DURING & AFTER? DESCRIBE WHERE & WHEN IT WAS, WHY IT WAS IMPORTANT TO YOU, WHO WAS THERE & WHAT YOU CAN RECALL ABOUT IT?

_____

_____

Positive Psychology - Methods to Boost Your Mood
Dr Martin Seligman is a pioneer in the area of happiness and wellbeing. He found people who wrote down 3 things they were grateful for each day, for seven days, reported greater wellbeing and a lift in mood.

TAKE SOME TIME NOW TO WRITE DOWN &
EXPERIENCE THE 3 THINGS YOU HAVE IN YOUR
LIFE RIGHT NOW THAT YOU ARE GRATEFUL FOR.
(NOTE, LOOK BACK TO CHAPTER 2 - JOURNALING
THE JOURNEY & INCORPORATE THIS EXERCISE
DAILY IF YOU PLEASE)

_____

_____

Practicing Optimism

Albert Bandura's "Theory of Agency" has three elements: First, you must project yourself into the future to have something to work toward. Second is self-regulation, which is the extent that you can regulate your thoughts, emotions and behaviour. The third is self-reflection, meaning, to what extent can you judge your capabilities (also known as self-efficacy).

Looking at the first element, if your lens is pessimistic when you project yourself into the future and you see negative outcomes, it would be more challenging to be at your best. When you have thoughts of worry about what could go wrong in the future it could be challenging to organize your life to pursue your personal best. If your negative self-critique is the primary judge of your capabilities, it might be challenging to stay in something long enough to get the benefits of your hard work. The Theory of Agency speaks to the importance of training optimism as a mechanism for organizing your life around finding your best.

Another way to train optimism is to work to find the opportunity in challenging situations. To become your very best, you'll need to stay connected to the challenges. What is something that has been challenging you recently, and how could you reframe your thinking about it to find the opportunity in it?

WRITE ABOUT THIS CHALLENGING SITUATION. WHAT
WORKED WELL ? WHAT IMPACT DID IT HAVE ON YOU?
WHAT CAN YOU LEARN FROM IT FOR NEXT TIME ?
HOW CAN YOU PRACTICE & IMPROVE THE AREAS
MENTIONED?

_____

_____

Optimism is a competitive advantage because it helps you stay cognitively open and flexible when you experience adversity or setbacks. How well do you adjust when you are in uncomfortable situations? Do you see your ability as something that can be developed, that effort leads to growth and mastery, that tough challenges are great opportunities? Optimists view obstacles as temporary, controllable, and linked to specific situations rather than permanent.

The way you talk to yourself (see Skill No. 6- Confidence- The Power of Language) will not only determine how you feel but also the range of options you are capable of seeing as you move forward. The good news is that, you can learn to change this mindset if you so wish.

How you interpret an event is under your control and involves three strategies.

Three Emotional Elements of Optimism
(Martyn Newman – Emotional Capitalists)
1. Look for the benefits from this situation.
Respond in a positive constructive way and reframe the situation in a positive context – identify the benefits, however remote they feel. Constantly review the best parts of your performance.
2. Seek the valuable lessons.
Stop focussing on mistakes. Examine how you performed and learn the lessons for future action and commit to new and improved actions. 'What can I learn from this situation that will make me better the next time I face it?'
3. Focus on the next task and seek out opportunities.
Clear your mind of negative emotions and focus on what is important now e.g. the next tasks to be performed – see the opportunities within the task. Reframe the issues into 'challenges to overcome'.

References:

Bandura, A. (2008). *Self-Processes, Learning, and Enabling Human Potemtial*, pages 15–49. Information Age Publishing.

Bandura, A. (in press). *The reconstrual of "free will" from the agentic perspective of social cognitive theory*. In J. Baer, J. C. Kaufman, & R. F. Baumeister (Eds.), Psychology and free will. Oxford: Oxford University Press.

Bandura, A. (2018). *Toward a Psychology of Human Agency: Pathways and Reflections Perspectives on Psychological Science 13(2):130-136*

Dweck, C. (2006). *Mindset The New Psychology of Success: How we can learn to fulfill our potential*. New York: Ballantine Books.

Newman, M. (2009). *Emotional Capitalists. The New Leaders*. Jossey Bass.

Race, P. (1993). *Ripples Model of Learning*.

Seligman, M. (2011). *Flourish: A Visionary New Understanding of Happiness and Well-being*. New York: Free Press.

SUMMARY POINTS - Chapter 4

- The starting point of the learning process must be a willingness to learn.
- Learning is the product of the activity of the learner.
- The 'doing' must be wanted, opportunities for 'feedback' must be actively sought and welcomed and opportunities for 'digesting' seized.
- Having a personal philosophy of continuous improvement is priceless.
- Be curious, read books, watch documentaries, listen to podcasts, ask questions. Be a student of your game and its leading lights.
- Your mindset is a way of thinking that determines your outlook and therefore drives your actions and behaviours.
- Individuals with a 'growth mindset' have huge levels of 'coachability'. They are 'mastery orientated'.
- Those with a 'fixed mindset' believe ability is a fixed trait. They avoid challenges, because challenge may result in mistakes and errors, being more probable.
- Mindset can be changed and developed. Most of us have different degrees of both 'fixed' and 'growth' and this can vary from situation to situation, or domain to domain.
- Optimism is a fundamental belief that something good is going to happy.
- Optimism is a mindset skill we can train and improve.

CHAPTER 5: INDIVIDUAL PRACTICE

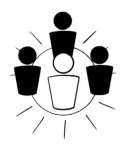

	STRONGLY AGREE	AGREE	SOMEWHAT AGREE	SOMEWHAT DISAGREE	DISAGREE	STRONGLY DISAGREE
YOU FEEL IT IS IMPORTANT TO REGULARLY 'PRACTICE TO GET BETTER' THROUGH INDIVIDUAL PRACTICE SESSIONS.						
CURRENTLY YOU USE INDIVIDUAL PRACTICE SESSIONS WITH THE PURPOSE & INTENTION OF GETTING BETTER.						
YOU KNOW HOW TO PRACTICE TO MAKE THE MOST OF YOUR INDIVIDUAL PRACTICE SESSIONS.						

I have posed these questions to those I coach countless times over the years. There is a trend to the answers. They all 'strongly agree' individual 'practice to get better' is important, but very few 'strongly agree' with the final two questions.

If our last chapter began with 'I have often heard it said that the best students are those who want to learn', the following two chapters could be captioned as, 'the best students are those who know how to learn.' 'Preparation delivers success' is a truism I like to share with those I coach. If you wish to be the best you can be, making a personal commitment to honing your craft is critical. Taking 'ownership' is key. To build skill, we need to take and sustain action. Action drives motivation and confidence follows.

Collective training is one thing, and in truth, is possibly the easy part. I hope this book will offer you many tools to help how you approach it in a positive manner and we will look at this separately in the next chapter. Individual personal 'practice to get better' is a different thing and in my experience is rarely optimised. Great opportunity lies here. For example, if you wanted to work on fielding a high ball in Gaelic football you might get two or three 'reps' in collective training, whereas if you spend five minutes on your own you might do 50 reps. However, making them meaningful, quality reps is critical and we will look at this shortly.

The reality is that every athlete can push their capabilities within skill execution, and one of the secrets to enjoying sport is to become more proficient in the fundamental skills of the game. Your skills are your tools. The outcome of performance in competition is simply a by-product of the effort you have made to prepare, relative to your ability. Everyone has the will to win, but not everyone has the will and know-how to prepare to win. The fundamentals require constant re-emphasis.

Many athletes fall into the trap of confusing mindless, aimless, 'practicing all the time' type routines, with 'maximum intensity and quality' type practice. All practice is not created equally. If you want to change you need to do something that changes you. Simply repeating a skill, even over a period of many years, doesn't build expertise. Once you reach a reasonable level of competence the skill becomes automatic and 'mindless practice' will at best, maintain your abilities but not improve them. If your craft is something you really want to excel in, you have to push past that comfortable stage and challenge yourself.

ACHIEVEMENT TRIANGLE

PEAK PERFORMERS ARE COMFORTABLE WITH BEING UNCOMFORTABLE. THEY ARE CONSTANTLY PUSHING THE ENVELOPE. — PEAK PERFORMANCE ZONE

WILLING TO RISK & GET UNCOMFORTABLE. IN FACT THEY ARE UNCOMFORTABLE MORE THAN THEY ARE COMFORTABLE. — HIGH PERFORMANCE ZONE

THERE ARE LESS PEOPLE HERE. MORE COMMITMENT, OCASSIONAL RISK. OCASSIONALLY UNCOMFORTABLE. — PERFORMANCE ZONE

THE COMFORT ZONE IS WHERE MOST PEOPLE OPERATE. THEY ARE SATISFIED & ALWAYS COMFORTABLE. THEY TAKE NO RISKS. — COMFORT ZONE

More isn't necessarily better- quality is critical. You have a limited amount of time and energy to practice so it is prudent to make the best use of it. Effort and strategy are key. Some athletes often fall into the trap of being 'too busy training to practice'. This is a time management issue and can be addressed (see Chapter 21). Individual practice is essential.

Though perfection is unattainable, aiming high allows you to surpass your own preconceived limitations. Run from your comfort zone. Aim for perfection; deliberately practice the core skills of your game. Get uncomfortable. Strive to be 'brilliant at the basics'. In the basics, attention to, and mastery of, tiny details are commonly overlooked. Do the simple things better! How close can you get to perfect?

As with most things in life, effort is important but so too is strategy. If you focus your practice, while maximising your application, with time, the repetition will create momentum and this momentum will produce improvement and better performance. The key to effective practice is to make it purposeful and deliberate. Understanding the demands of your sport and the role or position you play, as well as learning how to properly analyse your performance (see Chapter 7), will help inform you of what parts of your game you need to focus on.

Deliberate Practice
Deliberate Practice is based on the research of K. Anders Ericsson. It refers to a special type of practice that is purposeful and systematic. For example, if you were a full back in rugby and high catching was something you struggled with, you would purposefully and systematically practice to address this. High catching would be one of your 'work ons' and could be done before or after collective training with the aid of a teammate or coach. Visualisation techniques (see Tony Óg's Skill No. 3) could also be used to assist the process.

Deliberate Practice requires focused attention and is conducted with the specific goal of improving performance. It differs from 'regular practice' in that regular practice might largely consist of mindless purposeless repetitions.

> "Excellence demands effort and planned deliberate practice
> of increasing difficulty".
> Anders Ericsson

The goal of Deliberate Practice is not to be enjoyed. Its only goal is to improve your performance. However, I feel this is not to say it cannot be enjoyed by those with the correct mindset and outlook. Satisfaction is to be gained through application and learning, and this should be embraced and viewed as enjoyable. Deliberate Practice requires sustained effort and concentration. It requires the learner to continuously challenge themselves, set goals and practice at the edge of their current ability. Too easy, and there will be no learning. Too hard, and there will no opportunity for feedback and improvement. Remember, when you do what is easy in life, life becomes hard; when you do what is hard, life becomes easy.

The greatest challenge of Deliberate Practice is to remain focused on improvement. The more we repeat a task, the more mindless it can become. Mindless activity is the enemy of Deliberate Practice. Feedback is essential. Measurement is one means of feedback. What we measure we improve.

Example of Deliberate Practice in Hurling:

Key Focus Skill- Striking off both left and right hand side. Secondary Skill- Catching
- Stand 7 metres away from a high wall and have two/three standard sliotars (not wall balls) at your feet (if one flies away you can resume with the spare ones).
- Do 4 x 1 minute blocks alternating left hand side and right hand side striking, catching the ball without taking it on the hurl as it returns to you from the wall.
- Only count the ones you catch. To begin, it can be ok if it hops before you catch it once you catch it without using your hurl. As you improve perhaps only count the ones that go directly to your hand (without touching the ground).
- Count your score for one minute and repeat 4 times in total each day. If time and energy allow do 2 sets of 4. It doesn't matter how many you get, what matters is you focus on getting better and trying your level best to beat your personal best.
- Remember the wall is a mirror and if you strike the ball on the sweet spot of your hurl it will come back to you.

The fact that you are 7 metres away from the wall using a standard sliotar means you must strike with conviction using 'strong hands' in a game-like manner. Useful and meaningful feedback from a coach or mentor is also important as it allows you to adjust, refine and become more specific on the areas you are working on. You can also video yourself and compare your technique to a player whose striking you admire. Using a model can be useful, as can videoing yourself.

Below are principles you can utilise to practice deliberately.

- Desire and Motivation- The natural inclination will be to give up. Motivation and self- discipline are key. Understanding 'why' you are doing it is crucial.
- Set specific, realistic goals - These give you the motivation to excel past your current abilities and help measure progress, thus driving meaningful improvement and sustaining motivation. Goal setting requires thoughtful planning, identifying areas for improvement and creating a specific plan of action (see Chapter 7). You can use your journal to track your progress.
- Get comfortable with being uncomfortable - Stretching yourself is the key to growth and improvement.
- Routine - Repeat and Persist. Consistent, intense bursts of effort are key to maintaining momentum in building expertise.
- Seek feedback from your coach, mentor or trusted peer (see Chapter 9) not just about how you are doing, but also about how to practice. This is essential to identify areas for improvement and gain meaningful insights on progress. Technologies, such as video can be used to aid the process.
- Find a model - You can find an athlete that is better at the skill than you are and use them as a model. YouTube can be a great place to find models.
- Recover! This is not 'practicing all the time', it is 'practicing to get better'. Relaxation and recovery (see Tony Óg's Skill No. 8) is crucial to offset the intense effort of Deliberate Practice to avoid mental or physical fatigue.

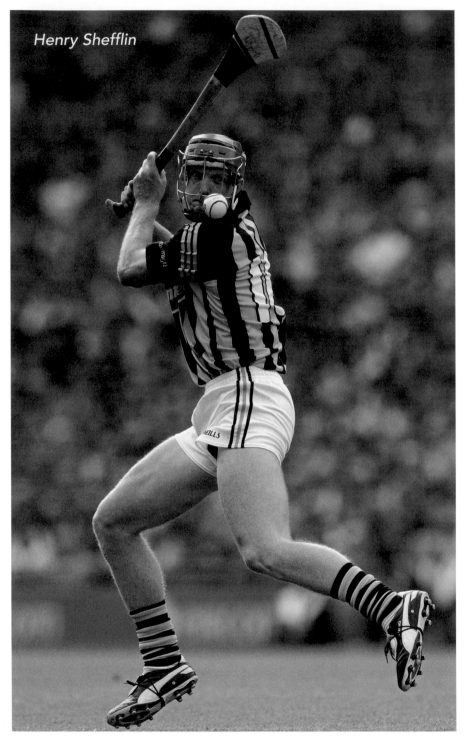

Henry Shefflin

CHAPTER 5

Henry Shefflin

Henry Shefflin is a former Kilkenny Hurler who won a record ten All-Ireland medals with Kilkenny as well as three All-Ireland Club titles with his native Ballyhale Shamrocks. His career tally of 28 goals and 485 points ranks him as the top championship scorer of all-time. He won a record-breaking eleven All-Star awards and is the only player ever to be named Hurler of the Year on three occasions. He was named RTÉ Sports Person of the Year in 2006 and inducted into the RTÉ Sports Hall of Fame in 2015. Shortly after retiring he went on to manage his club Ballyhale Shamrocks for two years where they we crowned All-Ireland champions on both occasions. He is viewed by many as the greatest hurler of all time. Here he shares with us the roll individual practice played in his success.

I played hurling. The technical demands of the game are huge. The simpler and more efficiently you can execute any of the skills, the more time and space you afford yourself on the ball. The more skills you master the more options you possess in the game. This makes you unpredictable and allows you to pose more complex problems to your opponent. Being able to execute the appropriate skill, as simply and quickly as possible, in as tight a space as possible is often the difference between success and failure.

Hurling is a team sport, but the team is made up of individuals. We train collectively, but will never reach our potential if we are not willing to practice individually. The players who commit to extra individualised practice are the ones you want on your team. The game needs time and if you want to maximise your potential you must be willing to give it time.

I was born and raised above my parents' public house in Ballyhale. You could say it was a strange place for an athlete to be raised but for me it was perfect. There was a squash court behind the pub and this is where I honed my skills as a youngster. In the winter months I would be inside the court with the lights on and in the summer I would be outside on its gable wall. The challenge was always to try and hit the bullseye targets my brothers had painted on the wall. This required focus and concentration. If I missed, the challenge was to figure out why. For me, there was nothing like honing my skills- it drove my love for the game. All I needed was a wall, a ball and a hurl and I was happy.

As a youngster I practiced a lot with my brother Paul who was just a year younger than me. We were very competitive and we would challenge each other, keeping scores and always looking for a winner. Wanting to be the best was something that always drove me on. This period of my life undoubtedly laid the foundations for the hurler I would become. My skills were developed, my wrists and the hands were hardened and strengthened.

Throughout my underage club career we usually played in the B and C grades of the competitions. I didn't really appreciate it at the time but this afforded me more time and space on the ball as the pace of the game was relatively slow. When I moved to secondary school in St Kieran's College there was a huge change in game-speed and a sharp rise in standard. This forced me to look at all areas of my play and improve my hand speed and indeed foot speed. Focused practice was given to both areas away from collective training. Counsel and feedback was sought from coaches and wise heads.

As I matured and joined the Kilkenny senior panel I became increasingly aware of the areas of my game that needed more targeted work. The higher the level, the greater the chance of any limitation in my game being exposed. My left side needed strengthening. I was too predictable in possession with my left side only a very distant second option to my right. I went after improvement with relentless practice on my left side. The more I practiced the more confident I became on it. I was no longer predictable. I had multiple options in possession.

I always loved going down to the pitch by myself. I felt connected to it. It felt like home. I had picked the stones out of it when it was a farmer's field and as a community we had brought it to life as a hurling field. It was a place that brought me to life. It was a place I was free with myself. For shooting practice I would bring twelve balls and scatter them randomly around the field. I would approach each ball individually with a 5 or 10 meter full speed run up, jab lift and then execute the shot. I used visualisation to make it as real or game-like as possible. Often, I would visualise the Cork half back Sean Óg Ó hAilpín breathing down my neck as I attacked the ball and took on the shot. I would count how many went over and as I walked in to gather the balls I would reflect on why I had pulled a ball on the near post or whatever. I was always asking 'why', always wanting to be better and always willing to do what it took.

When I joined the Kilkenny senior hurling panel DJ Carey was the team free-taker. At that time DJ was a hurling god. He helped me greatly *not only in the area of free-taking but also in giving me an example of what a good teammate was and how you could influence and help those around you. We would practice together and he would offer me guidance and feedback.*

My individual free-taking practice would go hand in hand with my individual shooting practice in the pitch in Ballyhale. In my early twenties, it would be over an hour down the field by myself on the evenings we weren't training. I genuinely loved it. It was here I honed my routine: place the ball correctly on a nice piece of grass with the rim of the ball pointing in the direction of the target. Set my feet shoulder- width apart about a foot back from the ball with the ball placed centrally between them. Take two deep breaths, check that my shoulder and hurl are in line with the target. Chin down, jab lift and follow through. Each free was given focused attention and none were taken lightly; the routine I developed and practiced ensured this. Again visualisation played a critical role. Although I was standing alone in a field in Kilkenny in my mind I was in packed Croke Park and the pressure was on.

In the later part of my career I began to work one-to-one with Bro. Damien Brennan. He was a unique and great man and became a mentor to me. We would discuss areas for improvement in my game and often practice things one-on-one where he would give me specific individualised feedback. The idea was to find an area for improvement, discuss it and practice it with targeted and focused practice. I found working with him extremely beneficial and would recommend seeking the guidance of a mentor to anyone who wishes to keep pushing the envelope on performance.

I loved collective training. I loved being with the lads, on the training pitch, giving it my all. I loved the energy of it. I also loved practicing by myself. It was a habit I created as a child in the squash court and one that continued to develop and evolved as I met new challenges and learned more about myself as a player and the demands of the game I loved. My advice to any youngster who wishes to both enjoy their chosen sport and reach their potential in it would be to commit to practicing away from the crowds in places where no one is watching. Know your strengths but be willing to attack your weaknesses. Practice with purpose. Hone your craft and have fun along the way.

I wish you well,
Henry Shefflin

A STRATEGIC APPROACH TO PRACTICE
Dr Phil Kearney

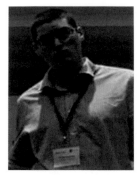

Dr Phil Kearney is a Lecturer in Motor Skill Acquisition and Coaching and Performance in University of Limerick. He is also Course Director of the Masters of Science in Applied Sports Coaching. I have asked Phil to contribute a piece in the area of practice. Below he explains a well-researched and proven method he uses to introduce athletes to a more purposeful and systematic approach to practicing what are termed closed motor skills.

Whether playing sport, practicing a musical instrument, learning to drive or studying schoolwork, understanding how to practice most effectively has great potential to accelerate learning and make more efficient use of practice time. However, as illustrated by the example from Gary Sice that follows, many athletes and players need help to learn how to make the most out of their practice sessions. For sports skills, the American psychologist Robert Singer introduced a five step strategy that could provide a framework for more effective practice. In particular, this strategy was designed for individuals attempting to learn closed motor skills: skills that are performed in a relatively stable environment where the learner can decide when to initiate the movement. Examples of closed motor skills include: the basketball free throw, the tennis serve, golf strokes, kicking for touch in rugby, taking a free in hurling or football, a vault in gymnastics, as well as many jumping or throwing events within track and field. So what are the five steps within the strategy?

- *Readying: The goal of the first step is to prepare for a high quality attempt; your body position should be suitably balanced, your mind free from distractions, thinking positively about how you will perform. This step often involves some preparatory action, such as a practice swing in golf, to help tune in to the body. In addition, simple breathing exercises or cue words might be used to control your arousal levels. It is important to stress that the optimal mental state to enhance learning (i.e., how relaxed or fired up you need to be) is likely to depend both on the individual and on the skill being practiced. The specifics of the readying step may be unique to each learner, but the goal is the same: you are ready to deliver a high quality action.*

- *Imaging:* In the second step, you imagine the desired action and/or outcome. As with readying, there is considerable flexibility within this step for an individual-specific approach. For example, you may use kinaesthetic (i.e., focus on feeling the movement) or visual imagery. If adopting visual imagery, you may rehearse the action from your own perspective (internal imagery), or as though observing yourself performing on television (external imagery). You may view the entire action, or you may pay particular attention to how one particular element of the movement looks or feels. Regardless of how it is achieved, the goal of this step is to have clearly established what you is trying to achieve within the attempt.
- *Focus:* During the third step, you focus your attention on one relevant cue, using this intense focus to block out potential distractors. For ball sports, you might concentrate on the seams of the tennis ball, football, basketball or sliotar. For track and field events, you might focus on the first checkpoint in your run up. As with the preceding steps, different individuals will focus on different elements; what matters most is that you narrow your focus to a relevant cue, thus "closing the door" on potentially disruptive thoughts.
- *Execute:* Expert performers can execute skills without conscious thought. Following the preceding steps will have primed you to do likewise. When everything feels right, "just do it", as the Nike advert advocates, without consciously thinking of or trying to control anything about the act itself or the possible outcome.
- *Evaluation:* In the final step, you engage with all available feedback to assess the performance outcome (e.g. did I score the point?) and the movement by which it was achieved (e.g. did I follow through like I was intending?). In addition, you should pay attention to the effectiveness of each step in the routine (Was I ready? Did I obtain a clear image? etc.), adjusting any procedure for the next attempt, if required. Undertaken correctly, the evaluation should be as detailed and mentally taxing as the performance itself.

Researchers have consistently demonstrated the effectiveness of Singer's Five Step Strategy for enhancing practice quality and thereby accelerating learning. Here are some key points to consider for any athlete/coach implementing this approach:

1. The Five Step Strategy is intensive; wait until the learner wants to engage in more structured, serious practice before introducing the full strategy.
2. The Five Step Strategy should not be implemented on every practice session. Sometimes you might be playing around with a

technique, exploring creative options. At other times, you might be trying to recreate a competition environment, challenging yourself to perform under specific conditions. In both instances, the Strategy is likely to disrupt your goals for the session.

3. *Most athletes will instinctively follow some of the steps outlined within the strategy. For example, Henry Shefflin has already provided an example of this in his account of practicing by himself, and working on his free taking: which of the steps can you find mentioned within his account? Start by identifying what you already do, and develop your strategy from there.*

4. *Although at first glance the strategy may appear to be formal and rigid, there is considerable flexibility within the 5 Step Approach to adapt each step to your needs and experiences while providing a clear framework to promote higher quality practice.*

5. *The strategy consists of a number of individual skills (arousal regulation, imagery, concentration), each of which may need to be practiced before being effectively utilised within the strategy.*

6. *Learners using this strategy will perform fewer repetitions within a set amount of practice time due to the increased time required to adequately prepare and evaluate; the higher quality of these repetitions will more than compensate for the reduced number.*

Best wishes,
Phil Kearney

CHAPTER 5

Gary Sice

Gary Sice is a former Galway and current Corofin Gaelic Footballer. He has been a central figure throughout the period which has seen Corofin become the greatest club team in history, winning 4 All-Ireland club titles in the past 6 years. Throughout his career he has moved from being an out-and-out defender to a scoring forward and a deadly-accurate free-taker. This has forced him to evolve and develop new skills that he would be required to execute in high pressure situations. Here he shares with us his interesting journey as a free-taker and gives us an insight into how he practices and prepares for the pressure kicks.

I took my first free in championship football at the age of 27 years old. It was the 20th of May 2012 playing for Galway in the first round of the Connacht Championship against Roscommon. Up until that point in time, I had never once even taken a free for my club Corofin, let alone take one at intercounty level. Alan O'Donovan was our free-taker in the club and he was prolific. Our Galway free-taker at the time was the deadly-accurate Michael Meehan, but he had gotten injured playing in our last league game against Kerry. Team management asked me would I take over the responsibility of the free kicks from the right hand side of the pitch. Only two years previously I had made the move from being an out-and-out defender at both club and county level to a half-forward. As far as free taking was concerned, it was fair to say I had my work cut out for me.

I spent the six weeks before the Roscommon game practicing frees in manner which I now know was less than optimal or indeed effective. I took on a huge amount of information in that short space of time. It would take me virtually the rest of my career to really understand it. As luck would have it I landed the first free against Roscommon and never looked back. I spent the next five years taking frees for Galway and in 2013 I took over the reigns as lead free- taker with Corofin. This was a time when, as a group, we were beginning to become increasingly focused on gains and improvement and were starting to build towards a very exciting period in our clubs history which would see us win 4 All-Irelands and seven county titles in a row.

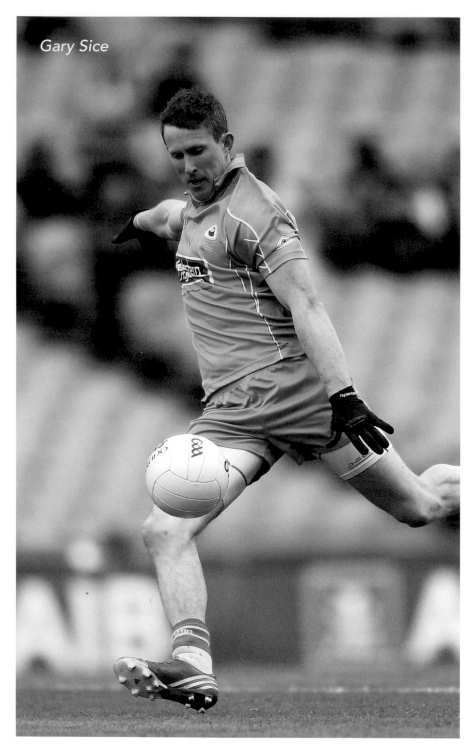

Gary Sice

When I began taking frees, nerves were an issue for me. I would put weight on certain 'important' frees and kick the situation and not the free that was in front of me. If I had missed one previously I would feel pressure for the next one; if the game was tight and the free was 'important', it would play on my mind as I set up for the kick. As I progressed and grew in confidence I got over this and was just …in the moment… in my routine. Nothing of what had happened previously or may happen in the next phase of play would bother me. I soon found the responsibility of free-taking added to my overall game; it drove my confidence. For me, free-taking became a part of my game I could control really well and it gave me the confidence to gain control over others parts of my game.

My free-taking routine has developed and evolved over the years. I have studied others and knowingly or otherwise have taken bits and pieces from them. For example, I fall into a semi-squat position as part of my routine. I can only presume I took this from former English rugby player Jonny Wilkinson. I read his book a number of years ago and being a left foot kicker his insights were of particular interest to me. His routine involved him cupping his hands and taking a semi-squat position.

My routine has evolved into the following: bounce the ball and catch it, wipe my right hand/ glove off my shorts, bring my hand back to ball, wipe my left hand/ glove off my shorts, bring my hand back to the ball, semi squat, three steps, kick.

If my routine is interrupted I go back to the start as if it changes, for whatever reason, I am in trouble. For example, I missed two frees over the course of last year's club championship. One was in the All-Ireland semi-final against Nemo Rangers after a heavy collision where I should have taken more time to recover and hence execute my routine better. The other was against Padraig Pearses in the Connacht final where I failed to deal with an interruption from an opposition player prior to the kick and lost focus. My routine is my comfort blanket and brings me to the place I need to be to convert a free-kick. It is bullet proof provided I have the practice done. I can be in any field in the country, playing any opposition in the country, in any minute of the game and it will be of no relevance to me. If my routine is strong, everything will be fine.

I take frees from the right hand side of the pitch on my left foot. In order to make the goals seem bigger I aim for the section between the black spot of the crossbar and the far post and target half way up the goal posts. Most of my free-kicks are taken in winter and so aiming half-way up the post gives me consistency across all weather conditions. My only real chance of missing is pulling the kick on the near post but as I have said, this only occurs when I deviate from my routine.

My routine has been developed and honed through hours of quality practice. I say 'quality practice', because without doubt, quantity is critical, but often quality can be overlooked. I aim to engage in meaningful, purposely practice where every kick is weighted similarly. In-season, I do two individual free-kicking sessions weekly. I also punch in numerous free-kicks at various stages before and after training. I find these particularly valuable. Before and after training there is 'interference' around the place. I often kick from areas on the pitch where people are gathered talking or stretching or whatever. Where possible I actively seek out these areas. For me it is a great challenge; can I switch on and off my routine at an impromptu moment?

My individual free-kick sessions look like a bag of balls and a definite number of kicks in my head before I head to the field- usually 40 or 50. I count them as I go, constantly reflecting and studying my kicking. I am looking for a 90% + conversion rate depending on the weather. A good strike feels effortless, it feels correct- it's a sensation. I often purposely pick bad days for my practice. If I can kick in the wind and rain I can kick any day. For upcoming games I try to do my opposition homework in advance and target areas in the pitch I feel we will get frees from. Other than this, my kicking sites are chosen at random. After every game I watch back the match footage on our team analysis app and critique each kick, often with input from my coaches. This allows me to learn as I go- any miss will be dissected and a remedy will be sought.

The more I practice the greater my scoring range becomes and the more my confidence grows and my routine is solidified. Some say practice make perfect but for me 'perfect practice makes (semi) permanent'. When the right type of practice is in the bank it will be there when I need. However it won't stay there forever and so I need to keep topping it up. For me, practice is reversible. Without my required dose my body shape and confidence suffer, the trajectory of the ball is effected and my scoring zone shortens significantly- my routine is weakened. I depend on 'quality practice' and it serves me well.

All the best,
Gary Sice.

As human beings we are designed to be improvable. While we may not all have the makings of a top-end elite athlete we can all learn more effectively, practice smarter and build or improve our skills. No matter your pre-existing skill level, improvement is there for you if you follow the above principles. In sport and indeed life you must learn to trust yourself, however I would also note that you must have a reason to trust yourself. You must earn the right to be proud of, and confident in, your skills. Cultivating excellence is not a quick process. It is a daily routine of meticulous preparation and repetition. Everything we do is practice; it is up to you to make it deliberate.

References:
Ericsson, Anders; Pool, Robert (2016). Peak: Secrets from the New Science of Expertise. Boston: Houghton Mifflin Harcourt. ISBN 978-0544456235.
Singer, R. N. (1988). Strategies and metastrategies in learning and performing selfpaced athletic skills. The Sport Psychologist, 2, 49–68.
Retrieved from: http:///www.humankinetics.com/tsp
Singer, R. N., & Cauraugh, J. H. (1985). The generalizability effect of learning strategies for categories of psychomotor skills. Quest, 37, 103–119.
doi:10.1080/00336297.1985.10483824

SUMMARY POINTS - Chapter 5

- If you wish to be the best you can be, making a personal commitment to honing your craft is critical.
- The fundamentals require constant re-emphasis.
- If your craft is something you really want to excel in, you have to push past that comfortable stage and challenge yourself.
- The key to effective practice is to make it purposeful and deliberate.
- Deliberate Practice requires focused attention and is conducted with the specific goal of improving performance.
- Understanding the demands of your sport and the role or position you play, as well as learning how to properly analyse your performance will help inform you of what parts of your game you need to focus on.

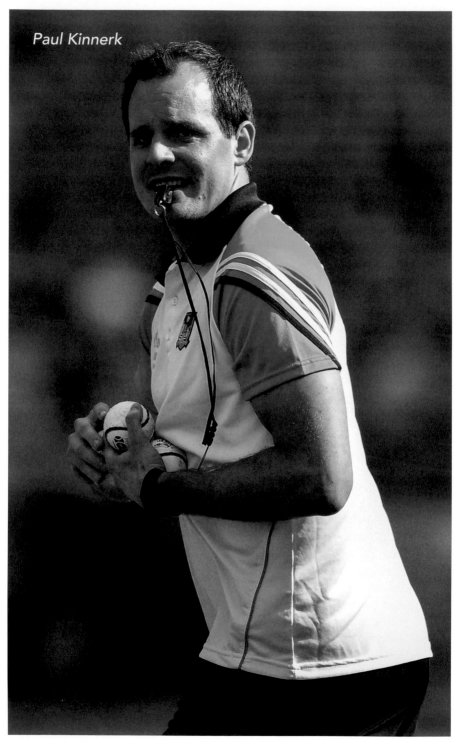

Paul Kinnerk

CHAPTER 6: APPLICATION IN TRAINING

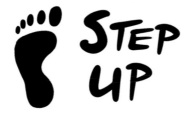

By Dr Paul Kinnerk

Dr Paul Kinnerk is a highly respected and accomplished GAA Coach. He is seen as a pioneer of innovative coaching practices within the GAA. His most notable accomplishments have been as part of the All-Ireland Hurling Champions Clare coaching team in 2013 and Limerick in 2018 where he remains as team coach. He has recently completed a PhD which focuses on game-based approaches to coaching in Gaelic Games. Other research interests of Paul include Sports Coaching Pedagogy in Team Sports and Game-Based Approach Pedagogies. Here he offers you advice on how to maximise your application in collective training sessions.

"Hard work beats talent if talent doesn't work hard", or "fail to prepare, prepare to fail", and the list goes on. Essentially, these sayings emphasise the importance of an athlete committing maximum efforts to their preparation for competition. Over the past 10 years I have been fortunate to work with some of the best athletes within our country. One prominent common attribute shared across these athletes is their ability to apply themselves within training sessions. This piece will share some of my experiences on coaching players over the past 10 years and identify areas within the coaching session where you can maximise your application to training.

Social learning is one of the great outlets that athletes have the opportunity to engage in, holding many benefits. However, in many settings, this form of learning remains an untapped resource by both coach and athlete. Athletes learn by engaging in conversation and listening to other athletes. In fact, some of the great forms of learning take place during debate; when one athlete comes forward with one opinion and is then positioned to defend that opinion, whilst also engaging with the thoughts of another athlete. The academic research refers to this as 'cognitive disequilibrium' and highlights high levels of engagement and learning occurring as a result of these interactions (Light, 2013). A point for reflection- how often do you engage in conversations with other players or the coach as regards tactical issues or game-plan, and how often do you really listen to others. Some of the healthiest sights I have witnessed on the training ground have involved players in conversations amongst themselves about a tactical problem between games or after the session. This form of social engagement is a way for you to test and develop your own knowledge as well as promoting your teammates to do so.

Another socially related form of learning can be achieved through requesting feedback (see also Chapter 7 and Chapter 9). There are two simple ways you may seek feedback. Firstly, you can ask your coach for areas to improve on. The coach is well placed to offer insight on specific areas of the game that could lead to improvement in your performance. However, many athletes do not avail of this feedback, and coach-initiated feedback can be infrequent in team based sports. Therefore, you must ensure to approach your coach regularly and request feedback on specific areas of your game to work on rather than waiting for your coach to initiate such conversations. In receiving specific feedback, the athlete is made consciously aware of a narrow area of the game to direct their attention and efforts. For novice athletes, this feedback may allow them to adjust a technical movement that enables them to improve the execution of a skill. For a highly skilled athlete, the feedback may encourage them to exaggerate a less developed side of their game that can be critical for performing at the highest level. The second form of feedback which I would encourage you to actively seek on a regular basis is from a teammate. Training games present an excellent opportunity to avail of such feedback. Within invasion game sports such as Gaelic games, soccer, hockey and rugby, players are typically competing against an opposite number or 'marker'. These opponents may hold great knowledge about aspects of your game; what you do well, what you do that puts them under pressure, what you do poorly. A true team player will be forthcoming with such detail if you request it. I have witnessed excellent feedback conversations between players during training games where they openly share feedback to their opposing marker. Feedback shared in this way can be powerful as it is 'live' and, therefore, enables the player to act upon the feedback in an upcoming play. The process of seeking feedback, reflecting and acting upon the feedback are effective means to maximise application within training and provide a targeted plan for improvement.

Developing understanding and meaning of the content within the training session can improve athletes' tactical knowledge and decision-making (Kinnerk et al., 2018). You develop understanding by engaging in a process of interpretation throughout the session. This process of interpretation should involve you reflecting and making sense of the practice tasks designed by the coach. You should strive to understand why certain conditions have been employed within a specific game. For example, in a Gaelic football modified game, the coach may use a condition that restricts players to wide channels of the field or a limited number of plays on the ball. In such cases, the player rather than simply abiding by such rules, should instead question their worth and make sense of how these conditions could be used (or not) to impact their own game. This level of critical thought and reflection is essential in developing understanding (Light, 2013). Moreover, you may develop understanding by making connections with content covered earlier within the session and previous sessions. For example, if a player is struggling with a tactical problem such as breaking down a packed defence within a modified game, it is likely that possible solutions to this problem were explored and discussed previously; either within the current session or an earlier session. Therefore, by engaging in a process of interpreting how previous content connects with the current scenario, the player is developing knowledge and tactical understanding to assist their decision-making with the game.

Training at high levels of intensity is a critical factor to enhance your performance during competition. Intensity must be smart and defined for you to maximise your efforts. The coach will play a significant role within this process by designing tasks and rest periods which facilitate a suitable stimulus for athletes. However, within many game-related tasks, the player is in control of the decision to run, to support, to track, and to 'work hard'. So, while 10 players may all take part in the same task, each player's level of involvement and intensity of effort will differ from player to player. I believe the players that perform at the highest level, train to their highest level within tasks in training. There are a number of easily applied methods which can facilitate your ability to train at a high level. Firstly, "self-talk" (see Chapter 12) is a skill which I constantly advocate during training. Self-talk refers to using internal dialogue as a means of producing a positive response. You may engage in positive motivational self-talk to assist you in making a hard supporting run, or sprinting after an opposing player to the maximum of your ability. This internal dialogue may prompt greater levels of effort than you may produce without using it. Secondly, you should become aware of what 'hard work' constitutes in your sport and your team's game plan. Physiological markers such as heart rate and Global Positioning System (GPS) data can be informative to help athletes focus. However, tactical markers such as number of possessions, tackles, support runs, defensive covers, and assists offer greater indications of intensity (see Chapter 7). Players should seek to become consciously aware of these markers and focus their efforts on achieving high numbers for these markers within all training tasks. For example, a player that is explicitly aware of the need to gain possession is likely to increase their efforts off-the-ball in order to get on-the-ball. This may involve the player making a greater frequency of supporting runs at higher velocity to lose their marker which of course leads to a higher intensity of effort. Critically, the player must hold themselves accountable in chasing these targets during training in an effort to achieve gains from an intensity perspective. Athletes that commit their efforts in this focused and process driven approach will maximise their chances of training at high intensity.

The final point I'd like to highlight in relation to maximising application within the training session involves you creating time for isolated skills practice. Whatever your sport, and whatever your position, technical skills that involve throwing, kicking, catching, shooting, striking, and controlling are likely to be present. While you will receive opportunities to execute technical skill within the main training session, efforts should be made by you to supplement the training session content with additional skills practice (see Chapter 5).

The time before training offers an excellent opportunity to engage in this type of practice. You should identify areas of your game that you wish to improve such as your weaker side and use the unpressurised environment before training to accumulate a large number of executions of the isolated skill. Moreover, you should use the time before training to engage in practice of skills deemed critical to your position on the field (see Chapter 7) even when you are highly proficient in such skills. For rugby, a hooker may use the time to practice their line-out throwing, in soccer, a defender may use the time heading the ball from corner kicks, in Gaelic football, forwards may use the time shooting, and in hurling, a half-back may use the time catching and batting high balls from a keepers puckout. The point being, you are in control of this time and should take ownership for organising tasks which are specific to your needs. This self-led form of practice is a common characteristic shared amongst many of our successful elite performers in sport.

This piece has highlighted that effective application within the training session is multi-faceted and not limited to the often ill-defined notion of "training hard". Effective application within the training session should incorporate high levels of social and reflective engagement to facilitate athlete's development of decision-making and tactical knowledge. Furthermore, progress in the critical components of intensity and skill execution can be developed through you taking ownership to develop these aspects of your game before and within the session. A meaningful commitment by you to developing these aspects of training should maximise your progress and participation within the session.

Best wishes,
Paul Kinnerk

SKILLS FOR DRAWING
ON YOUR INNER STRENGTH
SKILL NO. 2 - CONTROL
By Tony Óg Regan

Why is this Important?

There is much in the 'outer world' we are not in control or aware of, that drives our mind and bodies into a state of panic, fear and anxiety. When you start to identify the things you can't control and focus your lens on the controllable factors it frees up your mind and attention (see also Chapter 11). This allows you be creative in new situations, gain new insights about your potential, form new thoughts and ideas and indeed focus on the things within your control. High performers in pressure situations are the best in their fields because they recognise that uncertainty exists in a lot of cases, but they focus on what they can do in that moment to influence their skills or decisions on that task at hand.

The four main things you can train in this world are: your mind, your body, your craft and your sport. Before you look at these, you must look at living in the uncertainty of what you can control, influence and not control at all. What you can control are things that are 100% in your control, what you can influence you have a certain degree of control over and what you have no control over is what you have absolutely no control over whatsoever!

LIST WHAT YOU CONTROL IN RELATION TO YOUR SPORT?

_____

_____

Here is what I came up with regarding CONTROL: my thoughts, my state of mind, my organisation, my energy.

LIST WHAT YOU CAN INFLUENCE IN RELATION TO YOUR SPORT.

_____

_____

Here is what I came up with regarding INFLUENCE: My skills, my opponent, the officials, my sleep, my hydration, my food, my equipment, my travel plans, my coaches, my teammates, and my performance.

LIST WHAT YOU CAN'T CONTROL IN RELATION TO YOUR SPORT.

_____

_____

Here is what I came up with regarding CAN'T control: The weather, the outcome, the venue, the time, the supporters, the media and other people's opinions.

How can I practice letting go of control? Mindfulness
A key skill to practice in being in control in the moment, is the practice of mindfulness. It is known from the field of psychology, that our thoughts and feelings influence how we behave. You can learn to manage your thoughts and feelings by practicing what are known as mindfulness techniques. We all have different responses under pressure. Through the practice of mindfulness, you become more aware of the helpful and unhelpful thoughts and feelings you have during pressure moments.

The first step is AWARENESS – What do I say to myself when under pressure?

The second step CHANGE – What is the thought or behaviour I wish to change?

The third step ACTION – What new thought, statement or behaviour will I execute to override this old way of reacting?

Examples: Trigger statements like "I got this" or "I love being in these moments". A physical behaviour might be deep breaths and reset body language with head up, shoulders back and hands on hips in a power pose (acting confident changes the physiological response we are having which influences our psychological response).

'Thoughts are not truths and feelings are not facts'

This is a good mantra to reinforce to yourself when you are not thinking or feeling your best in pressure situations. We know that a thought can fire an electrical signal or a response through our bodies which we may deem as unhelpful to our performance in the moment. It is about switching your point of attention to something inside (like your breath or a sensation or a thought) or outside you (like a point in front of you e.g. a ball or a target like the corner of the goals). Below is a short, 90-second training technique that helps prime your brain and mind to be more present, more focused, more grateful and calmer.

Morning Mindset Training
On awaking, keeping your eyes closed, take one large inhale and one larger exhale – this sends a signal to the brain all is ok.
On the inhale, breathe in for 4 seconds through your nose, pause at the top of the breath for 4 seconds, exhale out through the mouth for 4 seconds and rest for 4 seconds. Repeat this as often as you like, until you feel present, grounded and calm.
Now think of someone or something in your life right now you are grateful for having. See that image in your mind and hold it for 5-10 seconds allowing those feelings to sink in.
Set an intention for today to feel joyful and energetic in your body, to be caring and kind from your heart, to be alert and thoughtful in your mind and to experience a lightness in being.
Now feel the points of contact with your body and the chair or bed. Open your eyes when you are ready.

Summary
Focus your time and energy on what you can control and what you can influence. Practice becoming aware of when you focus on things outside of our control and let go of them through a simple breath to redirect your attention. Ask two simple questions:

1. *What circle am I in right now: the circle of control, the circle of influence or the circle of no control?*
2. *What can I do right now that is in my control regarding this situation?*

The ability to live more consistently in the present moment is what helps to separate average performance from great performance. This allows them to make better decisions in the key moments. In modern life we are living with the distraction of social media, gaming, TV, Internet and noise. We are on our phones for 3-5 hours a day. We are diminishing our ability to hold our attention.

At the start of 2000 we could hold our attention on a single thought for up to 12 seconds. In 2013 that figure had dropped to 4-5 seconds. In the last 7 years the levels of technology use have increased year on year. In the sporting environment what effect is this lack of attentional control having on our performance? How easily distracted do you become by external stimuli like supporters, weather or your opponents? How easily can you access 'no mind' where you are free from internal distraction, completely absorbed in just being in the moment you have right now?

The skill of the mindful performer to become aware of this internal or external distraction and refocus in the moment is going to be one of the most important skills to train now and in the future. Make this a daily practice to RECOGNISE when distracted and RETURN to the PRESENT MOMENT.

See also - Skill No. 4- Composure & Skill No. 7- Commitment

References

Kinnerk, P., Harvey, S., MacDonncha, C., & Lyons, M. (2018). A review of the game-based approaches to coaching literature in competitive team sport settings. Quest, 70(4), 401-418.
Light, R. L. (2013). Game sense: Pedagogy for performance, participation and enjoyment. New York, NY: Routledge.

SUMMARY POINTS - Chapter 6

- Athletes learn by engaging in conversation and listening to other athletes.
- You must ensure to approach your coach regularly and request feedback on specific areas of your game to work on rather than waiting for the coach to initiate such conversations.
- You should actively and regularly seek feedback from a teammate.
- Self-talk refers to using internal dialogue as a means of producing a positive response and is a skill that should be developed.
- You should become aware of what 'hard work' constitutes of in your sport and team's game plan.
- Before the beginning of training is an excellent time for you to engage in isolated skills practice.
- When you start to identify the things you can't control and focus your lens on the controllable factors it frees up your mind and attention.

CHAPTER 7: PERFORMANCE ANALYSIS

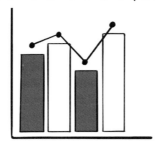

One of the most important challenges of the coach is to connect those they coach to the sport at hand. A question I always ask myself is: how can I help those I coach grow their love for the game? To truly master one's craft, there must be love.

> "The most important difference between champions and others is the love and passion for the game".
> Rafael Nadal

A genuine love of the game is needed in order to reach your potential, because the journey will be filled with struggle and setbacks. If the joy and love aren't present, you will burn out and fall away.

> "The game of basketball has been everything to me...
> It's been the site of intense pain and the most intense feelings of joy and satisfaction. It's a relationship that has evolved over time, given me the greatest respect and love for the game".
> Michael Jordan

With a view to nurturing love of the game in those I coach, another question I always ask myself is: How can I help make them 'students of the game'? It is only then that they can truly pursue excellence. The goal is to develop 'loving students of the game'. In order to enable you to become a 'loving student' of your sport, it is important that this book offers you some tools and skills required to study and learn your sport, self-analyse your performance and create your own 'Personal Improvement Plan'. I have asked David Morris and Mark McAreavey to help you here. The majority of the piece is targeted towards athletes in team sports, but in reality, analysis is a principled based practice and as such, the same principles apply to both sporting arenas.

(Please Note- Preparing to Perform is also an important part of this area, and this will be looked at in detail in Chapter 11.)

By David Morris and Mark McAreavey

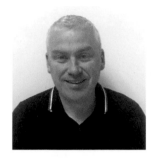

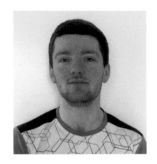

David Morris has been an ever-present Coach of the famed Corofin Senior Football team throughout their recent history, which has seen them winning 4 Club All-Irelands over the last 6 years. He is also a GAA Level 4 Performance Analyst and has worked with many successful intercounty teams. He is co-founder of 'GAA Insights' which provides detailed data analysis for a wide range of intercounty hurling and football teams.

Mark McAreavey is an ISPAS Level 4 Performance Analysis Consultant with Avenir Sports, currently working with a number of intercounty Gaelic Football teams and the Northern Ireland Senior Men's Football team. He has worked with Northern Ireland Netball for over 6 years, helping them achieve their highest ever world ranking of 8th. He was Team Northern Ireland Performance Analyst at the 2018 Commonwealth Games, working mainly with swimming and netball. He is also an Associate of the Sports Institute Northern Ireland and has worked across a range of other sports including: Hockey, Hurling, Rugby, Swimming and Table Tennis.

"Do the best you can until you know better.
Then, when you know better, do better".
Maya Angelou

Performance Analysis - An Overview
Performance Analysis can provide athletes (and coaches) with unbiased information that helps them understand both the demands of their sport and their performance. The goal is to analyse information, draw insight, and act on it. If we break this down, it is important that we analyse the right information, draw the correct insights and act appropriately to get the most benefit from the analysis. If we can do these three things correctly, we will improve performance.

On its own merits, analysis cannot achieve anything. It must be part of a performance system and be underpinned by quality practice, and a commitment to improve.

The Evolution of Performance Analysis

In recent years, performance analysis has evolved, with technological advancement to the forefront finding new, advanced ways to engage and improve the performance of athletes and teams. Some years ago, the role of a Performance Analyst was to 'click and count'; simply consisting of clicking to start recording a game and counting basic statistics. Thankfully, the days of a whole team sitting down to watch a full game together, and pausing to highlight a mistake, time and time again, are resigned to the past.

Through the advent of technology and improved training for analysts, this traditional form of analysis has now been replaced by a more player-centred approach. Today, the role of Performance Analysts has evolved where they now require more expertise in tracking data from the various systems, and increasing its accessibility for players and coaches. Data, as well as video, is now available for coaches and players to interact with during, and immediately, after the game. Many analysts are now qualified and certified and the quality of their delivery is more relevant and suitable to a learning environment. We know that learning can take many different forms, but the most effective learning is achieved by those that can teach others, closely followed, by practice by doing. Examples of how elite-level teams currently operate with regard to involving the player in the analytics process include:

- *Players facilitating analysis sessions sharing what they see: what went well and opportunities to improve.*
- *Coaches presenting scenarios to players on tactics board, and in training games, for them to solve in a limited timeframe.*
- *Injured players joining the analysis team to develop their game understanding and awareness.*

As well as this, players can log and view wellness behaviours and scores, monitor sleep patterns and training loads (GPS) and view video, selecting only the relevant clips to them, all through their smartphone. In many sports, they can also view videos of their direct opponent, in advance of the game. With all of this data available, it is fair to say that the player has become a Performance Analyst.

"Once he had that little bit, he wanted more.
If the greatest player of his generation is looking for an edge,
I think other people would be wise to follow".
Shaun Battier on Lebron James

Tactical Innovation

Of course, the above journey has not just come about because of technological and learning advancements. Nowadays teams rarely go out simply to play each other; most come with a strategy for the challenge that awaits them. Opposition analysis has become the norm, with detailed match-ups and playing systems being utilised to nullify perceived opposition strengths, and capitalise on perceived opposition weaknesses. In many management teams, a significant amount of time is spent analysing the opposition and drafting a 'game plan'.

Innovation is everywhere in sport. Soccer is now far removed from 4-4-2, and we see clubs hiring experts to analyse and improve areas of the game such as throw-ins. Set-plays in rugby have led to a surge in copying NFL playbooks. Gaelic games have evolved to take learnings, and tactics, from many sources.

Reading the Game

In addition to teams having different tactics, many teams will also adapt their tactics in-game in order to gain a competitive advantage. It is now up to the opposition to adapt quickly, to turn the game back in their favour. Traditionally the analyst, or coach, would have to spot the change in tactics, come up with a plan to address it, communicate the plan, and then ensure that all players follow the plan. Wouldn't it be much more efficient for the players to be attuned to this and change the tactics for themselves in-game?

One of your challenges going forward will be to learn how to analyse or 'read' the game as it unfolds in front of you and communicate it to those around you. You will need acumen and awareness to identify the issue, figure out a solution, and communicate this to your teammates so you can all adapt and respond together.

Analysing Your Opponent

Another skill, which is worthy of note here, is the ability to analyse your direct opponent in-game. As noted, in more elite-level teams with a professional analyst, individualised opposition video footage and data is often provided pre-game to allow players: study habits, look for trends, and establish strengths and weaknesses of their direct opponent.

Below is a sample data graph that might be shown by the analysts in a pre-game presentation. It shows the shooting habits of the top three shooters on the opposition hurling team. How might you use this information to approach marking each player?

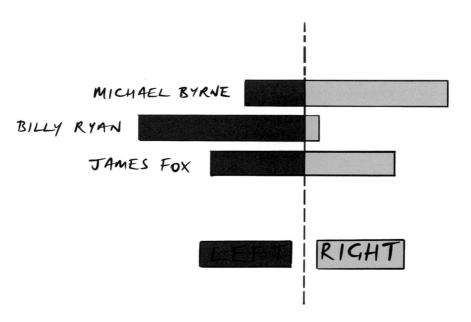

Whether this resource is available to you or not, it is still prudent to analyse your opponent in-game and use the information to strategise how you can best approach the challenge they pose. For example, after the first few phases of play, you may establish that your opponent is physically weaker and slower than you. Armed with this information, you may decide to take them on in a foot race, when the opportunity affords itself. Similarly, after a few possessions you may observe that they are predominantly dependent on one side and there is a trend in their pattern of play. This information allows you to strategically position yourself in tackling and out-of-possession scenarios. Developing this ability to analyse and strategise in-game is something you should be continuously mindful of. In-game awareness is a critical skill.

Self-Analysis

What follows is a guide to self-analysis for the athlete, who does not have the support of professional analysis. The aim here is to offer you the tools and skills required to analyse your own performance and create an ever-evolving 'Personal Improvement Plan' that can inform your individual practice (see Chapter 5) as well as your application in collective training (see Chapter 6) and ultimately improve your performance.

Firstly, it must be noted that there are many avenues available to you already that you may not be attuned to. Coaches, assistants and mentors are all useful resources (see Chapter 9). Indeed, although not a probable option until recently, video is now becoming more readily available, and will continue to do so. As you move forward, you will no doubt have increased access to video, and so your personal analytics skills can become a huge potential weapon in your search for improvement.

When you talk about performance, you can ask 3 important questions:
1. What are you trying to achieve? (Goal)
2. Where on the journey are you now? (Current State)
3. How do you get from Current State to Goal? (Close Gap)

The GROW model, designed by Sir John Whitmore, is a simple method for goal setting and problem solving and provides a useful framework for you. The cycle never ends, it just resets as you adjust your goal in order to continue your development.

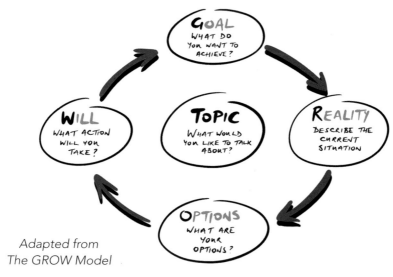

Adapted from
The GROW Model

Know Your Sport- Be a Student of the Game

If we return to Question 1 we ask ourselves: What am I trying to achieve? What is the goal?

In order for you to understand your performance, you must first understand your sport, the demands it places on its participants, and your role within the game, and the team.

By now you have probably been playing your chosen sport for many years. You are likely to have watched it played countless times, either live or on TV. Yet if somebody asked you to sit down and write out a list of qualities and skills that the best teams perform consistently well, could you do it with any degree of accuracy?

Case Study

Darragh is a 14 year old who loves soccer and wants to understand the game at a deeper level. During the 2018 FIFA World Cup he decided to do exactly this. He sat down with a pen, and journal, and watched France as they took on Croatia in the final.

As the game unfolded, he made a note of every positive quality and skill the French team showed. By the final whistle, and with France winning 4-2, he had a list of over 20.

His list read as follows:

- PASSING THE BALL
- RECEIVING THE BALL
- OFF THE BALL MOVEMENT
- SCANNING
- CROSSING
- FINISHING/SHOOTING
- COUNTER ATTACKING
- PENETRATIVE PASSING
- DRIBBLING
- TACKLING
- DEFENDING CROSSES
- PRESSING FROM THE FRONT
- SET PIECE DELIVERY
- 1 v 1 ATTACKING
- SWITCHING PLAY
- OVERLAPPING RUNS
- 1 v 1 DEFENDING
- AERIAL DOMINANCE
- SHOOTING FROM DISTANCE
- PLAYING OUT FROM THE BACK
- DEFENDING DEEP

Darragh now had a deeper, and more knowledgeable appreciation of the game of soccer. He was a student of the game. He knew the key qualities and skills of a top team. He knew what it is they do well and with continued study he could refine this knowledge. He was some way to having a goal to work towards.

This is a relatively easy exercise to carry out, regardless of your chosen sport or discipline, and will help to paint a really good picture of the demands of your sport. Of course, not all successful teams play with the same style. For example: The All Blacks play a vastly different style of rugby to France and Liverpool's 'heavy metal football' under Jurgen Klopp, is significantly different to Pep Guardiola's Manchester City 'tiki taka' philosophy. For this reason, the above exercise needs to be performed a number of times, while watching various teams, or individuals, compete to give you a more comprehensive view of the key qualities and skills displayed. The key message is to actively and consistently watch your sport being performed by the elite teams and players. Success leaves clues.

This is exactly what Darragh did, he continued to study various teams. However in order for the information he had collected to become truly useful, and relevant to him, he would need to further refine it.

Know Your Role

Taking the qualities and skills (or ones relevant to your sport) listed above is a nice framework for finding areas of your game to improve. Now, question how important and relevant are they to your position or role within the team? For example, in rugby, an important trait of a successful team may be tactical kicking. However, the significance of this to a fly half, as opposed to a hooker, is vastly different.

Your next step is to examine your specific position and role within the team. One of the simplest ways to do this is by analysing a favourite player who plays that position. List the most important qualities and skills they exhibit. This task may be best performed live as you look to fully immerse yourself in the role of the player in your position, not just when they appear in the video. Sometimes the most important actions of a player in a game go unnoticed and are selfless for the betterment of the team. For example, a player who makes a run which creates space for their teammate to score may not get the credit for the score, but without their run to drag the opposition out of position, the score doesn't happen. Again, not all players will play the role, or position, in the same manner, so it is important to perform this exercise on a number of occasions, analysing a different player in that position each time.

If we return to Darragh he now has a list of the key qualities and skills of the top players who play in his position of central midfield:

- **PASSING THE BALL**
- **OFF THE BALL MOVEMENT**
- **RECEIVING THE BALL - CONTROL**
- **DRIBBLING**
- **FINISHING / SHOOTING**
- **TACKLING**
- **SCANNING**

These points of reference are commonly termed 'Key Performance Indicators' or 'KPIs'.

Darragh now has a starting point, a goal to work towards and he can study how the best players effectively carry out these qualities and skills and what particular actions within each of them are most important. He can use the top performers as models (see Chapter 5).

For example, Darragh noticed that the majority of top midfielders are constantly scanning (regularly checking their surroundings) during the game. He then looked more closely at the skill over a number of games and what it was that the best players were actually doing. He found that expert scanners would check their surroundings approximately 8 times in the 10 seconds before they received a pass. He noticed that as a result of this they were better at pass completion especially in the attacking third of the pitch.

The message for you is to get to know in detail what constitutes good execution of the key skills of your position. It is then that Question 2 becomes relevant: Where on the journey are you now? In other words, what is your 'current state' in each of these areas?

Establishing Current State

Your ability to objectively come to sound conclusions about yourself will be the real differential. Some athletes can overestimate their abilities, while others can underestimate them. Here, the advice is to be as true to yourself as possible. Don't be too hard on yourself, don't be too easy on yourself. Know and understand why you are doing this; the sole purpose is to improve.

Scoring Yourself

Numerical rating systems normally consist on a 1-5 or 1-10 scale. However, a scale which is a small, even number such as 1-4 is often more thought-provoking and useful as it forces you not to pick the middle option making each number significantly different in definition. In a 1-4 scale the terms: 1 – Very Poor, 2 – Poor, 3 – Good, 4 – Excellent, can be attached, simplifying the decision and allowing for clearer ratings.

You can also define these four terms in relation to the quality or skill being studied and decide the appropriate option. If for example, Darragh was scoring his ball control when receiving the ball using the aforementioned 1-4 scale, here are some examples of what each number could symbolise:

1. A number of bad touches which often leads him to lose possession.
2. A number of touches which make the second touch be a form of recovery and allows the opposition to gain a better position.
3. A number of touches which effectively gather possession, but changes the speed of the attack for his team
4. A number of touches which allow him to gain an upper hand on his direct opponent putting them on the backfoot.

Darragh then took his KPIs from above and established his 'current state' using the suggested 1-4 scale. He scored himself as follows:

- PASSING THE BALL - 3 OUT OF 4
- OFF THE BALL MOVEMENT - 3 OUT OF 4
- RECEIVING THE BALL - CONTROL - 0 OUT OF 4
- DRIBBLING - 3 OUT OF 4
- FINISHING / SHOOTING - 1 OUT OF 4
- TACKLING - 0 OUT OF 4
- SCANNING - 0 OUT OF 4

Next he plotted his scores on a simple graph to help visualise his scores.

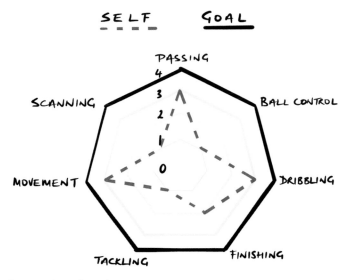

Cross Referencing for Accuracy

This process can be completed in conjunction with a mentor or coach (see Chapter 9) who can provide an alternative insight into your abilities using the same rating system. This leads you to a place of self-discovery as you try to understand what causes the difference in opinion in these areas. For example, why does your mentor or coach rate you as 'poor' in an area which you think is 'good?' What are their expectations in this area and how does that differ from your perspective?

The Work Begins

Darragh must now focus his attention on Question 3: How do I get from Current State to Goal? (Close Gap) And so the work begins and in truth never really ends. He is now equipped with his own 'Personal Improvement Plan'. He can pick three key qualities and skills to focus on for the next four weeks and this gives him a very clear direction as to the areas of his game that require the most focus in individual practice (Chapter 5) and team training (see Chapter 6). In Darragh's case he chose control, tackling and scanning which were his three perceived weakest areas at the time. Self-awareness is the key to individual improvement.

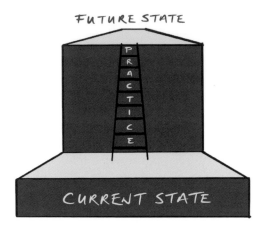

Performance Analysis - The Power of Reflection

The very same process as described can be used to analyse your performance post game. Using your Key Performance Indicators KPIs and scoring system you can create a Personal Performance Analysis Tool (see Darragh's below) and then you can score yourself in each KPI when reviewing your performance either from memory or match-day footage. Match footage is obviously best because it will allow you to remove the emotion of match-day and effectively evaluate your performance; however, if this is not available, recall from memory will suffice. Be clear and concise in your summaries of what success is in that quality or skill and rate your performance in line with these metrics. Again, the above process can be completed in conjunction with a coach or mentor (see Chapter 9) who can provide an alternative insight into your performance using the same rating system.

Darragh's Personal Performance Analysis Tool

	GAME 1	GAME 2	GAME 3	GAME 4	AVERAGE
PASSING THE BALL					
OFF THE BALL MOVEMENT					
RECEIVING THE BALL - CONTROL					
DRIBBLING					
FINISHING / SHOOTING					
TACKLING					
SCANNING					

I MUST START _____

I MUST STOP _____

I MUST CONTINUE _____

More importantly though, by monitoring these scores over a 3 or 4 game period, you can further refine and establish a clearer direction as to the areas of your game that require the most focus in individual practice (Chapter 5) and team training (see Chapter 6). In other words, you can continue to 'grow'.

Darragh's Completed Personal Performance Analysis Tool

	GAME 1	GAME 2	GAME 3	GAME 4	AVERAGE
PASSING THE BALL	3	3	2	3	2.75
OFF THE BALL MOVEMENT	1	2	4	4	2.75
RECEIVING THE BALL - CONTROL	1	1	2	2	1.5
DRIBBLING	4	4	3	3	3.5
FINISHING / SHOOTING	3	1	2	4	2.5
TACKLING	1	1	2	1	1.25
SCANNING	2	2	1	2	1.75

INSIGHTS I HAVE DRAWN:

I MUST START WORKING ON MY FOOTWORK TO IMPROVE MY POSITIONING IN ORDER TO EFFECTIVELY EXECUTE A TACKLE.

I MUST STOP BEING SO INCONSISTENT WITH MY FINISHING.

I MUST CONTINUE TO WORK ON MY SCANNING AND RECEIVING THE BALL.

Continuous Improvement- The Next Level

The mindset should be one of 'continuous improvement' and striving to get to the 'next level'- a relentless pursuit of improvement.

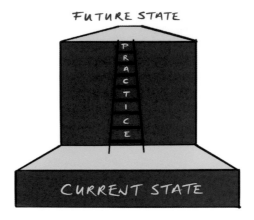

Keep Asking...Why?

You may have uttered something along the following lines to yourself, "I wasn't great today. We lost and I missed a number of shots." If so, you're not alone, indeed many players, even those performing at a very high level, assess their performance as so.

By asking 'why' we get to the fundamental areas which need improvement in order to lead to greater performance. You can't have true awareness without curiosity. See below an example of this process for Ava, a netball goal shooter, self-reflecting on her own performance:

- *My shooting was poor today. Why?*
- *I shot from a lot further than I normally would so my shooting wasn't actually that bad. The shot location was a problem. Why?*
- *I was receiving the ball mainly at the edge of the shooting circle rather than under the goalpost. Why?*
- *My teammates weren't confident in passing to me under the goal post. Why?*
- *The defender was quite loose and confused the space. This led to my teammates being indecisive and me coming closer to them to receive the ball. Because of this I found myself further from the goal. Why?*
- *I didn't make it clear I had the appropriate space to receive the ball. I should have made it more difficult for the defender and used my body to shield an area for me to receive the ball. I need to work on my body positioning to allow my teammates to play a better pass.*

Without this reflection process, Ava may feel she needs to work on her shooting when the real issue is in the build up to the shot, rather than the skill execution. The lesson here is to constantly challenge your beliefs about yourself.

Analysing Other Areas of Life

Whilst we have talked about analysing your performance on the pitch from a tactical and skill perspective, this type of self-appraisal can be carried out on any aspect of your life. As you look to make improvements in any facet of your life, consider what success in this area would look like, examine where you are now and how you would close the gap on success. Below is an example of a lifestyle rating system Kate, a 17 year old GAA underage county player, created using her own definitions. She uses this to ensure she is making the correct lifestyle choices whilst balancing the requirements of her sport, school, work and social life (see chapter 21).

	_1_	_2_	_3_	_4_
Sleep (see Chapter 20)	I had a lot of disturbed sleep throughout the week with no set routine.	I didn't get the minimum sleep required every night and could improve my sleeping pattern significantly	I got the minimum sleep required every night but could improve my schedule to improve my sleeping pattern.	I got adequate sleep every night, going to bed at a regular time and made sleep a priority for recovery, especially after physical exertions.
Recovery (see Chapter 20)	I didn't put any recovery protocols in place during the week.	I implemented a recovery protocol but was inconsistent in this during the week.	I implemented a number of recovery strategies throughout the week, but could've done more planning in this regard.	I placed recovery as a high priority, making sure to appropriately plan for upcoming sessions and making time for active recovery.
Nutrition (see Chapter 20)	I didn't monitor my food intake and didn't plan my meals. I ate poorly.	I didn't monitor my food but planned meals of reasonable quality for most of the week.	I monitored my intake of quality food but could improve my planning, especially after training and matches.	I monitored my food intake of quality food, planned my nutrition and adapted to other events in my life.
Time Management (see Chapter 21)	I struggled to manage things in my life and missed/ forgot to do a number of tasks.	I managed to complete nearly all tasks but was acting mostly reactively and some tasks were completed later than required.	I planned my week in advance but didn't complete everything I would like due to a number of unexpected events occurring during the week.	I adequately planned my week. I completed all tasks as required and felt in control.

The Individual Athlete

While this chapter has been written with the individual within a team sport environment in mind this same process of self-reflection can be implemented within an individual sport, and perhaps with even added importance. Within an individual sport, you commonly do not have as big a support network around you. As a result, the importance of self-analysis and providing personal feedback to aid performance is integral.

Gavin Maguire, an international table tennis player and coach, speaks of how he implements this process. "Journaling after matches was an important part of my analysis and this practice allowed me to be clear on where I needed to improve and helped me deal with situations better as they arose in the future." This exemplifies how you can build up a knowledge of your own performance through reflecting on how previous situations arose, noting how you reacted and focusing on how you wish to improve on this in the future. However, this isn't just about reflecting on what went wrong, for Gavin it was also about reinforcing what he did well to recreate "point winning tactics".

The Eternal Student

Two soccer coaches previously mentioned in this chapter, Pep Guardiola and Jurgen Kloop, employ relatively new philosophies of playing and emphasise the need to continually monitor tactical innovation within the game. Both are students of their game and you can be one too. This chapter has introduced you to some simple concepts you can utilise and harness to create a 'Personal Improvement Plan' and a pathway of continuous improvement for yourself. In truth performance analysis is a relatively simple process and those who are the most effective at it, simplify it best. Your challenge is to get to know your sport and your role within your sport. You must then learn to honestly and appropriately appraise your performance and take from this, useful insights that will help you to 'get better at getting better'.

Best wishes,
David Morris & Mark McAreavey.

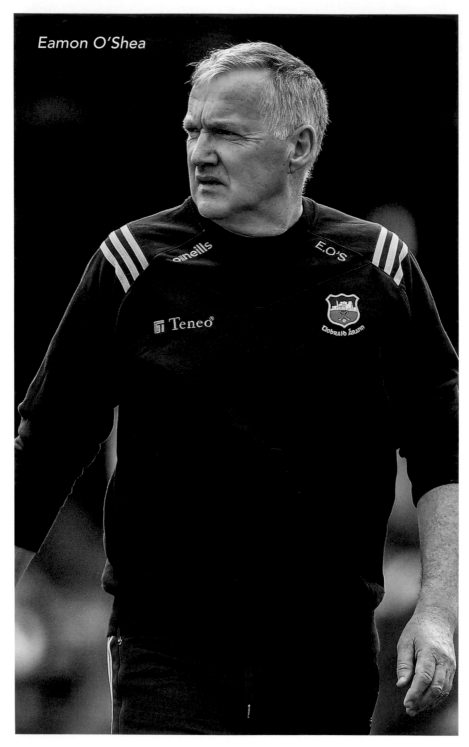

Eamon O'Shea

CHAPTER 7

Eamon O'Shea

Eamon O'Shea is Performance Director to the Tipperary Senior Hurling team, having previously served as both coach and manager. He is seen by many as a thought leader in hurling, coaching and player development. He is a Third Level Academic Professor by profession and brings a unique level of intellect and thought to how both athletes and coaches should approach their craft. I have asked Eamon to share with you his insights into how you can become a student of your game and examine your performance with a view to improvement.

The chapter you have just read is all about performance. That's what most coaches talk about nowadays- the need to improve performance. When I was your age - a long time ago now - it used to be more about winning, but winning is not always under your control, while performance generally is. That's why it is important to think a lot about performance - where it comes from and how to maintain it. My sport is hurling, but many of the ideas I will be discussing apply equally to other team sports and to individual sports as well.

The first thing to say is that performance is strongly related to the enjoyment you get from being involved in sport. It seems simple, but you need to enjoy what you are doing, and be challenged in that doing, to feel good about being involved in your chosen sport. So, what does that mean in practical terms -- quite literally it means that playing sport should make you feel happy and give you a sense of freedom and fun. And normally that's why we do it and keep doing it. Therefore, make sure you periodically check in on whether you are still enjoying your sport? Does it make you feel good? Even now, in older age, I take out my hurley and strike the ball on to the wall or into the nets almost every day, just to get that feeling of enjoyment and freedom I had in my teenage years from doing the same thing. The feel of the ash in my hands, the sound of the ball off the hurley and the sight of the ball In the air still brings a sense of calm and wellness unmatched by most other things in my life.

One of the key things when starting out in sport is learning the craft of the game you have chosen. For me, it starts with touch. The hurley is integral to the hurler - an extension of their limbs and sometimes their personality- an organic relationship between brain and muscle. The golfer has a bag of different clubs, each having their different uses depending on shot and distance to the pin, but the hurler has only one hurley and every inch of timber is important for shot selection. Of course, the hurler is no different in that regard to the squash player or the tennis player who rely on their relationship to the racket in their hand. Similarly, for those of you who play any type of football- get to know the relationship between boot and ball. Footballs are more generic, not as specific as hurleys, but can be as temperamental. Therefore, you need to interrogate the nature of the football, every part of the circumference and its inner workings. My message is, whatever game you play, get in tune with your instruments - using all of your senses in the process.

Becoming one with your sport does not mean the game should define you, or take over every aspect of your life. Sport is just one part of your life, one among many expressions of your personality and accomplishments. Treating your sport with respect is a two-way street- it must also treat you with respect. Success or failure in sport should never define you as a person. One of your goals should be to enjoy your sporting achievements and learn from your failures. You will have many more of the latter, so resilience is important, allowing you to bounce-back from days when things do not go well. You can learn and practice resilience, just like you learn the technical aspects of your sport. The things that are not in your control have no relevance, those that are in your control can be addressed. Having the right people around you and listening only to people who value you as a whole human being can be a great help in dealing with setbacks. Your immediate circle of friends often determine the atmosphere and ambiance of your sporting life, including your performance. Make sure you choose those friends wisely and that you remain independent and strong in what you want to achieve in sport.

Reflection is an essential element in maximising your performance in sport. Reflection is different to brooding. I have seen many athletes beset by negative mind-sets and poor behaviours after failing to deliver a good performance. Reflection helps you to come to terms with good and bad performances. Therefore, think through good performances as much as poor performances. Visualisation (see Chapter 11) is an essential prerequisite to reflection. It allows you to think through your relationship to the game before you play and facilitates using all of your skills in a positive and effective way. Visualisation allows you to engage in deep practice where you can become immersed in your training environment and skill development in a deliberate and methodical way. Be attentive and present in all your training sessions, with all of your senses tuned to the activity going on. Stay firmly in the moment, even if that moment is not obvious to anyone else. Whatever the challenge, whatever the conditions, the moment is all you have – be present for it. Strive to get to the frontier of high skill and high challenge in your training. It's not easy to find that point and, even when found, it does not last for long, but that's the ultimate performance experience. Seek it out through practice and more practice.

In summary, here are a few points that have guided me through my playing and coaching life and may be of benefit to you, especially in relation to performance:

- *Play your sport for enjoyment, freedom and fun.*
- *Make sure you do many different things in your life besides sport – you have many different talents and attributes.*
- *Set clear, achievable and time-limited sporting goals.*
- *Train with concentration, intention and purpose.*
- *Engage all of your senses in practice, as if learning a craft.*
- *Stay in the present moment during practice and games, because that is the only place we truly live.*
- *Build resilience and perspective to help you deal with set-backs in sport.*
- *Be yourself and good things will inevitably happen in sport and life.*

Eamon O'Shea

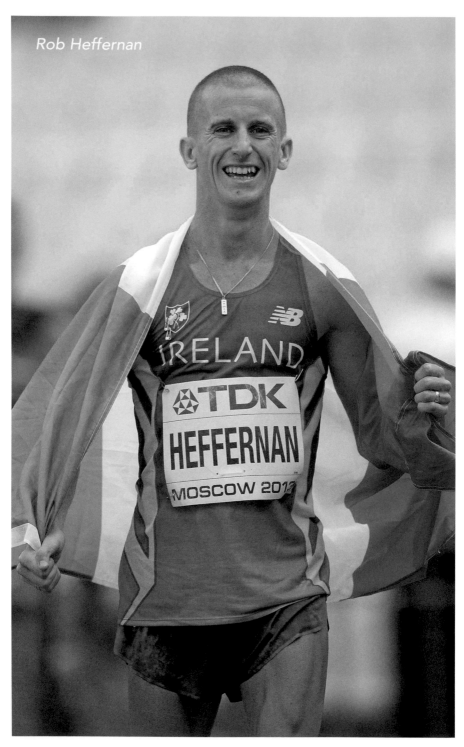

Rob Heffernan

CHAPTER 7

Rob Heffernan

Rob Heffernan is a retired Irish race walker, whose career was defined by continuous improvement. This culminated in him winning a World Championships and an Olympic and European Medal. Nothing came easy for Rob, everything was earned the hard way. His story is one of passion for his sport and determination and drive to be the best he could be.

My sport of Race Walking is a mentally and physically brutal discipline. Knowing what's important and how to strive towards it, putting in the correct work load and peaking at the right time is all part of it. Many athletes have the ability to get themselves into really good shape, but doing so for the day of a championships, is completely different.

Race walking is a very measurable sport. Get from Point A to Point B as fast as you can. At a fundamental level it is as simple as that. It is a primitive endeavour. Develop an ability to endure pain, injury, grind, monotony, the list goes on. There really is no substitute for hard work and graft. It is the cornerstone upon which everything is built.

Is doing more always better or is quality key? Is there a balance and if so where is it? Sometimes it's hard to know because sometimes the smarter we get, the more clinical we become and we lose an element of the required rawness and doggedness. Race walking is a raw game where the dogged prevail. Anyone that knows it, knows that. This rawness can never be taken from its core. There must be a hunger deep inside the athlete, a drive, a want. The fire must burn and burn bright.

When I look at the list of the chapters in this book I really feel I could contribute to all of them. Mindset, deliberate practice, dealing with setbacks are all part of the game, but training smart and hard is certainly critical. Knowing and loving the game, being an apprentice of your craft and knowing how, what and when to practice in order to get better is key. I feel my career is a story of continuous improvement that led me to being a student of race walking and occasionally a master.

I qualified for the European Junior Championships in 1997 which at the time came as a massive shock to those around me. This opened my eyes to a bigger world and ignited my desire and motivation to get better at my event of race walking. I set my focus on a dream of going to the Olympics in Sydney in 2000. I accepted a college course which would facilitate my training and entered the European U23s Championships in 1999. I finished last and was set to retire. Self-doubt can cripple you.

Shortly afterwards, I went on holidays to Spain and while I was there the World Championships were taking place in Seville. I took a train to Seville to watch the Men's 20K Walk. Ilya Markov won the race. I had met him earlier that year and was completely inspired watching him win. I returned home with renewed vigour and trained like an animal. Good old fashioned grind- pound the road! The following year I broke every Irish record: 3k, 5k, 20k, and 35k and went to my first Olympics in Sydney after setting some incredible times as a raw kid. My only ingredients were passion and hard work, there was no subtlety or nuance to my training. I look back at a young Rob Heffernan, who obviously had a massive talent and think, 'He should have been educated better'.

I got my 'peak' horribly wrong in Sydney and finished 28th. There was no detail in my preparation. I felt I had had a disgraceful Olympic Games. I wanted to get better; the hunger was there and I was willing to do whatever it would take. I returned home and trained really, really hard that winter. I knew there had to be more to it though. I ended up emailing Robert Korzeniowski, the gold medallist from the 20K and 50K in Sydney. It was clear to me that it wasn't enough to simply want it and to train as hard as possible. I told him my goals and shared my training plans and how I did things. Not long after, I informed my then coach I was moving on from him and jumped on a plane to South Africa to train with the double Olympic champion. I wanted and needed to learn from the best.

This was the true beginning of my education on what it would take to be elite and to realise my athletic potential. I started observing Robert daily. I studied his every move in and out of training: how he warmed up, what he ate, how he recovered. It was a slow process but from simply being in that environment I improved immensely. I went to the World Championships that year and ended up finishing 14th, fourteen places better than in Sydney. Korzeniowski turned to me after the race and basically said that my performance wasn't up to scratch and that I was prepared to do a lot better. Even though I was the number one performing athlete in Edmonton for the Irish team, he said it wasn't good enough and that I should have done better.

Robert was a guy who had self- actualised and become the best athletic version of himself; he had won everything, done everything in the sport. I had to take it on board and start evaluating myself, my preparation and my performances. I was digging deeper in search of answers. I was learning my craft. The following year I went to the European Championships and finished 8th, just 11 seconds off a medal. I was progressing and training harder than ever and pushing my limits but in hindsight there was still a primitive element to my training. It wasn't specific, personalised or detailed enough.

For the next four years I was either injured or sick or disqualified. It was a devastating period in my career and I struggled both physically and mentally. I was injured with stress fractures for the World Championships in 2003. In 2004 I was disqualified in the Olympic Games in Athens and in 2005 I was in 8th position in the World Championships when I was disqualified with 2 ½ k to go. 2006 was a washout as I missed the whole year with stress fractures. For me it seemed that the harder I tried the worse I became.

During this period I met my wife, Marian, which put me into a really stable and happy environment at I time when I was losing all hope. Things started to turn. Robert Korzeniowski became my full-time coach and everything I did from then on was with a specific purpose. I began to study the game of race walking closer and closer. Training was blocked by lactic and heartrate. Everything we did on a daily basis was done for a reason. I was still training incredibly hard but I was beginning to train smarter. We would plot competitions throughout the year to quantify how well our training was going. Competitive and training performances would be analysed and the findings used to further plan preparation. I was beginning to become engrossed in the detail of the learning process and loved it.

I finished 6th in the 2007 World Championships in Osaka. The following year I went to the Olympics in Beijing. Robert was still coaching me. He was also coaching Ilya Markov and Paco Fernandez, the number one and two in the world at the time. In truth, although I was certainly training better and smarter I had been thrown into that group as a sparring partner for the other two. I ended up finishing 8th in the Olympic Games after breaking all the Irish records that year however I still wasn't happy that I was training and preparing as well as I could. I felt my preparation wasn't individualised and tailored enough to my needs.

It was time to re-evaluate my situation. My wife Marian and I had set our focus on winning a medal in Beijing. I felt Robert only viewed me as a training partner for the boys. Paco had only finished 7th and Ilya finished 16th and ended up retiring. The next year was disastrous. The energy was gone from our training group. I felt Robert didn't genuinely believe that I could be a medallist. I felt I had exhausted all of the learning I could from him. My progress had stalled- new stimulus was required. After the 2009 World Championships, where I finished 14th, I made a decision to finish with Robert.

I returned home and built my own team around me, using much of what I had learned from Robert. However, now my training would be more individualised, ever more detailed and the main focus would be on me. This forced me to be a lot more accountable. I had to justify the decision to move. I was becoming increasingly fascinated by the training process and finished fourth in the European Championships in Barcelona in 2010. This ended up being a bronze medal because one of the Russians was subsequently caught for drugs.

2011 followed a similar format. By now, I was attracting more sponsors and my funding had increased. I was able to invest more in my programme. I was becoming increasingly professional: the better performance analysis which saw every facet dissected, assessed and debriefed, detailed training logs with more specific training plans, clearer more measurable goal setting, more intelligent performance preparation and increased access to professional expertise. With the increased investment came more responsibility and more pressure to perform but I enjoyed that part. By now I was a highly self-aware athlete who was completely performance focused. I was really getting to know my game and how to be prepared to be at my best.

I went to the World Championships in South Korea in 2011 and three days before my race I had to come home because my mother died suddenly. This put my whole life into context. Afterwards I became even more matter of fact about my training. I began to optimise video feedback which in turn improved my confidence, mental preparation and motivation. I went to the Olympics in London in 2012 a prepared athlete. I finished 9th in the 20k which was a phenomenal result and I won a bronze medal in the 50k (which was fourth on the day and subsequently made bronze, again due to a doping violation).

I was ready to retire after London but Marian felt there was more in me and that it was only now I was realising my potential. She came on board as my coach and took over all of the external responsibilities. All I had to do was eat, sleep and train- a laser like performance focus. The 2013 World Championships were approaching in Moscow. I knew if I had the same motivation, drive and detailed preparation as I had in London, I could go into the hotbed of world race walking of the Russians who were doped, and regardless of me not being doped I could challenge them on their home turf. It was a massive motivation for me. I went to the World Championships in Moscow and won gold. This was me at my peak. All the variables had come together. It was relative mastery of my craft.

The next year I wanted to become invincible. In truth I probably got the balance wrong and ended up with a double hernia in the European Championships in Zurich. The following three years I was getting older but managed to finish 5th in the Worlds, 6th in the Olympics and 7th in the World championships before I decided to bow out. I was losing my desire and love for it. I didn't want it anymore. The edge was gone and I was done.

Today, I coach athletes and much of what I have discussed above is central to our process. We train hard, but smart. We use measurement, training with specificity and analyse our performance to inform our training. I aim to make those I coach students of the game of race walking. If I can help make them this, then they can make themselves the best they can be.

Best wishes,
Rob

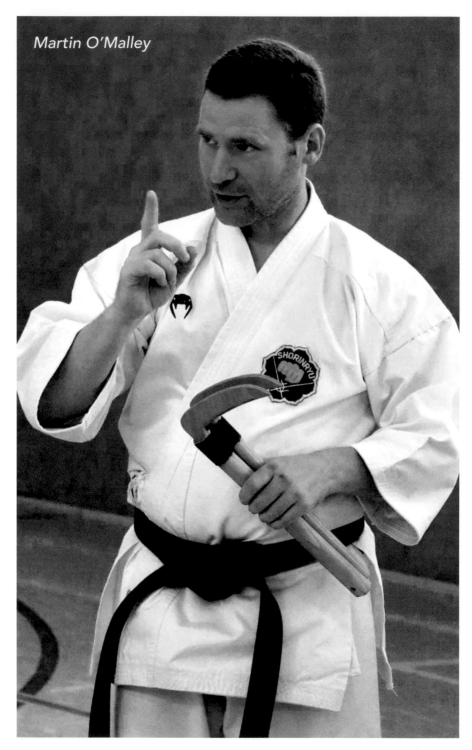

Martin O'Malley

CHAPTER 7

Martin O'Malley

Martin O'Malley is a Fourth Dan Martial Arts Instructor with over 20 years coaching experience. He has coached numerous national and world champions across the Martial Arts of Karate, Kobujutsu and Savate. Martin has taught Martial Arts across the world and trains annually in Okinawa and has received many awards for his work in Martial Arts in Ireland and beyond. Here he shares with you his learnings in the area of performance.

Improving performance is the goal of every athlete. Some do it better than others. Without doubt, the coach plays an important role, but you, the athlete, are the main driver. No one can want it for you. To achieve the rather vague goal of improvement, you should first start by setting some clearer goals; decide what, or who, it is you want to become, and where in sport you want to go. Create a clear vision for yourself. In order to do this to any degree of accuracy, you will need to study your sport and get to know what it demands of its participants. You will need to become a student of your game. There are many means to this, and this book will have taught you those.

Your next step is to determine where you are in comparison to your vision. Establish your strengths and weaknesses, or more appropriately your opportunities for improvement. Establish your current reality- ask some learned and trust people to appraise you. In doing this you now have a starting point, and a destination, and you can begin to plot a course between the two. Start where you are. Use what you have. Do what you can. Learn as you go. Discipline, diligence and effort will drive you towards your vision. Exhibit a ferocious and intelligently applied work ethic directed towards continuous improvement.

Many athletes try to hide their weaknesses. They are not honest with themselves about where they are starting from, or where they are on the journey. Consciously or otherwise, they want to self- preserve. The first rule of performance analysis, and improvement, is you must not fool yourself. Maybe you are not as physically strong as you'd like or certain skills are not as sharp as necessary... that's OK. It's OK to have those weaknesses, it's OK not to be perfect so long as you want to improve and are willing to do what it takes. In sport, you are either going one of two ways; you are either getting better or you are getting worse...you never stay the same. Being mature and honest enough, to really want to improve is a great gift. Without proper self-evaluation, true success is impossible. The training that follows this process should be directly connected to the vision you have created for yourself. Advice, coaching and guidance should be sought from wiser, more learned others. Every avenue that offers improvement should be investigated. Practice should be performed with precision and intent.

The next element of improving performance is learning how to perform. In order to analyse your performance to any degree of accuracy, you must first establish that you have competed to the best of your ability, and given your all. It is only then you will have an accurate gauge of where you need to improve. I have seen it many times, athletes failing to give their best in competition, and this leaves them with an unclear path, on how to improve their performance. There are tools and skills that will help you learn how to perform to the best of your ability, and again this book offers you many of them.

The cycle or process now becomes: practice, perform, analyse performance, establish learnings, practice using learnings, perform, repeat. The endless pursuit of getting better by establishing the truth and working from there. Developing an 'after action review' is key, something along the lines of:

1. What happened?
2. Why did it happen?
3. What do I need to do?

There is no shame in being beaten. If you prepare to the very best of your ability, if you truly give it your all on the day and are beaten, it is because that person (or team) was better than you (or your team) that day – just that day, not every day. Never run from defeat; soak up its lessons. Know that you can plan how to improve to meet, and overcome, the next challenge. Similarly never get too carried away with victory. The truth is, if you can learn to treat victory and defeat in the same manner you will place yourself on an unending cycle of improvement. Improving performance is the goal of every athlete. Some do it better than others.

Best wishes,
Martin O'Malley.

SUMMARY POINTS - Chapter 7

- Performance Analysis can provide you with unbiased information that helps you understand both the demands of your sport and your performance.
- Analyse or 'read' the game as it unfolds in front of you and communicate this to those around you.
- Analyse your opponent in-game and use the information to strategise how you can best approach the challenge they pose.
- When you talk about performance, you can ask 3 important questions: What are you trying to achieve? (Goal) Where on the journey are you now? (Current State) How do you get from Current State to Goal? (Close Gap)
- Actively watch the best teams in your sport.
- Actively watch the best performers in your position.
- List the key skills and qualities required in your position (KPIs).
- Establish your 'current state' with regard to your KPIs.
- Create a 'Personal Improvement Plan' and target areas for quality focused practice.
- Reflect on your performance in your KPIs over the course of a number of games and use this information to refine your 'Personal Improvement Plan'.
- Keep asking- Why?
- Be an 'eternal student' of your game and performance.
- It is important to think a lot about performance - where it comes from and how to maintain it.
- Performance is strongly related to the enjoyment you get from being involved in sport.

CHAPTER 8: BEING A TEAMMATE

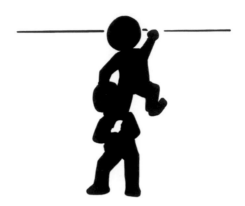

As I have stated from the outset, this book attempts to speak to all youths across every sport, individual and collective. Most, if not all, sports have a team element or at least a collective training environment. This chapter will look at 'mateship' and what it means to you, and for you, to be a good teammate.

It can be said that people make places and places make people. The environment we are surrounded by drives our behaviour but once again, people build those environments. In Chapter 3 we have seen that we are our character and values in action. 'You must be the change you wish to see in the world' was a great lesson from a man of peace, Mahatma Gandhi. The big question for you to consider is: What influence do you want to have on your teammates and team training environment? Again, I return to one of my central coaching philosophies of raising self-awareness. You must appreciate that one of life's great truths is that through others, we become ourselves.

The famous American basketball coach, John Wooden, said of those he coached "You don't have to like them all, but you have to love them all". I believe if you wish to be a good teammate the same is true of your relationship with your teammates. To paraphrase Mark 12:31:

"Love thy teammate as thyself".

In team sport, we stand on the shoulders of our teammates. The team is the star, more so than an individual player. Team sport is about the group coming together and sharing experiences in the hope that it will turn into something special. The good player improves themselves. The great players improve those around them. They improve the team and the team environment.

If you want to be truly great, you have to work as hard at being a great teammate as you do at being a great athlete. One way you can make yourself of value to the team is to make the players around you more valuable. Can you inspire through your words and actions? Can you be a positive influence? Can you be the light? Can you embrace the character traits of a player who wholeheartedly commits themselves to the group effort?

'In unity there is strength' is a phrase I use with every team I am involved with. Your connection with your teammates can be built and strengthened through sharing enjoyable experiences and love. This love can be shown in many ways and indeed sometimes it can be 'tough love' where you directly, yet respectfully, challenge the behaviours and standards of your teammates. Respect here is key; you must be coming from a place of love. Loyalty, both on and off the field, to and from those with whom you play with, is absolutely necessary for genuine success.

In team sport you really must appreciate that you will only be successful as an individual, if the team functions well. Personal interest, often erodes the unity of the group. You need unity, you need a 'we are all in this together' type mentality. This is not to say some of your motives can't be personally orientated. There is nothing wrong with this. You can care for others but be driven by self-interest.

In a youth team environment the best players, and the most socially outward, are usually the most popular among the group. They are chosen first for teams in training, picked first when partners are being chosen for drills, sat beside on the team bus etc. In poor team cultures, the weak (by this I mean either technically or socially) are often treated poorly on numerous levels. They are often the last to be thought of, socially ignored, blamed for losses and so on. Bullying type behaviour can be prevalent. All societies (and thus by extension teams) can be measured on how they treat the weak. Obviously, you can't control the team environment, but you can certainly influence it and hold yourself to your own standard of behaviour. Can you lead the way? This takes huge levels of maturity and self-awareness but will really set you apart as a teammate and leader. If your team environment is weak or socially immature it will take time for your example to be noticed and valued. As with most elements of performance, patience and consistency is key.

HOW DO YOU FEEL **ALL** MEMBERS ON YOUR TEAM
SHOULD BE TREATED ON & OFF THE FIELD?

_____

_____

_____

When looking at the varying qualities (both personal and performance) of a teammate I could give you a list of answers, however I will leave it to you. My question is, what are exceptional, acceptable and unacceptable characteristics and behaviours of a teammate? Another way you can categorise behaviours are: leader behaviours, neutral behaviours and drain behaviours.

"Only the guy who isn't rowing,
has time to rock the boat".
Jean – Paul Sarte, French Philosopher and Playwright

EXCEPTIONAL (LEADER) CHARACTERISTICS & BEHAVIOURS OF A TEAMMATE.	ACCEPTABLE (NEUTRAL) CHARACTERISTICS & BEHAVIOURS OF A TEAMMATE	UNACCEPTABLE (DRAIN) CHARACTERISTICS & BEHAVIOURS OF A TEAMMATE.

WHAT MIGHT YOUR TEAMMATES CURRENTLY SAY ABOUT YOU AS A TEAM MEMBER?

_____

_____

WHAT DO YOU HOPE YOUR MANAGEMENT & TEAM MATES WILL SAY ABOUT YOU AT THE END OF THE YEAR?

_____

_____

AS A TEAMMATE; WHAT DO YOU WANT TO BE KNOWN FOR? WHAT IS YOUR VISION FOR YOURSELF AS A TEAMMATE?

_____

_____

(Note; this particular question may be best suited to the front or back of your journal. This will allow you access it easily and take a moment daily, or weekly, to read and review).

Being a good teammate means you must be very aware of your influence on the team. Occasionally, it even means doing what's right for the team although it may not be what's right for you. It can mean being the best player for the team, not the best player on the team. To paraphrase the former American President John F Kennedy:

"Ask not what your teammates can do for you. Ask what you can do for your teammates".

Good teammates are only interested in finding the best way, not in having their own way. Two question you can use to guide your behaviour as a teammate could be:

WHAT CAN I DO TO HELP MY TEAMMATES SUCCEED?

_____

_____

WHAT CAN I DO TODAY TO MAKE MY TEAM BETTER?

_____

_____

Your challenge is to grow and develop as a teammate and make yourself more valuable in, and to, your team environment. Your character and values will drive this. Be the best teammate you can be.

Kieran Donaghy

Kieran Donaghy is a former Kerry Gaelic Footballer. He won four All-Ireland Senior Football Championship medals with Kerry, as well as three All-Star Awards and a Footballer of the Year award. He is also a long-time basketball player. In 2003 and 2008, he helped the Tralee Tigers win the Superleague. Top level basketball faded away in Tralee thereafter. In 2015, Kieran brought two rival clubs together and created a team called the Tralee Warriors. In the club's debut season, 2016, they won the Champions Trophy, defended it in 2017 and landed the prestigious Irish Super League for the first time in 2019. He is an athlete who plays with his heart on his sleeve, bringing colour and entertainment whenever he performs. I have asked him to share with you his insights into what it means to be a good teammate.

Many people know me as a Gaelic footballer- the big lad who played on the edge of the square for Kerry. However, Gaelic is only part of my sporting identity. Basketball is another passion of mine and it is the sport which has taught me most about team-ship and the influence of teammates. I am a natural extravert. I enjoy meeting people and social interaction. I love being part of a group; part of a team. I love the team environment. Lads coming from every walk of life and uniting with a common goal and purpose. Playing together, winning and losing together, sharing experiences. I have lived a great sporting life and continue to do so.

I played point guard in my teenage years. The job of the point guard is to run the team. They are the on-court coach, running the plays, the main source of communication and direction. They must also frequently communicate at an almost peer-to-peer level with the coach; you are really his or her conduit to the team. These interactions both require and develop confidence in the individual. You develop the ability to articulate your thoughts around the game and communicate with a coach who has vastly more experience than you.

Basketball is a sport where five players depend on each other to survive and thrive. The five attack together as well as defend together. There is no place for a passenger; no place for someone who isn't pulling their weight or contributing to the team. The weak link will be isolated and

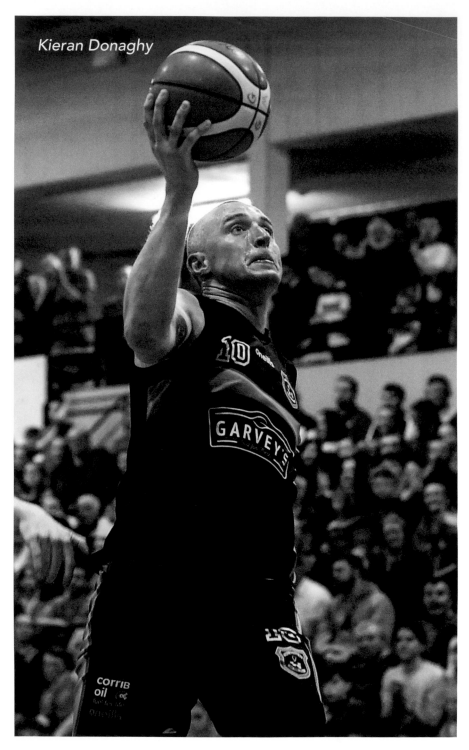

Kieran Donaghy

exposed to a far greater degree than in other sports with greater playing numbers. The panel is made up of only twelve. There is little room for cliques or groups. The unit must be compact, together, unified. The point guard plays a huge role in connecting the team. Often the role requires you to drive lads around the court. Empathy is an important skill in this; some need to be told directly and abruptly, while others need an arm around them and a kind work. Knowing the needs of your teammates and being able to communicate with them appropriately is a key skill.

The point guard is the orchestrator and their crew look to him/her to guide them. For me, the ultimate point guard was Steve Nash. He was a two-time NBA Most Valuable Player (2005, 2006) and an eight-time NBA All-Star. He is on record as giving 239 'high-fives' in one game. That was a phenomenal level of encouragement and positive interaction towards one's teammates and came after both scores and misses, fouls and rebounds. He was always there for his teammates: to congratulate them when they did well, refocus them after an error and pick them up when they fell to the floor. Indeed, on the subject of 'high-fives' and 'touches', I recall scientists at UC Berkeley releasing a study some years ago which claimed that the teams in the NBA which were the 'touchiest' were typically the best ones; with the LA Lakers and Boston Celtics being the most 'touch orientated' teams. This came as no surprise to me; all things being relatively equal, the team that is the most united will win out every time. Good teammates make for united teams. When everyone cares about each other, the unit is solid.

It must be noted that the physical environment in which basketball is played in lends itself to communication. The court is relatively small, so physically we are in close proximity to each other. We don't have wind and rain to contend with and it can be easier to concentrate as the field of play and its surroundings, are less vast than say a football field. The levels of intra team communication is off the charts in basketball. You are continually talking your teammates through the game and the language of the game is very exact and detail orientated. The very nature of the game of basketball and the traditions which surround it teaches you about team-ship on a daily basis. I feel it has moulded me and I have brought this style or 'way of being' to my football. In general, on field communication in Gaelic football is nowhere compared to basketball. Certainly 'touches' are not a 'thing'. The vastness of the playing field doesn't lend itself to it organically and therefore the players aren't given that same opportunity to develop these skills. In many ways basketball has taught me how to be a good teammate and what it means to be one.

I think we can learn from rugby too. I had the pleasure of watching the great Munster team of 2006 train in UL one day. I was blown away by their level of on-field positive communication. Some GAA teams have incorporated this into their game, but more can learn from it. In rugby, when a player wins a dirty ball in the ruck, or causes the opposition to give away a penalty, you see guys rushing to congratulate them. This form of positive reinforcement creates energy for the giver, the receiver and the team in general. It also acts to drive the point home to the opposition. I was big on this as a player and like Steve Nash I used to get in my 'high-fives' or 'pats on the back' for good measure.

In order to be a good teammate the 'we' must always come before the 'me'. Throughout my career I have always tried to make the right decision for the team, give the ball to the man in the better position and understand the power of my influence on those around me. I have always aimed to give everything to the group; create energy, bring life. Taking my learnings from basketball and my role as point guard I have always tried to provide what I felt the team needed in the moment: stand up to one of the opponent's 'tough guys', celebrate a score, track a run, a word of encouragement or direction. In essence, I have made a career by making those around me better players. It is not something I have had to contrive. Basketball has given me the developmental opportunities and it is a skill that has come naturally to me. I have an in-built desire to keep everyone around me going.

Sport is all about skills and certain skills come easier to some than others. I believe being a good team is a skill and because of this it is something you can work on and develop. Granted it comes easier to some than others but a simple question you must ask yourself is, 'what type of teammate do I want to be?' And follow it by answering the next question which is 'what do I need to do on a consistent basis to be that teammate?'

Common wisdom tells us that actions speak louder than words. I think now to those I played with, who I consider to be great teammates; many spring to mind. Aidan O'Mahony was a man that would put his body on the line in order for Kerry to win. He did this from the very first day he put on the famous green and gold jersey to the last; whatever it took - until the death. He would also be the one to ring a young lad he thought was struggling. Gooch was another great teammate. He was the most gifted player I ever teamed up with. He could have tried to score 1-10 in every game and had the skills to do so, but his decision making was always team orientated. He would regularly turn down a simple point scoring opportunity for himself, instead making a slip pass to pursue a possible goal chance for the team. Kerry winning was always to the core of his decision making, and that's all you want in a teammate.

Declan O'Sullivan was another true team player. He was dropped as captain in 2006. I took his No. 14 jersey and went on to have the summer of a lifetime winning Player of the Year. Declan was in my ear all that summer; I was nervous at times and he would reassure me. He offered advice when it would have been so easy to do the selfish thing and hope I had a stinker so he could take my spot back. He stayed positive throughout and got his reward in the end when he started the All-Ireland Final in Croke Park that summer. He led by example throughout his career and ended it by 'dying on his shield' to help us win that important All Ireland title in 2014. By then, the cartilage in both his knees was virtually non-existent.

It is easy to be a good teammate when things are going your way; however, this is not a true test. I experienced a similar faith to Declan's as team captain in 2015. I was dropped for the All-Ireland Final and was gutted; gutted deep inside. I was told I wasn't playing four days before the team was named. I cried in the car after I got the news. I was heartbroken in work and around the house. However, when I was around the team, I was positive; happy to ensure fellas weren't edgy around me. I learned that from Declan in a way. Good teammates put the team before themselves; every time and twice on Sundays. Looking back, I feel I dealt well with it. I quickly reframed the challenge and put my energy into focusing on how I could support the team and play my part in bringing home Sam Maguire. Take it from me, when all is said and done, lads remember the self-centred ones, the ones who moan when things aren't going their way, the ones who suck the energy out of the group. Who wants to be this type of a teammate?

I was once told by a great leader of men, "What I want are good teammates; men who lead by their actions, who call me out if I'm slacking and encourage me when I'm down". Simple words, but so true. As a young athlete, you have it all ahead of you and you can choose the route you take. Choose wisely; bring energy to the group, look out for your buddies both on and off the field of play, think of the 'we' much more than the 'me'. Give to the team and the team will give to you.

Best wishes,
Kieran Donaghy

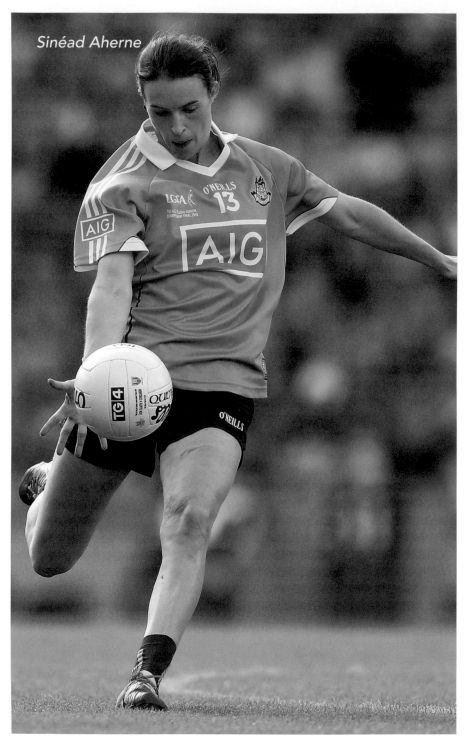

Sinéad Aherne

Sinéad Aherne

Sinéad Aherne is a Dublin senior footballer. In 2017, 2018 and 2019, she captained Dublin as they won the All-Ireland Senior Ladies' Football Championship. In 2010, when Dublin won their first All-Ireland title, she was both player of the match and the top scorer in the final with 2–7. In 2018 she was named the TG4 Senior Player's Player of the Year and received her seventh All-Star award. She has also represented Ireland at International Rules. Here she gives us a personal insight into 'teamship'.

"We are all in this together"; words that have recently become a call to arms for Ireland in facing down COVID-19. It is the sense of appealing to the collective spirit; a binding unity, and a recognition that we cannot act in isolation if we are to beat this, just as much as we can't thrive in isolation as human beings. Though we have had to try. As a footballer, a captain, and a teammate, this has been a difficult adaptation, and one that makes the privilege of being a teammate shine through for me. Even for individual athletes in these times, the need for a coach, a mentor, a family member or a friend to be your team has been keenly felt.

As individuals, we thrive in the collective, the environment we live in and which as a team, can be created from within as well as shaped from outside. When my days are done and the jersey is hung up for good, it will be the moments of experiencing the dressing room banter, the epic celebrations after big wins, and even the commiserations with teammates of big losses that I will miss more than the prizes themselves. That exact winning moment of euphoria we strive for in competition fades quickly and it is the sense of the journey, rather than the destination that lasts longest in my memories.

We all have the opportunity to be the most important person on the team. Good culture on a team is about valuing every individual as part of the collective, not just on the pitch. I've played on teams where people have been hugely influential to how successful a team is without getting a minute of championship action. This is simply because they value the team and the team values them: their energy, their engagement, their positivity, their competitiveness to push the collective, even if the reward doesn't come back to them as directly as the effort deserves. Success as a team isn't about the tiny percentage of time you spend in competition; it's the hours of teamwork on the training pitch, the bonds built on social nights, the laughs in the dressing room.

Being a leader to your teammates involves an awareness of those around you and how you can make their experience better, whether that's spotting that they've had a bad day at work, that they're struggling with their game, that they've passed a big exam, and reacting to that to make it into a shared experience. You don't have to be the most vocal person or the most outgoing or the best player. Becoming captain of the Dublin team, that's the biggest thing I took out of it that I would pass onto a younger player – to develop that awareness of what the group needs, and to recognise that what you put in, we all take out. There must be a realisation that 'this thing' only works if we share the same values, and we want to improve individually, but for the benefit of the team. Statistics on assists, events around the ball and tackles made, aren't the first thing that gets reported on from games. However, they are the heartbeat of the team, the work rate and what you must be willing to put in for your teammates.

I promise you the sense of having met the obstacles on and off the pitch, being supported through injury, helped up the hill (literally in the case of Magazine Fort), ultimately achieving a shared success as a team, but mostly of figuring it out together is one of the greatest satisfactions of all.

For the strength of the pack is the wolf, and the strength of the wolf is the pack.

Yours in Sport,
Sinéad Aherne

SUMMARY POINTS - Chapter 8

- The good player improves themselves. The great players improve those around them. They improve the team and the team environment.
- Loyalty, both on and off the field, to and from those with whom you play with, is absolutely necessary for genuine success.

CHAPTER 9: UNDERSTANDING & COMMUNICATING WITH YOUR COACH

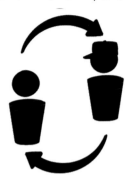

I am a coach. I know how challenging and tough of a job it is. I also work as a coach developer, so I continuously meet and work with coaches. Most of them are good people, who want to serve well and improve. Some are excellent, they are hungry to learn and improve; while others simply don't know how to improve. Being honest, there is a real lack of structured support for the volunteer coach. This is a shame as I believe volunteer coaching is one of the noblest vocations of all.

Throughout your sporting career you will come across many types of coaches. Indeed, you will come across coaches who are at different stages in their coaching journey. Always remember the coach is on a learning journey too. When I look back at the coach I was (and occasionally still am) I am embarrassed. I simply didn't know better. I urge you to take personal responsibility; you can learn from every coach and training environment, both the good and the bad, but only if you have an open mind.

Leadership is a mighty challenge and one that can bring out the best, and the worst, in people. Understand that your coach is human and don't expect them to be perfect. Some coaches assume leadership roles long before they are ready or prepared, and indeed others, are never prepared to lead. Some people find themselves in roles they are simply not suited to, nor have the required competencies for. Some coaches come from a more old school mentality where they are the boss and the athlete's role is to be subservient and obedient. They fail to see that 'obey and command' is no longer an optimal form of leadership.

Every coach is different. Aim to understand your coach and where they are coming from. Learn to become comfortable with reasonable and constructive critique; develop a growth mindset towards it (see Chapter 4). Listen to learn as opposed to listen to justify or defend. When we are defensive, we are incapable of taking on new information that can make us vulnerable, leading us to losing out on learning opportunities. Appreciate that sometimes coaching communication is about rupture and repair.

The role of the coach often includes making judgements and decisions. These decisions lead to consequences and can result in athletes being dropped, substituted and other scenarios that, while not ideal, are all part of sport and the challenges it poses that you must to learn to overcome. I always explain to athletes as they grow and develop, that they must learn to adopt what I call a 'no entitlement mentality'. By this I mean, they must appreciate that you are not entitled to: start a game, get a full game, win etc. These are things you must continuously earn. An 'entitlement mentality' is having a state of mind whereby you think you are owed something, when most others around you would beg to differ. Always remember, entitlement is the enemy of performance. You must earn everything, every day.

In dealing with your coach I urge you to assume good intent on their behalf. Try not to make it personal or take it personally. Look for feedback (see Chapter 6 and 7). Ask pertinent questions. Put your hand up, not out. Talk to them and engage with them. Ask them, how are they? Their job is ultimately to care for others so as a coach it is always refreshing to have someone care for you. Be patient with them, they have a tough job.

The vast majority of coaches in Ireland are volunteer coaches. Remember 'coach' is only one hat they wear. Many have demanding jobs, spouses, children, families, friends and lives outside of coaching. It is only reasonable to assume they come from a broad range of backgrounds and will have a broad range of experiences that has brought them to where they are. As with all walks of life, there are coaches who have low levels of self-awareness and self-mastery. In everything we do in life, there are: things we know and do, things we know and don't do and then things we don't know and therefore can't do. Some coaches simply don't know what they don't know and because of this they present as incompetent, egotistical and lacking empathy.

It is likely many coaches are more stressed than you can appreciate. Give them a break if they aren't perfect or if their tone isn't fully in line with what you'd prefer. Again, always try to presume good intent on their part. It is most likely they want what is best for you, although some struggle to articulate this. If you feel your coach is being consistently and unjustifiably harsh on you and you are confident enough to discuss it with them, find the right time and explain to them how this is effecting you. Alternatively discuss the issue with a trusted and respected adult and maybe they can help you work towards a solution.

Look your coach in the eye, thank them every day after training or competition whether it has gone your way or not. Set your own standards of behaviour and long term it will stand to you. If you want something clarified, choose the right moment and ask respectfully. Ask them to help you- seek their feedback. Communicate! If you have something you want to discuss with them privately, ask them for a quiet word. Never forget the best athletes are those who want to learn and improve. Don't fall into the trap of being too shy to ask for feedback or help and be ready to take it whether you feel it is accurate or not. Accept that their opinion of you will likely be based on what they see of your application and effort in training and competition over time.

Finding a Mentor
One piece of advice I would offer would be find a mentor (see Chapter 7) who can provide calm, measured, agenda-free advice and feedback to you. A person that can act as a sounding board to your learning. Indeed this might well be your coach, or it could be a selector or helper in the team environment. It could also be a parent or trusted adult in your life. If needs be it could be a trusted peer. Surround yourself with wisdom and those who want what's best for you.

"Blessed are those who find wisdom".
Proverbs 3:13 NIV

Feedback is critical, as is constructive critique. Your mindset must be one of continuous improvement and a mentor can be invaluable here. Ask them to watch you in games and competition, take on board their feedback and work towards improvement. We all need a go-to person that keeps us focused and honest- an accountability partner. Share challenges with them. Allow them help you find your way.

WHO WOULD BE A GOOD PERSON TO ACT AS A MENTOR

& TO ASK FOR FEEDBACK ?

It is beyond the scope of this book to cover every scenario you may encounter in your dealings with your coach. I have asked Dr Ian Sherwin to provide some further insight into the area from his research into coaching practices and his years of experience in both coaching and coach development.

Dr Ian Sherwin

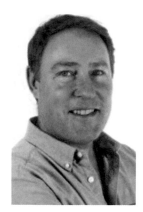

Dr Ian Sherwin is a Lecturer in Sports Coachin and Coaching Science at the University of Limerick. Ian's research interests focus on coach and athlete development. His recent work has investigated coaching behaviours and their impact on the coach-athlete relationship and athlete participation.

Ian has over 30 years coaching and coach development experience, including 13 years working for the Irish Rugby Football Union (IRFU) and Munster Rugby. Ian continues to coach rugby in a local school and is on the development and competitions committees of his local tennis club.

Realist Evaluation (Pawson and Tilley (1997), is a theory that studies how social interactions are conducted and why and how the consequent results evolve. Youth sport is a great example of such social interactions, many of which are often beyond the control of the participants. An advancement of this theory is, Critical Realism, which was used by North (2016) to try to explain what motivates the coach to behave in a particular way. This short piece will seek to give you an insight into the coach, as well as advising you in your interactions with the coach and how you can positively influence the training and playing environment.

It is important to appreciate the complex nature of coaching when trying to interpret and understand coaching practice. Human interactions are influenced by many factors and illicit a huge variance in human behaviour. The complexity of coaching, with challenges and specific situational issues unique to each group dynamic is great. In youth sport, the majority of coaches are volunteers who give up their time to help out. Even if the volunteers have attended formal coach education programmes, the research would indicate that these programmes don't always meet the needs of the coaches (Sherwin et al., 2017). The key message for you is to work with your coach and respect the fact that they are still learning too.

As such, it would be simplistic to compartmentalise coaching in two distinct categories. However, within these two categories we can locate the familiar characteristics of a variety of coaches, and this in turn may help you understand your coach at a deeper level. The first category is the Autocratic Coach whose practice is characterised by the coach leading the decision making and, overall, taking a dominant and directive approach to all exchanges. The autocratic coach will also determine the rules, standards and disciplinary procedures in the group. Crucially, this type of coach typically lacks empathy towards the athletes and relationships are hierarchical in nature with the coach at the top. In contrast, the Democratic Coach encourages athlete participation in decision-making and has an interactive communicative approach to all aspects of the sports programme. The democratic coach easily builds relationships with the athletes, demonstrates empathy, and has a broad appreciation for the athletes' wider environment beyond sport. The graphic below, taken from Lyle and Cushion (2017) depicts the two extreme ends of the coaching spectrum.

AUTOCRATIC COACHING PRACTICE

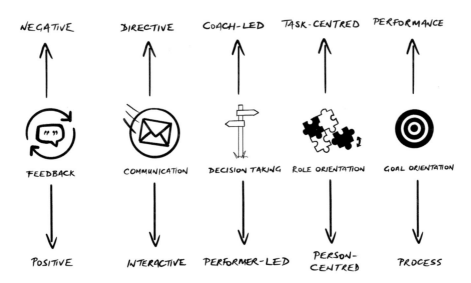

NEGATIVE	DIRECTIVE	COACH-LED	TASK-CENTRED	PERFORMANCE
FEEDBACK	COMMUNICATION	DECISION TAKING	ROLE ORIENTATION	GOAL ORIENTATION
POSITIVE	INTERACTIVE	PERFORMER-LED	PERSON-CENTRED	PROCESS

DEMOCRATIC COACHING PRACTICE

Adapted from Lyle, J. & Cushion, C., (2017).

Between the extreme examples mentioned here, a number of other coaching styles can be found. These styles are frequently influenced by the context in which the coaching takes place and, unfortunately the perception of what constitutes a "good or successful coach". In youth sport this is particularly important as a successful coach is often *determined by the number of games or trophies the athlete, or group of athletes, with whom the coach is connected, has won. In this context, the outcome is the determining factor and this is neither an accurate or fair means of measuring success. Research from Williams and Kendall (2007) shows that if you only measure success on the outcome it becomes difficult to understand why the particular outcome was achieved. Failing to understand the process that led to the outcome leads to a repetitive coaching regime that will not address the athletes' developmental needs. The coach's perspective is wrong and so their focus is not one of development rather, it is results orientated.*

This type of coaching can also be referred to as 'conquest coaching' (Wilson and Burdette, 2020). Unfortunately 'conquest coaching' has a number of negative consequences including decreases in athlete motivation, self-confidence and drop-out (Gearity and Murray, 2011). When the objectives and expectations of either side of the coach-athlete dyad are not compatible, the relationship will break down. The consequence of this situation is often one or the other leaving the environment. One possible solution to this is to set agreed goals for the group at the start of the year. Goals and objectives help to show progress in a more intelligent manner than merely winning and losing. It is quite acceptable that you and your teammates suggest such a beginning of year practice in the absence of the coach doing so. It is possible the coach has not thought about it or doesn't have the required confidence or skill-set to lead such an activity. It is likely the coach will welcome such a suggestion from you and if the activity is managed correctly at the start of the year and reviewed intermittently thereafter it may provide the clarity required for the coach to focus their attention on smarter and more controllable inputs. This will help you, your teammates and your coach to have a clear focus on progress and learning throughout the season ensuring that "outcome and trophies" are not the only objective.

The focus of youth sport should be on the development of the person through the sport and positive coaching behaviours. In the book co-authored by Tony DiCicco and Colleen Hacker, the former cites Benjamin Franklin "Any fool can criticize... and most fools do". DiCicco tells the story of a coach who always yelled, constantly found faults and highlighted errors in team review sessions. So much so that the athletes lived in a constant state of fear that negatively impacted their performance. Despite the fear and worry, the two co-captains approached the coach asking if they were going to be cut from the squad at the end of a tournament only to be told that they were the foundation on which the future squad would be built. Their response to this feedback was, "if you're not going to cut us...why are you yelling at us so much". The coach took this feedback on board and from then on adapted his coaching to focus on reinforcing good practice and highlighting demonstrations of technical quality. The coach named this aspect of coaching as "Catch them being good" which is also the title of DiCicco and Hacker's book. The lesson for all athletes here is to talk to your coach, even if you are apprehensive about doing so. During these conversations you can bring up your concerns, and if they are supported by possible solutions, you will probably find the coach to be receptive. The manner in which you approach the coach should be with an open mind and non-confrontational. It would be naïve for you to believe that coaches must only focus on giving positive feedback (general non-specific verbal or non-verbal statements aimed to be supportive towards the athlete, e.g., "well done", "good job" - Cushion et al., 2012). Research tells us that corrective feedback (statements which include information that specifically aim to improve the athletes' performance at the next attempt - Cushion et al., 2012) rather than positive feedback in isolation will enhance technical and/or tactical performance. Furthermore, corrective feedback is known to lead to increased athlete self-motivation and perceived competence (Badami et al., 2011).

You must learn to expect, value and actively seek corrective and specific feedback. The prudent athlete quickly figures out the coach behaviours and that includes feedback that does not add to their learning. For example, if a coach only says "well done" you don't really know what you've done well! The advice here is to simply ask for more corrective feedback. If you find that progress is not being made in your performance it's a good idea to ask the coach specific questions to help you get back on track. It is also important that you give feedback to the coach on what you're experiencing during the session so that the coach can give appropriate feedback to help you learn.

The athlete must understand the influence of their own mood on the coach and indeed the training environment. For example, you may be experiencing an excellent run of form and present to training in a jovial mood. This mood has the capacity to translate across the training squad, even to the coach, thus acting as a calming influence over the running of the session. Furthermore, you must also learn to appreciate the challenges the coach may have incurred in life on any given day. For example, a coach may arrive at a training session having spent two hours in traffic. This is a frustrating experience that may have a negative *impact on the mood and the performance of the coach in the training session. In this case, patience and understanding will be really helpful to the coach. The lesson here is that you should appreciate that your mood and levels of understanding and empathy have an influence on the mood of your environment and those in it.*

In youth sport, you, the athlete must come first. You are the ones playing the sport, not the coaches and therefore your developmental needs should be prioritised. Getting to know and understand your coach will help develop a strong relationship. This relationship is built on respect for each other and the roles you have within the sporting environment. Athletes will always have an influence on the coach. A positive approach and attitude towards training from you will help cement your relationship with the coach. Setting goals that are designed and agreed by you (and your team) and the coach, at the start of the season and reviewed regularly during the season will help monitor progress. Finally, the relationship you have with your coach should allow for open, two-way communication that encourages input from both you and your coach.

Yours in Sport,
Ian Sherwin

References:

Badami, R., Kohestani, S., & Taghian, F. (2011). Feedback on more accurate trials enhances learning of sport skills. World Applied Sciences Journal, 133, 537-540.

Cushion, C., Harvey, S., Muir, B., & Nelson, L., (2012) Developing the Coach Analysis and Intervention System (CAIS): Establishing validity and reliability of a computerised systematic observation instrument, Journal of Sports Sciences, 30:2, 201-216, DOI: 10.1080/02640414.2011.635310

DiCicco, T., Hacker, C., & Salzberg, C., (2002) Catch them being good. Viking Penguin, England.

Gearity, B. T., & Murray, M. A., (2011). Athlete's experiences of the psychological effects of poor coaching. Psychology of Sport and Exercise 12: 213-21

Lyle, J. & Cushion, C., (2017). Sports Coaching Concepts: A framework for coaches' behaviour. 2nd Edition. Routledge, London.

North, J. (2016). Benchmarking sport coach education and development. Advances in Coach Education and Development: From Research to Practice, 17.

Pawson, R., & Tilley, N. (1997). Realist evaluation. Changes.

Sherwin, I., Campbell, M. J., & MacIntyre, T. E. (2017): Talent development of high performance coaches in team sports in Ireland, European Journal of Sport Science 17(3) 271-278 http://dx.doi.org/10.1080/17461391.2016.1227378

Williams, S. J., & Kendall, L. (2007). Perceptions of elite coaches and sports scientists of the research needs for elite coaching practice. Journal of Sports Science, 25(14), 1577-1586. doi:10.1080/02640410701245550

Wilson, C. H., & Burdette, T., (2020) In "Coach Education Essentials: Your guide to developing sport coaches" Eds Kristen Dieffenbach and Melissa Thomspon; Human Kinetics, Champaign, Il.

SUMMARY POINTS - Chapter 9

- Coaching is a complex area.
- In youth sport, the majority of coaches are volunteers who give up their time to help out.
- Assume good intent on your coach's behalf. Don't expect them to be perfect.
- Talk to your coach and engage with them. Get to know them and learn to appreciate where they are coming from.
- Goals and objectives help to show progress in a more intelligent manner than merely winning and losing. You can play an active role in this process.
- Learn to become comfortable with reasonable and constructive critique.
- Actively seek corrective feedback from your coach. Ask pertinent questions.
- Appreciate that your mood and levels of understanding and empathy have an influence on the mood of your environment and those in it.
- Find a mentor who can provide calm, measured, agenda-free advice and feedback to you.

CHAPTER 10: PLAYING FAIR & COMMUNICATING WITH THE REFEREE

Sports are defined by their rules and laws, and we can have no games without referees. If you are serious about being the best you can be in sport, your ability to execute the skills of your game within its laws or rules, as well as your ability to communicate with the referee, are critical areas you must consider.

It is all too easy to deflect and blame others, and often in these cases the referee is the easy target. Many athletes have spent their whole career challenging referees and denying wrong doing on the field of play. Surely they would have been better served putting their time and energy into focusing on improving their technical execution and learning to work with the referee in the spirit of fair play and healthy competition.

'Play fair' is a simple statement, but it is nonetheless a challenge that demands much of you. Personal responsibility must be taken in this area and you must lean on your values and character qualities (see Chapter 3) to guide you. My hope is that the insights that follow can be helpful and lead you in the right direction.

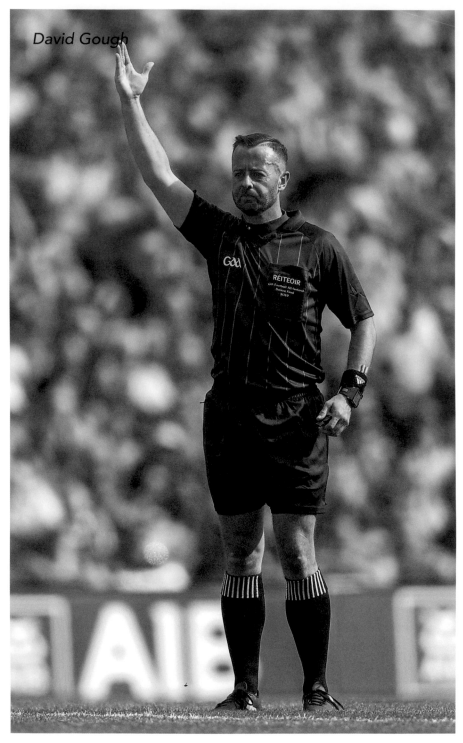

David Gough

CHAPTER 10

David Gough

David Gough is widely recognised as one of the most respected Gaelic Football referees having refereed the top four competitions in the GAA Calendar; All-Ireland Finals at minor, U21, club and senior intercounty. Below he shares his insights into the demands and challenges of refereeing and advises on the best way to approach both your relationship with the rules of the game and the referee. This is a principled based piece and so the thinking and messages hold true across many sports.

It can be said that a game is not a game without a set of rules. These rules must be implemented and enforced by someone. In competitive sport we can have no games without referees. This is one of sport's insurmountable truths. The role of the referee is to control the game in accordance with the playing rules. Your relationship with the rules of the game you play and your interactions with the referee may be something you have given little or no thought to. My goal with this short piece is to give you an appreciation of the value of knowing the rules and communicating appropriately with the referee.

Refereeing is something that comes quite naturally to me. I have a huge interest in the rules and the language of the rules. I spend a lot of time reading the rules and reflecting on them to help me understand how to implement them. The language of the rules is very prescriptive. The rule book is difficult to read, difficult to understand and difficult to implement.

From a psychological perspective referees are told to never expect the perfect refereeing performance. We must accept that just like the players, we will make mistakes. However, we have the added burden that the consequence of a mistake on our behalf can have significant impact on how the game evolves thereafter. The only real comparable in a playing sense is a goal keeping error. Refereeing is a high stakes game.

At any serious level of sport, referees implement a set of rules which they have an in-depth knowledge of. Often those we deal with; players, management, fans and indeed pundits simply don't have that same level of knowledge. Referees get their knowledge of the rules, from the rule book itself. Almost everyone else doesn't; they get them second-hand from a person who most likely has attained them second-hand t best. Often I give talks to squads of players and on average two of a panel of 30 will have read the rule book. In order to referee at inter-county level I must get 94% in a 50 question, 30 minute exam. From my perspective the inequality between the referee and everyone else often lies in the lack of knowledge of the rule book. In short, most people don't understand what we as referees are trying to implement. They become frustrated due to their lack of knowledge of the rules.

I use a three-step process in communicating how I implement the rules: firstly I say what I have seen, secondly I link or apply it to a rule and thirdly I implement the rule. An error of judgment is to be expected, for example, I may feel it wasn't a foul when the evidence suggest it was. There are reasons for this such as my viewpoint may be blocked or my attention may be else. To be human is to error. Errors of fact are different and should not happen. An error of fact is when the rules are implemented incorrectly such as awarding a penalty for a technical foul that does not occur inside the small rectangle. No matter the decision the old adage that a free will never be overturned is something you should learn to appreciate and accept. In rule it is not provided for; once a free is awarded it cannot be overturned.

All referees receive the same training and strive to implement the same set of rules. What makes us different is our personalities. We are all human and because of our life experiences we deal with various scenarios in different ways. We hear the word 'respect' frequently used and the reality is we all have different definitions and understandings of the word. What might be acceptable to some referees might be unacceptable to others and again this is something you should learn to appreciate. From my perspective what is totally unacceptable from a player towards any match official is: any form of physical or verbal abuse, any invasion of personal space or constant challenging of decisions and authority.

I am presuming that in reading this book you are striving to participate at a reasonable level in your sport. Therefore, I can assume you are striving to learn how to interact with the rules and communicate with the referee in a manner that is expected at the highest level of your sport by the best referees and officials. I would advise that firstly you should always assume good intent on behalf of the referee. It is too easy to convince yourself that the referee has a personal vendetta against *you or your team and when you go down this road you are giving away control and abdicating responsibility. You will never know what mindset a referee will arrive in on any given day. This is something that is outside of your control. Another uncontrollable for you is the referee's decision making. What is within your control however is your reaction. From a personal perspective how you communicate with me will dictate my response to you. Below are a few simple pointers for you.*

- *Play inside the rules- this is very simple advice but in order to do this you must know them. Learn the rules and learn the skills required to play within them.*
- *It is important to appreciate that it is not the job of the referee to allow the game 'flow'. The game flows when players play within the rules.*
- *Use the language of the rulebook when communicating with the referee. The referee will appreciate this and it is most likely you will receive a favourable response.*
- *Tone of voice and body language are critical in all forms of communication in all walks of life not least player/referee interactions.*
- *Own your actions and take responsibility for the consequence of them. This will serve you well in the long run as it will lead you to the truth.*
- *Ask questions in a respectful manner and expect a respectful response, although occasionally you will have to accept the response you are given even though you may not like it.*

All games and sporting environments depend on the relationship between the players, the rules and the referee. If your aim is to be the best you can be in sport, I would advise that you take the time to learn the rules of the game, take the time to develop the skills needed to play within the rules of the game and remember, that just like you, the referee is human and will make mistakes.

Best wishes,
David Gough

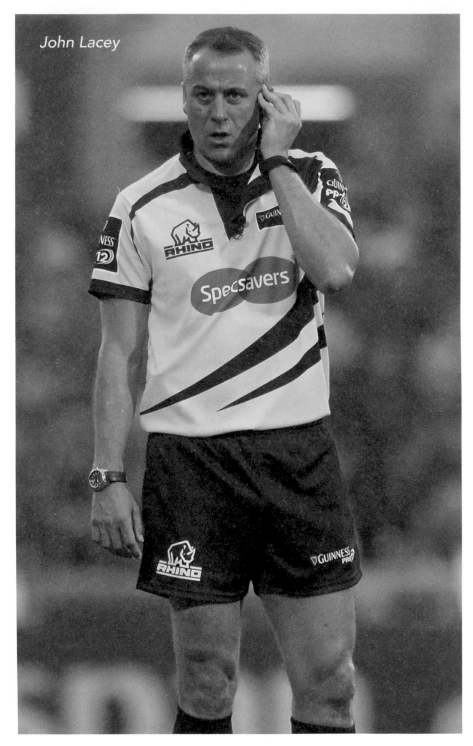

John Lacey

John Lacey

John Lacey is the IRFU High Performance Referee Coach and Talent ID Manager. Now retired from refereeing at professional level, he refereed the 2013 Pro12 Grand Final, as well as the 2015–16 and 2016–17 European Rugby Challenge Cup Finals. He also refereed at: Six Nations Championship, Rugby Championship and Rugby World Cup level.

As a non-rugby person I feel there is much other sports can learn from the game of rugby regarding how both players and coaches interact with the referee, and indeed vice versa. I have asked Johnny to give you an insight into this, which I hope will prove both interesting and useful to you.

Rugby is a physically brutal sport. Although the object of the game is simply to place the ball in the opposition's scoring zone, it is nonetheless an extremely complex and multifaceted sport. There are no rules in rugby, but laws...and plenty of them. Rules are defined- black and white, whereas laws are there to be interpreted in order to keep the game flowing. With this said, it must be noted that where a law is infringed, and this has a material effect on the game, it must be penalised. Rugby is a sport which has a great tradition in the laws of the game.

In rugby, a code of ethics is traditionally instilled in its participants from the very beginning. Players, coaches and referees must all learn to live by the core values of the game. The IRFU Spirit of Rugby lists: Respect, Integrity, Inclusivity, Fun and Excellence as its core values. It is becoming of all associated with the game, to turn these words into tangible and obvious actions and behaviours. As a rapidly expanding sport in this country, it is the duty of rugby traditionalists to pass on these values to newcomers to our game, and ensure they are both upheld and reinforced.

In rugby, the relationship between the player and the referee is critical to ensure the game is fair and safe, and provides for a good spectacle. This relationship is a two-way street. The game is in the care of all participants. The team is represented on the field of play by its captain and they are entitled to speak to the referee when appropriate. Articulate use of language, tone of voice and general demeanour from both sides enhance this captain/ referee relationship, and so the game is improved. In professional rugby, the captain now uses the captain/

referee relationship as a 'pressure tool' to put on the referee, and if done so in the correct manner, this is perfectly ok.

Rugby Law states that the referee's role is paramount for the safety of the players on the field. As a result of this, it has evolved that communication between all parties has become central to the refereeing process. In domestic rugby at all levels, the referee will enter the team dressing room pregame to check the legality of studs and discuss various issues with coaches and players such as what they might want from the front rows around the scrum, etc. The coach is also entitled to interact with the referee pre-game where they can discuss concerns about elements of the opposition's style of play. In professional rugby, this line of communication to the referee is open in the week approaching a game and can be via phone or email. At international level, all parties meet the day before the game. An example of an interaction in this scenario would be that the coach may express concerns about the legality of a certain element of the opposition's play and may ask for the referee's thoughts on this, or for it to be clarified. The coach may reinforce their position through the use of video evidence, and it is up to the referee to draw their own conclusion.

Pre-game video analysis on the part of the referee has become commonplace. In the IRFU at professional level, our referees are extremely well prepared ahead of the game. They will have established what type of attack and defence the teams play and any relevant statistics around trends in technical penalties, etc. As a group of referees, we are improving our understanding of the 'Rugby DNA' of each team and this can inform and influence our on-field positioning, allowing us to place ourselves in the optimal position to make the correct call. We are increasingly better prepared, and this work can also inform our pre-game interactions with the team coach and captain.

In professional rugby, the coach is not allowed in the technical zone. Only medics and water carriers are allowed here. There may be some scope for the coach to get a message to the referee through these people and, if on investigation, the message proves accurate the referee will often respect it. Alternatively, if the information provided proves inaccurate, this may affect any further potential interactions between the two.

In all successful player/coach-referee interactions, the governing principle is the improvement of the game. There can be no games *without players or referees. This is also almost always true of the coach. Rugby is a sport that aims to provide a positive disposition in the interactions between all parties. This is grounded in respect for the laws and can only be upheld through open and positive communication. It is better for all involved if we treat each other fairly and get along.*

Yours in Sport,
Johnny Lacey.

SUMMARY POINTS - Chapter 10

- 'The game' is in the care of all participants.
- Learn the rules or laws of your sport.
- Develop the skills required to play within these rules or laws.
- Take personal responsibility for your actions and always seek the truth.
- Using the language of the rule book, communicate with the referee in a manner which you would like to be communicated with yourself.

CHAPTER 11: PREPARING TO PERFORM

In competitive sport, the main reason we train is to perform when it matters most - in competition. This becomes more important the older you get, and the more competitive your sporting endeavours become. The aim of performance preparation is to optimise readiness to perform when it matters most. The goal is to arrive with determination, purpose and energy - in a state of preparedness. Your aim is to show up as the best version of yourself. It is important to appreciate you cannot function optimally, either physically or mentally, unless your emotions are under control. You must develop a sustainable and intelligent process which leads to composed performance.

You can have all the self-belief and confidence imaginable, but without the necessary focus and concentration on the sporting field your performance will be erratic and inconsistent. The best athletes can attend their focus to what they need to prioritise in the moment. The practice of achieving this performance focus begins long before the whistle is blown or the game begins. How you think about competition will influence how you feel and perform. You must first become aware of what you are thinking leading up to competition. Are your thoughts affecting how you feel and act on game day? Again, deciding what you can control, and influence, is a good way to focus on what you want to do, and what you can do. It is a good way to 'control the controllables', and readily prepare yourself to perform. Remember, the most you can do is to create the best possible conditions for performance.

PERFORMANCE FOCUS

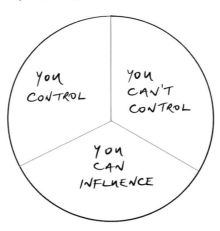

What are you focused on prior to competition?

Below are some of the areas you can control, you can influence and you can't control prior to competition (see Skill No. 2 – Control).

YOU CAN CONTROL	YOU CAN INFLUENCE	YOU CAN'T CONTROL
SLEEP	YOUR TEAM MATES (WITH GOOD PRACTICE, COMMUNICATION & SUPPORT)	THE RESULT
HYDRATION		THE WEATHER
REST/RECOVERY		THE DATE, TIME & VENUE
DOWN TIME		
NUTRITION	YOUR COACH (WITH APPROPRIATE FEEDBACK & SUPPORT)	YOUR OPPONENT'S PREPARATION
SKILLS PRACTICE		
MENTAL PREPARATION		
EQUIPMENT		
STRETCHING & MOBILITY	THE OUTCOME	
KNOWING YOUR ROLE		
KNOWING GAME-PLAN		

The Wheel of Preparation

A useful tool to use for mental and physical preparation ahead of a game is the 'wheel of preparation'. It is suggested to use it between 7 to 10 days out from a game. The 'wheel of preparation' is a simple yet effective tool and one you can create yourself with a blank page of paper and a marker or pen. Alternatively, you can create it in your journal - see sample below.

1. Draw a circle as per diagram and divide into segments (there is no 'right' or 'wrong' amount of segments – between six to eight is usually good).
2. Each segment is representative of an element of preparation for the game ahead. Fill out what you see as key elements you can control e.g. hydration, nutrition, visualisation work, self-talk routines, knowing the game plan, knowing your own role and KPI's (see Chapter 7), mobility, sleep, skills work.
3. Shade in each segment to represent where each one is at, ahead of the game – fully shaded means you are 100% prepared and this element is in a good place.
4. In any element there are gaps, identify simple specific actions you can take in the next week to improve your preparedness in this area e.g. action: get one hour more sleep per night or do five to ten minutes deliberate skills practice daily.
5. Come match day the aim is that most, if not all (please don't fret if it's not perfect…this not about being perfect it's about getting better) areas are fully shaded and you are well prepared in the areas which are within your control. You are now relaxed, prepared and ready to perform.

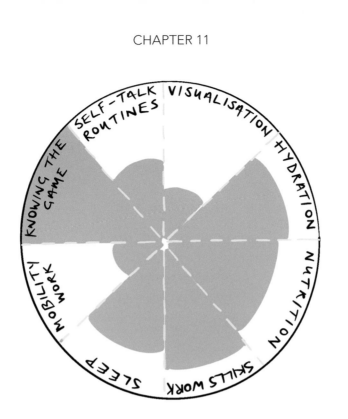

Often, young athletes leading into competition focus on areas that are outside of their control. This can lead to anxious thoughts and feelings, and these can lead to nerves and anxiety that affect performance. In Chapter 7 we have looked at the types of performance goals you can set and the processes involved in achieving the goals. These will enhance motivation, confidence and focus on the key actions and behaviours that lead to strong performances. The outcome of the game should only be a very small measure of success.

Having a clear action or process focus is crucial. For example:

"I can control my effort, my attention, my communication, my scanning, my striking, my tackle technique, my support play and movement. I can influence my opponent by how I make runs, tackle or position my body. I can influence the referee by communicating calmly and clearly and by playing the game in a fair and honest manner".

Degree of Controllability

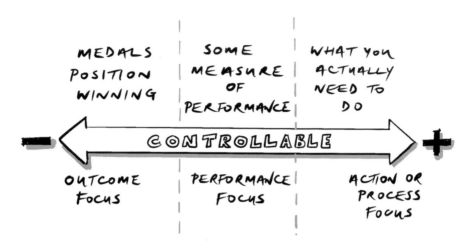

Questions to Consider

1. What is in my control in the lead up to competition that helps me deliver my best performances?
2. What is outside my control in the lead up to competition that interferes with my performances?
3. How can I overcome these interferences?
4. What are my performance focus goals for the challenge ahead?
5. What are the actions, behaviours or processes I must execute during competition for greater performance?
6. What are the outcomes I would like to achieve by completing these process and performance focused actions?

CHAPTER 11

David Gilllick

David Gillick is a retired International Track and Field athlete. He is one of Ireland's most successful sprint athletes, becoming an Olympian in 2008, finishing 6th in the 2009 World Championships and topping the podium on two occasions at the European Indoor Championships in 2005 and again in 2007. He specialised in the 400 metres where he holds both the Irish indoor and outdoor national records. He competed in all major athletic championships over a 13 year career. Here, David shares his insights into preparing to perform on the biggest stage.

Looking back on my career as an athlete, there are a few things I did that really helped my performance both mentally and physically.

I trained hard, I was motivated, determined and focused. I loved the training process, the recovery, eating right; however, one area I really needed to look after in the run up to competition was dealing with nerves, doubts and my inner voice. It took a bit of work. I had to put my hand up and ask for help. I was physically in the best of shape with the talent to compete at the highest level, but I needed to make sure I brought my head in line.

Sometimes, nerves got the better of me. Ahead of competition I would be anxious, over thinking things, restless, unable to eat and not focused on the task, losing track of my preparation and race plan. What I needed to do was remind myself of my success, the work I had done and the fast times I had run. Sounds easy, but how many of us actually look back at the moments we excelled, overcame obstacles and challenges? I had to learn and, I did. I learned to reprogram the way I thought. When the nerves got a hold prior to a big championships, I would smile and think 'nerves are good, they tell me that I care, and if I care I'll perform'. I began to welcome the nerves. They told me I was ready.

I would sit down with a pen and paper and briefly write down all the negatives, all the stupid thoughts that would come into my head regarding the upcoming race. The things that had never happened before but for some reason I think might happen. I would simply write them down and rip up the page or go into the garden and burn it. I

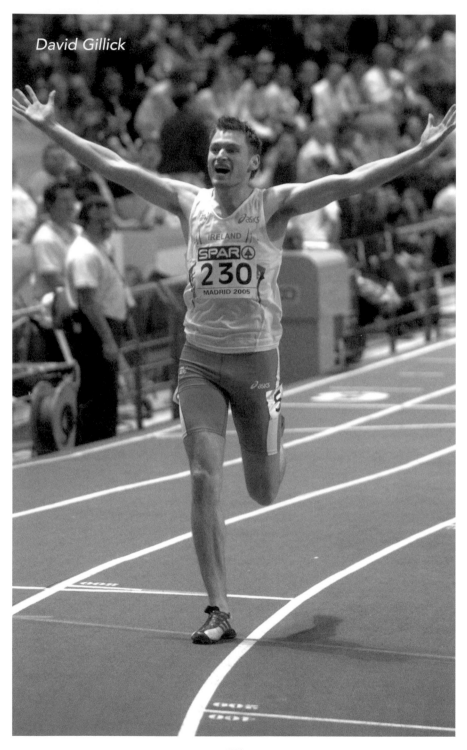

David Gillick

would get those thoughts out of my head! Then I would write down all the facts: the times that I ran in previous races, all the training sessions I had done and the other skills I had developed that I knew would drive my performance. Those were the facts- the real facts!

I also began to look back at my big successes in races and championships. I downloaded all the videos and pictures and made a little video with a song that inspired me. I kept it on my phone and would watch it in the days and hours prior to a race. It lasted about 40 seconds and showed me excelling and performing. It was powerful! Watching it filled me with confidence and self-belief. Any doubts I had suddenly disappeared, I was flexing my 'confidence muscle'.

Visualisation was something I became aware of and began to use regularly. In the days prior to races, I would visualise my race, every detail: track, crowd, competitors, smells and sounds. If I had an image or if I had previously competed at the venue it helped. I would simply lie on my bed or sit in a chair and close my eyes. I would go through all aspect of the competition, from the warm-up track to the call room, lacing up my black and yellow spikes, pulling on my race vest, walking out onto the track, setting my starts blocks, doing some practice starts, looking at the crowd, hearing the noise, smelling the tartan from the track, hearing the race starters voice as he's says "On your marks" and then running every metre of the race, picking my points on the track to relax and attack. I would do this numerous times in the days leading up to competition and then stop the day before; it was my way of telling myself 'the computer is programmed- I have been here before'.

When I retained my European title in 2007 it was like déjà vu, it honestly felt like I had been there, in the race, in the stadium, before. I had visualised every aspect of this race in my head many times, and I believe it helped me in the close moments of the real race to remain calm and collected. It allowed me to attack and win in the last 10 metres of a 400 metre race.

Backing yourself and believing in yourself is so important. I look back at my career now and I wish I realised how good I was when i was competing. Preparing to perform is a critical skill you can develop and I wish you well in your journey.

Best wishes,
David Gillick

CHAPTER 11

SKILLS FOR DRAWING
ON YOUR INNER STRENGTH
SKILL NO. 3 - VISUALISATION AND
THE POWER OF THE SUBCONSCIOUS MIND
By Tony Óg Regan

Why is this important?

In the lead up to big events, it is natural for your mind to wander into thoughts, images, or feelings about the event ahead. We all run through some version of what it will look like, feel like and sound like on that day. You can practice 'Mental Rehearsal' of what you want to do, what you want to say, what you want to think, feel and move like.

In your everyday life and in your performance life, do your thoughts and images help you create the realities you would like to live? Do your thoughts and images ever interfere with your chances of performing and achieving what you set out to do?

When we begin to focus our attention and mental images in helpful and positive ways, we begin to consistently create better thinking, feelings, and images around our performance and ourselves. Through using 'Visualisation' you can prepare yourself long before the event, in how you would like to perform and respond to events as they unfold. This will help you become a more composed, resilient, confident and focused athlete.

The big positive from using visualisation consistently and correctly is that it allows you to deal more effectively with challenges. You will learn to better handle and deal with, the emotional distress and disturbance that sometimes occur before, during or after that event. This will allow you to focus better on the moment or task in front of you. You will get a sense of having been there before and experienced this situation. It will feel like no big surprise to your mind and body anymore.

*"I am prepared, I relish these moments and opportunities.
I focus on one moment and one play at a time. I know most of the time good things will happen when I focus in this way".*

The reason this works so well in a performance context, and in any area of life, is that the subconscious mind, which we operate from 95% of the time, cannot distinguish between an imagined and real experience. Both feel equally real, for the mind and the brain. When you imagine, think, feel and move through our performance in this way, your brain firing neurons and lighting up a new neurological pathway in your b of thinking, feeling, seeing and doing. You create a whole new circuit, a whole new way of 'being'. Your thoughts, feelings and images have enormous power to change your personality in any setting. You need a certain number of successful experiences to create an integrated set of nerve cells in your brain to perform a skill at a high level with consistency. Nerve cells that wire together, fire together. When something is practiced repeatedly, those nerve cells develop a stronger and stronger connection, and it gets easier and easier to fire that network.

Video Imagery

Watching elite athletes perform the skills you require and visualising yourself making the same shots and executing the same skills hundreds of times can have the same effect on your brain. You can correct technical errors and improve performance skills effectively using this method also. Creating some of your best moments on video clips and watching consistently will fire the same neurological circuits as actually doing it physically. It will build confidence, reduce anxiety around performance, improve motivation and create a sense of excitement around previously worrying situations. You can use both mental, and video imagery, to learn new skills and improve overall performance in pressure situations.

Developing your imagery skills:

1. *Start with simple, familiar images or skills. For the next 14 days, practice for five minutes a day, on waking or just before bed. It is the best time as our mind is most lucid and creative. Before training is another effective time to rehearse this.*

2. *Imagine the place where you usually train – what it looks like, sounds like, smells like and feels like. See your teammates interacting, go through your warmup, feel the surface underneath your feet and the equipment you are using, feel the weight of it. Imagine and feel yourself doing the skills of your sport such as jogging, weaving, passing, catching, kicking, etc. As you move through the session, increase the intensity and difficulty of the skills.*

3. *Building this up to 10-15 minutes each day is your goal. Doing short periods of mental and video imagery of high quality is key. The more vivid and accurate our images and feelings and the more effectively you perform that skill, the stronger the*

chance you have of replicating that situation in real time events.

4.   *With this daily practice, your visualisation skills will improve considerably, your imagined performance situations will feel even more real. Using a piece of your game day equipment and rehearsing the moves without a ball, is even more effective. This allows your body to feel the shot.*

See Appendix for a template of a visualisation script I would use to improve mental rehearsal before competition. You may find it useful to adapt it to fit your sporting context and record it onto your phone to listen to.

Eddie Brennan

Eddie Brennan is a retired Kilkenny Hurler. Throughout his 12-year career with Kilkenny he won eight All-Irelands and four All-Stars in what was a glorious period for the county. He also won two Senior Kilkenny Club Titles with his club Graigue-Ballycallan who he has represented until very recently. After his Kilkenny career ended, Eddie moved into coaching and management. He is currently the Laois Senior Hurling Manager. Here, Eddie shares with you how he prepared to perform.

15 v 15, plus subs and a referee- that's a lot of variables. In terms of bringing consistency to your game, it is challenging to say the least. During my early days as a county hurler I played some good games and plenty of poor ones. At a time when the inside line played their position you were heavily dependent on the supply of ball, not to mention the quality of it. You simply accepted the good days with the bad ones. I wanted to hit 8 out of 10 performance wise for each game. As an inside forward my role and function was to score. If I didn't I had failed, simple as that.

It wasn't until maybe 2005 and into 2006 that I started to do some digging into developing insights into performance and proper preparation. I unearthed terms such as, "control the controllables" and 'visualisation' and began to appreciate that I needed to differentiate between 'performance' and 'outcome'. I began to read many sports books seeking nuggets of information, little buzz words or phrases that could help. I found Jonny Wilkinson's Autobiography and Phil Jackson's 'Sacred Hoops' really insightful. Understanding that scoring wasn't the only form of a measurable work-return was a crucial first step in building a routine of preparing to perform.

For me, there are two parts to preparing to perform. Firstly, the routine I developed that led into games and secondly what is known as visualisation. While both are directly connected and overlap, I will explain both separately from my personal experiences.

My preparation routine became standardised and cyclical for the week leading up to all championship games from 2006 to 2011. Planning

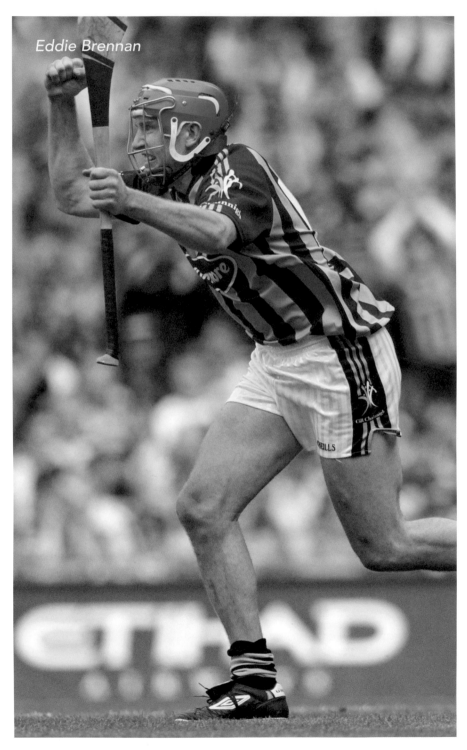

Eddie Brennan

ahead and developing habits meant I was ready to perform. I began to appreciate that there is a massive difference in, preparing to perform as opposed to preparing to win; understanding that the result was an outcome that was the consequence of a collective performance and as such something I couldn't control, only influence. For me developing a routine that had me in the right place mentally and physically was crucial.

It is very important for you to understand that developing a routine doesn't happen overnight; it takes time, trial and error and unfortunately does not guarantee a big performance. However, it does reduce the poor performances and allows you to take control of being in the right frame of mind to do the business.

The week of a match involved balancing being busy enough to avoid too much time to allow for overthinking and having time to work on my touch, flexibility and training. I preferred to work all week. Having too much time to fill was something I liked to avoid. We trained Tuesday and Friday and I would have ball alley work every other day. The week of matches was about getting fresh and fully charged up so training was light. I still liked to go hard at the touch-work on a Tuesday night, always with the same guys who worked each other hard. The touch had to be flawless and the mind concentrated. Friday night was a lot more relaxed with maybe 30 minutes collectively before the team was announced. For me, there was always 30 minutes of shooting and touch work before training. Repetition of shooting from all positions polishing up the 'muscle memory' and knowing I was ready.

The Saturday prior to games involved a similar routine: work and then down to Robbie Lodge for some physio and a stretch out, followed by dinner and some light ball wall work. From 2006 to 2011, I worked in my job with An Garda Síochána at the Electric Picnic Music Festival each Friday and Saturday before these All-Ireland finals. Some might think this strange but, for me, it kept my mind occupied enough without over taxing me.

Sunday morning it was up early, a walk and a few pucks followed by a good breakfast then on to the bus. Second back row beside Michael Rice, being entertained by the crew in the back seat all the way to Santry for our pre-match meal and then on to Croke Park. Same few tunes on the IPod and togged out in the same seat with the same few lads either side. It was repetitive and ultimately allowed a consistent familiarity to ensure I was in the right place mentally to perform. While it might sound a fraction OCD it wasn't rigid or superstitious to the point of paralysing me if something wasn't in place. It was repetitive enough to facilitate being ready but also allowing wriggle room for the unexpected. If a box wasn't ticked on my routine it didn't cause any distraction or stress but having all markers hit meant I was in the best possible place to perform.

James McGarry had a saying "play the match over in your head". He was talking about what we now know as 'visualisation'. It was a statement I lived by and relied upon heavily for much of my career. During work or walking the dog or driving to training or simply chilling out in front of the TV were opportunities to play the game over in my head. Picturing likely scenarios I would encounter became commonplace. What if the corner back wins the first two balls? What if I can't get my hands on the ball? How can I work my way into the match to influence it. What if my marker starts into me, mouthing or digging? How do I deal with it? I would go through all these scenarios in my head and my confidence in being able to deal with them would rise. More importantly what I found as a result of my visualisation work when these scenarios occurred during matches I was able to deal with them without getting rattled. 'Keep patient', 'maintain focus', I would use my trigger words.

In the run up to the 2008 All Ireland Final we received word that Waterford were planning to target some of us with 'special treatment'. I was due to mark Eoin Murphy, a 'hurling cornerback' who played from the front. I incorporated the expected 'special treatment' into my visualisation and scenario work. 'What do I do if he hits me? Strike back or ignore?' If something happens that you weren't expecting or haven't prepared for it can have a huge effect and may be enough to throw you off your game for 15 or 20 minutes. My thinking was if he started trying to physically impose himself on me before the throw in my focus would be on the first ball. Sure enough the messing started after the handshake and continued until I got my hands on the first ball, nailed a point and never looked back.

What is your understanding of a contribution and how to work your way into a match? Forwards are there to score? Well yes that's true, but there were other ways to contribute. Brian Cody wanted mean, hungry, ruthless workers. He knew we could hurl, but unless you grafted relentlessly, scoring wouldn't suffice. I envisaged hunting down defenders who beat me to the ball and turning them over. Bring a defender right out to the side line. Create an opening or space for a *teammate to exploit. Standing a defender up and not allowing him to break the tackle. Winning a puck out with a clean catch and offloading to a better placed teammate. These were all the different scenarios I would see in my mind's eye and plan how I would try to deal with them.*

I firmly believe the game is 90% in the head. Therefore, preparing to perform is undoubtedly a crucial component. By developing a flexible routine players can take control of their performance to a greater degree than many realise. Ultimately, it's how quickly you can build and develop these skills that will expedite those consistent performances. Top players do this even though some may not consciously realise it. You would be naive to think the best players, across all sporting codes, just turn up and things happen for them. Find what works for you.

I wish you well,
Eddie Brennan

SKILLS FOR DRAWING
ON YOUR INNER STRENGTH
SKILL NO. 4 - COMPOSURE
By Tony Óg Regan

Why is this important?
We all know what it feels like to be over-excited, overwhelmed, nervous, anxious or so wound up on occasions that we're not able to perform to our potential. Consistent performance happens in the present moment and it's a skill to find the right level of physical and mental activation: not too relaxed and not too fired up.

Depending on what you're going to encounter, the body begins to activate based on your thoughts and perceived level of importance of those events. Sweaty palms, increased heart rate and shortness of breath and butterflies in your stomach are all signs of internal activation. How do you interpret this? Is it nerves or is it excitement? When you view it as the body getting ready to perform, you begin to recognise these signals as performance time. You are excited to challenge and test yourself, to see what level you can reach. The only limits on your performance are the ones you put on it yourself. Do you go out with the intention to play great and act from a place of love of the challenge, or do you go out to avoid (taking risks, making mistakes, letting others down, etc.) and act from a place of fear? Below you will learn how to regulate your internal activation, or what we call composure, which will help you stay in the present moment and perform at your best.

Yerkes-Dodson Model Adapted from Yerkes- Dodson Model

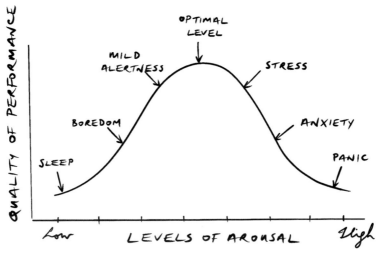

The Yerkes-Dodson Model of activation and performance is a scale that can be used to find your optimal level of activation to perform at your best. One on the scale you may find is, on waking each day where you are sleepy and drowsy, and your level of performance would be at 1/10. However, if on waking you hear an intruder downstairs, your activation may shoot up to nine or 10 where your arousal is high, and you hit the panic zone in relation to your performance.

THINK OF YOUR BEST PERFORMANCE IN RECENT MEMORY
WHAT LEVEL OF MENTAL & PHYSICAL INTENSITY
(AROUSAL) WERE YOU AT?

WHAT NUMBER WOULD YOU PUT IT AT? _____

NOW CONSIDER;

WHEN YOU ARE WARMING UP, WHAT NUMBER DO YOU
WANT TO BE AT? _____

WHEN YOU ARE PERFORMING AT YOUR BEST, WHAT
NUMBER ARE YOU AT? _____

At 9/10, there is too much blood flow to the heart, legs and head. There is too much over-activation, cortisol is released into the body. When you are activated, you can go into fight, flight, freeze, or flow. Athletes love their heart pounding on the sweet spot of activation. Small changes in physiology can make a big difference to legs, arms and body temperature. When we sweat it can help us to cool down our bodies.

5/10 is perceived to be the best level for optimal intensity and performance. You are not under or over activated. You are ready to ACT. You face the challenge and find a solution to the next task.

The important things you need to understand:
1. *Where am I on the scale when I am at my best?*
2. *What is my current level?*
3. *How do I increase or lower it?*

Techniques to Increase and Decrease Levels of Arousal
When you need to activate your brain and body there are several techniques you can use. If I was a soccer player, I could solo a tennis ball

or work with a partner passing two footballs over and back, in order to stimulate concentration and decision making and focus on the here and now. Listening to upbeat and high tempo music can stimulate strong emotions and raise your intensity levels. Physically, you can do some squats, burpees and sprints to raise your heart rate. Communicating strong and powerful statements can motivate and raise your emotions and intensity. Watching clips of past performances or sporting heroes can raise excitement and intensity levels. Raising the intensity and frequency of your breathing can increase or decrease arousal levels in the moment. Imagining a calm and composed start to the situation or event you are in can evoke a response in the moment too.

One of the most important tools to anchor you in the present moment and generate calm and composure is how you use your breath. When you get the technique of the breath right, you find a calmer state on a regular basis. Taking a deep breath is one of the most powerful "reset" buttons you have at your disposal.

When you are in a 'threat state' you are often breathing from your chest. When you are in a 'challenge/performance state' you are usually breathing from your stomach. It is natural for your brain to perceive many situations as a threat and induce this 'stress response' quickly. This pumps adrenaline and cortisol around your body faster. This is what drives up your activation on the scale. You need to be aware of your self-talk (see Skill No. 6) in these situations and develop your system of breathing from the belly to induce the relaxation response.

Here is a short abdominal breathing exercise:
1. *Hand on your belly – inhale a short breath in and follow up with two smaller ones again.*
2. *Let gut hang out.*
3. *Exhale slowly out through the mouth or nose.*
4. *Repeat the phrase 'I am calm, I am ready' after each exhale.*

The longer exhale is paired with relaxation in your brain. This tells your over activated threat detector system everything is 'ok'. The breath is connected to your brain, heart, lungs, etc. so it is a vital tool for your central nervous system to calm down when it gets over-activated.

Training this calm technique will help you to perform at your best in critical moments. If you train this consistently, you can use it in any stressful situations such as exams or public speaking.

Training Calm Exercises:
10 deep breaths in 3 different environments
- *A quiet and relaxing place at home*
- *When out for a gentle run in the park or before a conversation that causes some emotion*
- *High pressure situation with an outcome at stake*

Other means of lowering stress/ arousal levels include: listening to slow or calm music, slow mindful movements, imagery, visualisation and mindfulness.

FURTHER REFLECTION :

1). WHAT ARE THE LAST 3 SITUATIONS THAT GOT YOU UP TO A "7" LEVEL OF ACTIVATION OR HIGHER ?

_____

_____

2). DESCRIBE WHAT IT SOUNDS LIKE, LOOKS LIKE & FEELS LIKE WHEN YOU'RE AT YOUR ABSOLUTE BEST OR YOUR "5".

_____

_____

Summary
Training calmness and composure is an essential tool in the performance environment. Your brain has a natural 'threat detection' system which can cause you to become over-activated in any environment at any stage. It is crucial to be aware of your activation levels and how to manage them and ensure you are at the optimal level of arousal/intensity to perform at your best in the big moments. The crucial element to remember is that your best performance moments happen when you are in a place called "No Mind" – this is where you are no longer projecting yourself into the future through a thought of what might happen (usually fear) or a thought from the past (your memory). This is present moment awareness. You can practice being in the present and being in 'No Mind' every

single day to grow the length of time you have between your thoughts. You do this by focusing consciously on your breath, by observing your thoughts without judgement and letting go, by becoming aware of your senses for a few moments each day e.g. the smell of cut grass, the breeze against our skin, the feeling of hot water against our body, the sound of the birds singing, your feet on the ground. These all help you to rebalance your attention on the present. The more often you spend time in the present moment the more consistent you will be in any area of your life. When you train your attention in this way you become more absorbed in the task and your execution and decision making in the moment become of consistently higher quality.

The thoughts you have, what you listen to, what you eat and drink, your sleep quality and quantity and your perception of the situation you are in, all drive a mental and physical response. Using the tools in this book will allow you to get to a more consistent performance level by utilising the appropriate tools for that situation. Identify the tool that works best for you and practice it in training, everyday life and in your performance, be it self-talk, breathing routines, visualisation, reset routines, trigger words, etc.
See also Skill No. 6 – Confidence- The Power of Language.

References
Corbett, M. (2015), "From law to folklore: work stress and the Yerkes-Dodson Law", Journal of Managerial Psychology, Vol. 30 No. 6, pp. 741-752. https://doi.org/10.1108/JMP-03-2013-0085

SUMMARY POINTS - Chapter 11
- The aim of performance preparation is to optimise readiness to perform when it matters most.
- Prior to competition, it is important to appreciate what you can control, what you can influence and what you can't control.
- Through the use of 'Visualisation' you can prepare yourself long before the event, in how you would like to perform and respond to events as they unfold.
- Developing a pre-competition preparation routine is a good way to bring consistency to your performance.
- Consistent performance happens in the present moment and it is a skill to find the right level of physical and mental activation: not too relaxed and not too fired up.

CHAPTER 12 : SETBACKS

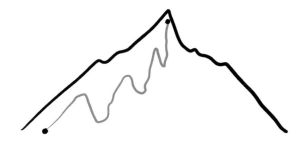

The struggle is the pathway' is a line I often use in my coaching. *There will be setbacks along the way'* is another.

Often I quote the former Irish Politician Terence MacSwiney:
"It is not those who can inflict the most,
but those who can endure the most who will conquer".

Resilience is the ability to bounce back from adversity and is a crucial quality to develop for sport, and indeed life. Things go wrong in sport and in life. Indeed, much of the story of sport is 'failure', so much so it can be said, that if you are not failing, you are not succeeding. Failing to master a skill instantaneously, reach a goal like a personal best or lose in competition are all part of learning. They are essential for true success, but it must be strongly noted that not all failure leads to success. Progress is never linear. The challenge is always to do what is right even when things are going wrong.

HOW TALENT DEVELOPS

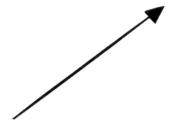
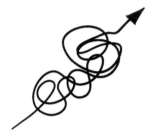

WHAT PEOPLE
THINK IT LOOKS LIKE

WHAT IT ACTUALLY
LOOKS LIKE.

Adversity can be an important stimulus for growth and development, provided you have the required skills to respond positively and the appropriate support around you. Always seek counsel in times of challenge, talk to trusted adults, coaches, mentors and peers. A problem shared is often a problem halved and the right words, from the right person, at the right time always helps to change focus and strengthen resolve (see Chapter 27).

Kanter's Law argues that 'Everything looks like a failure in the middle'. 'Expect things to go wrong', may appear negative, or pessimistic, on the face of it, but it is extremely prudent advice. Setbacks are certain but can often be unexpected.

CHAPTER 12

Bundee Aki

Bundee Aki is an Irish International Rugby Player. He has won a New Zealand Super Rugby title with the Chiefs in 2013 and a Pro12 title with Connacht in 2016. In 2015–16 he was named Pro12 Player of the Season. He also won a Six Nations Championship with Ireland in 2018. He has an interesting story to tell and here he shares the obstacles he had to overcome to build a life for himself as a professional rugby player.

My journey to playing for Connacht and Ireland has taken many twists and turns. I was born in New Zealand. At birth, I was named Fua Leiofi, but was called Bundellu after the doctor who delivered me. The nickname "Bundee" was given to me by my rugby coach as a child and it has stuck ever since. From a young age I loved the game of rugby and all I wanted to do was play.

As with most journeys in life, my path hit a bump in the road which saw me quitting rugby for a period. In my late teens I became a father and, with this, brought responsibility. I took a job in the bank in order to financially support my new family. Shortly afterwards, I was invited to New Zealand U 20 trials and managed to balance the first two stages of the three stage trial process with my work commitments in the bank. I was actually late for the second trial due to missing a flight after work but despite this, I still made it through to the third and final trial. This brought more scheduling conflicts for me. Work wouldn't allow me any more time off so I was forced to make a tough choice. I had to choose between my job and my dream. I chose my job because I had a young family who were depending on my income from it. It was a tough call but one I felt I had to make. I then chose to walk away from rugby completely and focus fully on my job in the bank and looking after and providing for my family. To support my family, I felt I had to sacrifice the thing I liked most, which was rugby.

I must admit that part of my decision to quit rugby at the time was that I was unsure as to whether I would make it as a professional or not. There were so many good young players surrounding me at the time. The bank offered me stability and a career path. Rugby came with no guarantees and a very uncertain career path. Due to my personal

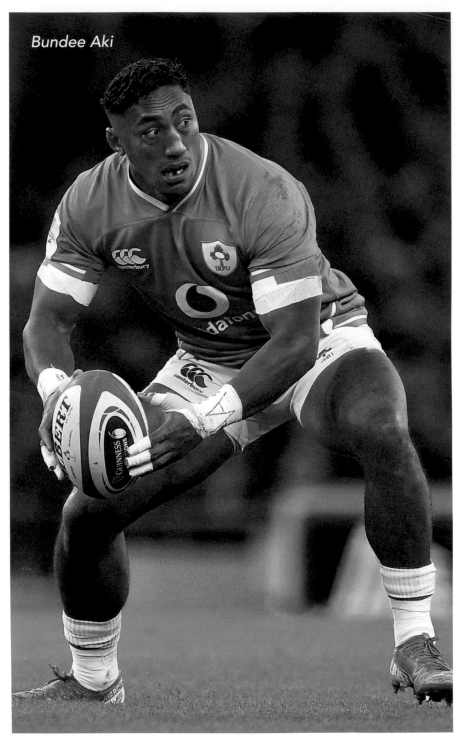

Bundee Aki

circumstances, I opted for stability. You could argue that fear played a part in my decision but my family's welfare had to come first.

Life in the bank went well and I soon found myself in a new branch with a new manager, Kalo Payne- Smith, who was a rugby fanatic. I kept a keen-eye on rugby and, watching my peers I had played with and against, I began to get a gnawing feeling that I was at least good enough to be there with them and that I could make it. My period in the bank was a time where I matured greatly. Having a stable family life helped with this also. For me, many of the qualities I would need on my second-coming to rugby were definitely developed during this period.

With no training or matches, a sedentary lifestyle as a bank official and a love of food, I sat at approximately 18 kgs over my current playing weight the day All- Black legend Tana Umaga came to visit me in the bank. At the time, Tana was Counties Manukua Coach and had heard about my playing potential from a number of sources. We talked in the bank and there and then he offered me a trial period with Counties. I was faced with another choice, the comfort and security of the bank or the uncertainty of rugby. I discussed it with my partner and my rugby-mad bank manager, Kalo. Kalo offered to be flexible with me in the bank and urged me to take on the challenge.

The trial period involved me training with the academy at 6 am in the morning. This would see me leaving home at 5:10am for a 35 minute drive to training. I would train at 6am and head straight to work in the bank afterwards. After work, I would go straight to training with a local amateur rugby club I had joined...I needed all the training I could get. I'd return home at about 9 o'clock at night. This was my routine for three days of the week and then on the weekend was more training and games.

Another big choice came for me and my family when Counties offered me a contract worth 15,000 NZ Dollars. This was significantly less than my job in the bank was paying and was far from an easy choice for me and my partner. This time I chose to back myself and follow my dream. I did so with a renewed drive and an increased level of maturity. My time had come and I was ready.

And so you can see that behind the big names in the big games are ordinary people who have overcome many setbacks and challenges and been forced to make hard decisions. I am now both happy and proud to play for Connacht and Ireland. I know I have many setbacks and challenges ahead of me in rugby but I also know I can overcome them. Had I not gone back to rugby I would have missed out on so much. I would have never known what could have been. My choices were difficult for me, I had a lot at stake and I had to overcome fear. I guess that's something we all have to overcome.

I wish you well on your journey,
Bundee Aki

Your focus must always be on how you respond to setbacks and adversity and how you can use it to fuel your subsequent effort and application. Mindset, self-talk (see Tony Óg's Skill No. 6) and other mental tools and supports we have discussed in the previous chapters, are crucial. Failure is an action and not an identity.

'Failure' can, and should, be productive. In order to grow you must struggle. A prudent way to look at setbacks is that they are happening 'for you, not to you'. The choices we make when we hit obstacles, define us. You can get bitter, or you can get better.

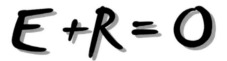

'Events plus response equals outcome' is another favoured maxim. You must learn to respond to things as opposed to react to them. Fundamentally, you need to be able to treat winning and losing in a similar manner. LOSS- Learning Opportunity Stay Strong. WIN- What's Important Now? Winning and losing is life's ultimate test of character.

When people develop resilience, they condition themselves to respond positively to setbacks and adversity. You can never hide from the fact that in times of adversity, you, and you alone, are in control of how you respond. Welcome your hardships like blessings, for they are laden with opportunity. Adversity can bring opportunity- how you respond to it can be what sets you apart.

In his book Atomic Habits, James Clear writes about a phenomenon of the delay between when we start working toward a goal and the time it takes before we are able to see measurable progress. He refers to this as the 'Plateau of Latent Potential'. It may also be referred to as having the ability to delay gratification. Clear uses the metaphor of the stonecutter pounding away at a rock with seemingly no progress toward his goal, only to finally break the rock with one swing and quotes Jacob August Riis:

"When nothing seems to help, I go and look at a stonecutter hammering away at his rock, perhaps a hundred times without as much as a crack showing in it. Yet at the hundred and first blow it will split in two, and I know it was not that last blow that did it - but all that had gone before".

Breakthrough moments are often the result of many previous actions which viewed incorrectly can be viewed as 'failures'. Just as the child learns to walk, the tripping leads to the walking and builds up the potential required to trigger a major change. Progress in any domain is rarely linear and often takes much longer than you expect. This can result in what Clear refers to as the 'Valley of Disappointment' where people are discouraged. Don't be discouraged. Plan, plot, learn and drive on in the direction of your goals. Never forget:

"Many of life's failures are people who did not realize how close they were to success when they gave up".
Thomas Edison

Persistence and strategy can change failure into extraordinary achievement. We cannot control the wind but we can adjust the sail.

Control the mind or it will control you. Often, it will seek to catastrophize things. Understand and appreciate whatever meaning is given to an experience, becomes the experience. What meaning are you attaching to setbacks or failures? This meaning can become self- fulfilling. You are not a robot so you can't expect to be super motivated all the time, and this is why clarity on who you are, and what you value is so important (see Chapter 3). It will act as your spotlight when times are difficult.

Develop your self-discipline. Self-discipline is the ability to do what is right and necessary when it needs to be done. Self-discipline means setting standards for yourself and living by them. It means being self-reliant. It is your decision, your choice. Move forward in the direction of your goals.

Again, your ability to ask yourself prudent questions is a valuable skill and again we return to the value of journaling (see Chapter 2). Can you ask yourself questions that will direct your attention to what's working, or what might work better, as opposed to what's not? These are what can be termed 'empowering questions'. 'How can I…', 'What can I ….' questions are powerful to change the focus from the failure or setback, or what didn't work. The right questions change your perspective and perspective is critical in times of challenge. If you can reframe and change the way you look at things, the things you look at will change.

Can you look at failure as feedback and can you learn from it? Appropriate questions give the mind direction and focus, and this is what it needs. They get you thinking constructively. Constructive thinking leads to positive feelings, positive feelings lead to action and this action leads to positive results. Successful people are successful because they have a mindset for success even during failure. Examples of empowering questions to ask in times of struggle or adversity are:

- What can I learn from this?
- How can I use these learnings in the future?
- Where is the opportunity in this?
- Why am I going to be better because of this?
- How can I progress from here?
- How far have I come (this is always important to acknowledge in times of struggle) and what do I now need to do to go further?

Another favoured quote of mine is:

"The first quality of a soldier is constancy in enduring fatigue and hardship. Courage is only the second.
Poverty, privation and want are the school of the good soldier".
Napoleon Bonaparte

When training and competing at a high level a strong commitment, discipline, and daily habits are required and can make the difference between success and failure. The higher you go, the tougher the challenges. Many days will follow a routine of sleep, eat, school/ work, eat, train, eat, and repeat. While family, teammates, close friends and coaches may understand the demands being placed on you, others may not. They will often question the reason, and motivation, behind choosing such a disciplined lifestyle.

Never forget the line from American architect Russell Warren:

"Obsessed is a word used by the lazy to describe the dedicated".

Some people will consciously, or unconsciously, try to pull you down for being different or committed. Aim to surround yourself with people who energise you. Never forget, unusual results begin with unusual behaviours and actions. If you have just suffered defeat in competition, performed poorly, picked up an injury, or even your self-motivation is simply feeling low, it can be a challenge to entertain and answer the typical "I don't know how you do it?", or "Is it really worth it?" narratives that people can often offer. It is only you that can answer as to whether it is worth it or not.

"If you want to improve, be content to be thought foolish and stupid".
Epictetus

As has already been noted, being crystal clear on who you are, why you chose to participate in sport and what you gain from it, are vital in holding your resolve and bringing you through your struggles and challenges. Having this knowledge and understanding can also help you to maintain motivation through what can sometimes appear a relentless season, packed with fixtures and competition. Once again, the practice of journaling is an excellent ally here.

It can be difficult, especially if sport becomes more serious, to keep it in the appropriate context. Throughout your youth, and indeed beyond, sport should be something that enhances your life, brings fun, excitement, challenges, friendships, opportunities, successful days and not so successful days. They are all part of the road to enjoyment, excellence and true success. Sport should leave you feeling better for having done it. Do not let it determine what you are or who you are. Sport is not your only identity (see Chapter 3). It's important to be yourself and to know yourself. As discussed in many of the previous chapters, having a broad and rounded sense of self-identity is helpful when aspects of your sporting life are not going to plan. It can help you on the road to recovery, whether due to injury, poor form or performance. As a well-rounded person you have the competencies required to help avoid the vicious cycle of low self-esteem which can be difficult to break. Once again, we return to one of the central themes of the book- character is the foundation of the athlete.

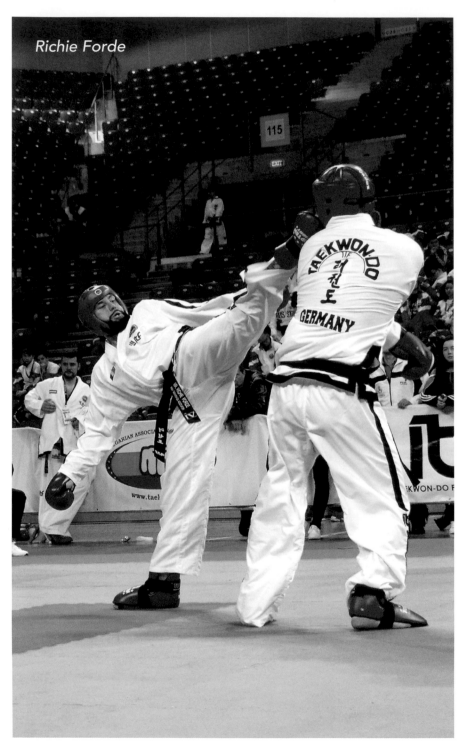

Richie Forde

Richie Forde

Richie Forde is an ITF Taekwon-Do 5th Degree Black Belt. He was a member of the Irish National Team from 2007 to 2017 and is a World & European Gold Medallist. He is currently Head Coach in East Cork TKD which is home to numerous National and European Medallists. This is his story of overcoming setbacks and failure.

I first made the National Taekwon-Do Team in 2007. Having had much national success, it was time to explore the international circuit. My first taste of the big stage was the 2007 European Championships. I lost in the first round and my championships were over. Later that same year, I travelled to Canada to compete in the World Championships. The result was the same; out in the first round. The following year came and having gained what I believed to be much experience I felt it was my opportunity to make my mark. The 2008 Euros & World Cup came along and again, I exited in the first round. The story repeated itself in 2009- first round and out!

2010 brought the European Championships in Sweden. Being honest, I didn't really have any great expectations, but I had that dream of being able to stand on that podium hearing Amhrán Na Bhfiann with the Tricolour around my shoulders. That vision was clear in my mind. On this occasion, unlike my previous outings I got my hand raised at the end of the first fight…and the second, and the third. I had landed myself into a semi-final and I was over the moon as I was guaranteed my first international medal! I came through that semi-final and was now at least guaranteed a silver medal.

After an extremely tough final, it ended in a draw. Extra time also ended in a draw and it went to sudden death. First score wins! The referee signalled to begin and my opponent launched towards me. I instinctively jumped in the air and landed a clean punch on my opponent's face. I fell to my knees with joy! I went from losing in the first round 3 years consecutively to winning my first fight & becoming European Champion in the blink of an eye. So what's to learn from this experience?

Disassociate the Results from your Passion
Looking back on it now I never really lost hope or felt demoralised with losing. Of course, I was disappointed but it never deterred me

or stopped me in my tracks. I think there is an important lesson to be taken from this and it is, you shouldn't relate your self-worth, or love for something, to results. Do it because you love it, not for any external reasons or recognition from others.

Seek Challenges
Another valuable lesson to take from this is how important experience, learning & challenge are when it comes to reaching your potential in any particular craft. We need to experience hardship of some sort and view them as valuable development opportunities that allow us to challenge ourselves and constantly push forward.

Patience is a Virtue
Those who persevere will be rewarded! Perseverance is one of the guiding principles of Taekwon-Do training. Setbacks are inevitable, it's about how we respond to them. How we perceive setbacks, is what makes the difference. Anything worthwhile should be difficult to achieve! Have a "why" which is strong enough to overcome any setback which may come your way.

I wish you well,
Richie Forde

SKILLS FOR DRAWING
ON YOUR INNER STRENGTH
SKILL NO. 5 - RESILIENCE
By Tony Óg Regan

Why is this important?

To lose at anything is to be human. Every living being experiences loss at some level. We can lose a game, a job, a loved one, a relationship etc. No one escapes the feelings from it or the experience of it. Even the greatest sports people have lost at different times in their careers. The key is that they have developed strategies to learn and grow from these life experiences. They use it to fuel their improvement in their chosen field. It can act as a catalyst for change in attitude, training, preparation and performance. They realise that they did certain things well in their preparation, practice and performance and certain areas they didn't do well in. These areas you did not perform in are not broken.

They can work well again. Some days your passing might be at a very high level and other days it may not. The key thing is to take RESPONSIBILITY for the things you can and improve and to LET GO of what you can't change; for example, the result, the blaming of external factors like the weather or the opposition or the referee. It is important to have a process in place to review your performances correctly (see Chapter 7). Writing about the experience, discussing it with a trusted mentor or coach, reviewing it through match recordings are all good resources to give us context around what happened.

Some key questions to consider:
- *Was I confident, under confident or complacent before or during the event?*
- *Was my focus and attention on what I was in control of?*
- *Was I clear on my role and responsibilities before and during the event?*
- *How did I respond when things did not go to plan before or during the event?*
- *What situations did I do well in and why?*
- *What situations did I not do well in and what would I do differently next time?*
- *What aspects of my preparation went well? What aspects didn't and what might I improve in my next session?*

The Three C's of the RESILIENT MINDSET

Challenge – *Resilient people often view a difficulty as a challenge to overcome. They tend to look at their failures and mistakes as lessons to be learned from and opportunities for growth. They tend not to view them as a negative reflection on their abilities or self-worth.*

Commitment – *Resilient people are committed to their lives and their goals. Commitment isn't just restricted to their sport – they commit to their relationships, their friendships, the causes they care about, their communities and their beliefs.*

Control – *Resilient people spend their time and energy focusing on situations and events that they have control over. Because they put their efforts where they can have the most impact, they feel prepared, ready and confident. Those who spend time worrying about uncontrollable events can often feel lost, helpless, and powerless to act.*

Exercise to Reflect, Recognise and Return

Think about a challenge you encountered in your life and overcame and write about the challenge you faced, the commitments you made and what you had personal control over in relation to that challenge. Write for 5 minutes on everything you can recall leading up to it, during and after.

1. *Reflect: What went well?*
2. *Recognise: What did not go well?*
3. *Return: What can you learn from that challenge going forward? What new statement can you reinforce to yourself based on this learning experience? Example: I am a resilient person; I see challenges as a great opportunity to learn and grow. This setback is temporary. When I am challenged in this way, I know it will push me to higher levels of performance. There is no limit to how far I can grow as a person and how well I can perform.*

CHAPTER 12

Kevin Doyle

Kevin Doyle scored 14 goals in 62 appearances for the Republic of Ireland. He was 19 years old when he first played for an Irish underage team, having failed to be selected at numerous trials throughout his younger years. He won the Football Association of Ireland Player of the Year Award in 2009 and represented Ireland in Euro 2012.

Kevin took the road less travelled for Irish players who reach the English Premiership, in that first he played for St Patrick's Athletic and Cork City in Ireland. Indeed, as a youngster, he picked up a serious foot injury the night before he was due to leave for a trial with Sunderland. At 21 years old he moved to English side Reading where he was named the Player of the Season in his first year. He was part of Reading's record-breaking promotion to the Premier League in 2006. In June 2009, he moved to Wolverhampton Wanderers for a then club record £6.5 million where he was named the Player's Player of the Season in his first year.

I have always been curious about the balance between the role that luck and hard work had to play in my career as a professional footballer. It is something that I have thought deeply about over the years. In that time, my opinion has swung back and forth between hard work having a larger influence and then back to luck being mainly at play. I think now after a few years away from the sport I have reached a settled conclusion that the role that luck and hard work play are both as important in their own right and one requires the other.

Did I have more luck than the twenty other sixteen-year-olds that my under age Wexford Youths manager Mick Wallace had in his squad? No, I don't think so. I feel we all had an equal opportunity to impress a man who would turn out to be one of the most important men in my career, namely Pat Dolan. Pat came to watch us all play, but I presume I shone more and showed more of the qualities and characteristics he was looking for in a player.

It was certainly a fair slice of luck that Pat was friends with Mick Wallace, but it was my years of hard work and discipline that made me stand out that day. Pat gave me my first professional contract at St Patrick's Athletic and ended up being my agent for my entire career. When Pat left St Pats to become Cork City manager I was the player he took with him. Was that luck for me that he got that job? Yes! At the time Cork City was the biggest club in Ireland and prepared me fantastically

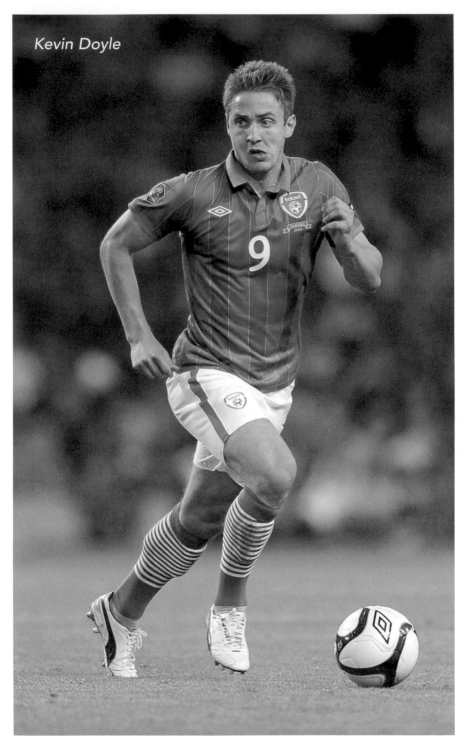

Kevin Doyle

for my years ahead as a professional footballer. Was it hard work and dedication at St Pats that made him bring me, and no one else, with him? Again, I'm certain it was.

When Pat left Cork a few years later and I moved to Reading. Was it luck that Dave Kitson, the then top striker in the championship in England, got injured a few games into the season and I got my chance? Again, yes it was. If he had stayed fit I would have been on the bench for the majority of the season, there would have been no international call up a few weeks later, no new contract, no Player of the Year Award.

I had prepared for that moment of luck- the break I needed. All the years of disciplined work when no one was watching, the long runs on my own in the woods of Curracloe, the countless setbacks and rejections, the injuries, the hours of practice by myself away from the training ground paid off. Prior to this point, my life had revolved around boring nights in when my college friends were partying, constant diet, years of ignoring doubters and naysayers who would be questioning my chances of making a career from the game, even if at times I may have thought they might be right. My inner desire and belief drove me and allowed me to stick to the plan even when things were tough and luck appeared to be against me.

I came on for Dave Kitson in that game versus Burnley FC, scored the winner and didn't miss a club game of any importance for Reading for the rest of my four years there. To many who knew no better, I was an over-night success. Little did they know the amount of ups and downs there had been along the way.

In conclusion, what I have settled on in my mind is that luck certainly plays a part but most people fail in putting in the necessary work and dedication to even realise they missed their bit of luck. I often wonder what the lads I played with for Mick Wallace's Wexford opinion would be on it.

Best wishes,
Kevin Doyle

SKILLS FOR DRAWING
ON YOUR INNER STRENGTH
SKILL NO. 6. CONFIDENCE - THE POWER OF LANGUAGE
By Tony Óg Regan

'The limits of my language means the limits of my world'.
Ludwig Wittgnestein

A confident athlete thinks about what they CAN DO and what they WANT to happen in their chosen sport. A less than confident athlete focuses on the things they don't want to happen. The great thing is you can grow your own confidence by the thoughts you choose to listen to, the language you use to yourself and others about your performance (your perceptions/interpretations), what you imagine happening (your imagination) and what you want to recall (your memory). These areas all feed into your 'strong self-image' as an athlete. If you can build a 'strong self-image', then mistakes that happen will wash through your mind very quickly. How you talk to yourself during mistakes or after defeats will either add or take from your strong self.

How do I grow my Strong Self- Image?
Our mind likes to create many stories. It is believed we work off our subconscious mind somewhere between 90-95% of the time. This is where we play sport also. The issue can be if the programme in your subconscious mind is faulty how does it affect your performance? It is believed we work off 50% half-truths in our subconscious. 'I am useless at my sport' might be a half-truth you need to address. When you make a mistake in a game, you may talk to yourself with language that damages your self-confidence. You miss a ball and tell yourself 'I am crap'. This is potentially another half-truth eating another piece of your self-confidence. How can you change this negative inner critic that is nibbling away at your self-confidence and impacting your enjoyment and ability to play at your best?

If your problem is that you are remembering all your bad shots and misses, then your confidence will suffer and so will your performance. You must unlearn this poor behaviour by allowing yourself to feel joy over the good plays; when you start to do this you cement them in your memory. Taking a moment in training or a game to appreciate tasks and skills you did well will slowly change your confidence in yourself. You will start to recall your better moments more regularly. Writing down your best moments after a session or game will start to change the context of how you played in your head. It will start to develop a new program in your subconscious mind; one that recalls and recognises your strengths and best moments, one that does not rehash your poor moments.

You have the power to develop a new program for your performance. You chose the words and images you want in your mind. You choose to see your best plays and speak about what you can and want to do. You start to override the faulty memory and subconscious programme with a new way of thinking, feeling and doing. You can become an unstoppable force.

Technique One – Self Talk

Self-talk is a very powerful method to improve self-confidence especially in stressful or intense situations. So, when you are talking to yourself during the game, try to encourage your effort or instruct yourself on what to do next. Focus on the process. For example, if you're a bit anxious after a mistake, say to yourself; 'Attack the next ball!'

Choose 1-3 phrases from the list below and build them into your training and matches as 'trigger words' or phrases to keep your confidence and focus high during important moments in the game. The use of trigger words is a powerful means to refocus or reset the mind on what's important in the moment.

- Use them after a mistake or miss in a game to get you back into positive thinking.
- Use them during breaks in play to reset your focus and concentration.
- Feel free to come up with your own ones.

The next play will be my best play.	I have the mind of a champion.
I start strong and finish stronger.	I love the challenges in big games.
I am a consistent and confident performer.	I am relentless on every ball.
I play with passion and intensity on every ball.	I stay in the present on every ball.
My concentration gives me the edge.	I have a ravenous hunger for every ball.

Technique Two – Affirmation Scripts

"Watch your thoughts, they become your words. Watch your words, they become your actions. Watch your actions, they become your habits. Watch your habits, they become your character.
Watch your character, it becomes your destiny".
Lao Tzu

Affirmation scripts can help to rewire your subconscious mind with a new program to develop the inner confidence required to perform at your best. You can use the examples below or develop your own scripts that can be read before training and matches in order to feed your subconscious with positive thoughts, words, images, feelings and actions about your game and become a more confident player every single training session and match. You can also record them on your phone and listen to them 4-5 times a week.

Mental Preparation

Starting today I will renew my attitude, my enthusiasm, and my commitment to pursuing greatness. I will honour my commitment to playing great.

I TAKE GREAT PRIDE in how thoroughly I prepare my mind before EVERY GAME.

I take 15 minutes to go over the next game in my mind. I prepare to think of STAYING IN THE PRESENT on every ball and I will have no concern for the result. I will have a CLEAR AND FOCUSED mind on EVERY PLAY.

Long before travelling to the match, I WILL KNOW WHERE MY MIND WILL BE FOR EVERY BALL.

I will be COMMITTED AND DECISIVE. I will be calm and relaxed. I will live in the present moment and PLAY ONE BALL AT A TIME until the game is over.

I will play my game and have no concern for or interest in anything anyone else is doing. I will respect and trust my game.

It is GREAT TO PLAY IN THIS MINDSET.

Knowing I have done all my mental and physical preparation. My game plan is laid out. I know my goal and this MAKES ME VERY CONFIDENT AND ALLOWS ME FOCUS AND TRUST MY GAME.

Skill Development Scripts
EXCELLENCE IN CATCHING
I AM A GREAT CATCHER OF THE BALL

The aerial ball is where the real game begins. I own the high ball. It is my favourite challenge on the pitch. It is where I separate myself from others.

I TRUST MYSELF to make great catches when they matter the most. I am great because I treat all of my catches the same. I have a GREAT INSTINCT for reading the flight of the ball. I am relaxed and confident when it is time to catch. I am totally focused on the ball dropping, I love the surge of confidence and power when I make my catches.

I am aware of where my man is before I make my jump to catch the high ball.

I commit myself to the ball. I wait until the last second before making my move. Nothing distracts me from this process.

I DEMAND of myself to relentlessly make every catch.

See Appendix for more Affirmation Scripts: Skill Perfection, Relentless Will to Win, Challenge and Adversity, I am a Great Player, Emotional Maturity. These can be read daily or recorded and listened to affirm and enforce positive performance behaviours.

References

Clear, J. (2018). Atomic Habits. UK: Random House.
Kanter, R. (2009). 'Change is Hardest in the Middle', Retrieved on 3.10.2020 from
https://hbr.org/2009/08/change-is-hardest-in-the-middl

SUMMARY POINTS - Chapter 12

- Resilience is the ability to bounce back from adversity and is a crucial quality to develop for sport, and indeed life.
- Failure is a part of learning.
- Progress is never linear.
- Adversity can be an important stimulus for growth and development, provided you have the required skills to respond positively and the appropriate support around you.
- Setbacks are certain but can often be unexpected.
- Fundamentally you need to be able to treat winning and losing in a similar manner. LOSS- Learning Opportunity Stay Strong. WIN- What's Important Now?
- Breakthrough moments are often the result of many previous actions which viewed incorrectly can be viewed as 'failures'.
- Persistence and strategy can change failure into extraordinary achievement.
- The right questions change your perspective and perspective is critical in times of challenge.
- Aim to surround yourself with people who energise you.
- Being crystal clear on who you are, why you chose to participate in sport and what you gain from it, are vital in holding your resolve and bringing you through your struggles and challenges.
- If you can build a 'strong self-image', then mistakes that happen will wash through your mind very quickly. How you talk to yourself during mistakes or after defeats will either add or take from your strong self.

CHAPTER 13: TALENT PATHWAYS & PROFESSIONAL SPORT

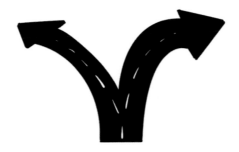

Sporting Talent Pathways aim to attract and recruit athletes who they believe possess the qualities required to excel in adult sport. The thinking is to surround these athletes with an environment which seeks to optimise every facet of their development. I have asked the following contributors to give you an insight into how talent pathways operate and what it is that their leaders are looking for from the athlete, up to and including professional level.

My hope is that having read the book to this point there will be nothing particularly new here only a reemphasising of the key messages and that the pieces below can give you a further appreciation of the qualities, skills and tools required to be the best you can be.

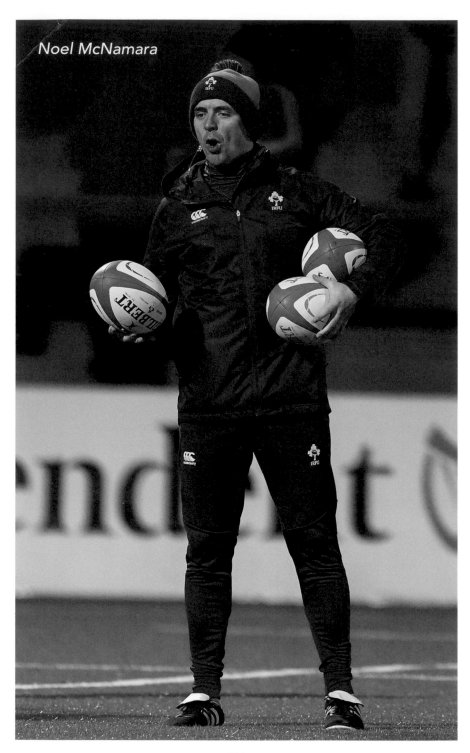

Noel McNamara

Noel McNamara

Noel McNamara is the Leinster Rugby Academy Manager. He is also the Irish Rugby U20s Head Coach. He has coached many age grade representative teams at Provincial and National level including the Ireland U18 Schools, Leinster U18 Schools, Leinster U19 and Leinster U20 sides. Here he gives his insights into talent development.

"Talent sets the floor, character sets the ceiling".
Bill Belichick

Winning in team sport is a people business. As a consequence, the identification, selection and development of people in the player pathway becomes critical for the long term success of any team. But this is not an exact science and there is no doubting the concept of keeping as many players as possible in the pathway, for as long as possible, to be as good as possible, will capture the best. The funnelling of young players towards the top level begins at higher age-grades, but the path should remain wide at each stage. Rugby is a late specialisation sport and there are many instances of players not selected on age grade pathway teams who go on and excel at the highest level. This has implications for how we identify and develop these players through our pathway and indeed beyond it.

Every player pathway starts with participation and moves towards performance as they progress. Regardless of what stage we are at within that, I believe that we should always start with the player.

What the player needs:
- *To be shown they are cared for and understood by their coach/ management and teammates. Connection is key here. It doesn't happen by accident and requires energy.*
- *To be given informed and appropriate feedback with the correct balance of support (praise) v challenge (stretch).*
- *A safe environment where people can take risks and be vulnerable in front of each other.*
- *Clarity on the expectations and an understanding that expectations have consequences.*
- *Time!*

What are the factors that influence talent development?
- *Genetics*
- *Training - purposeful practice*
- *Coaching – Environment*
- *Initiative*
- *Birth date*
- *Geography*
- *Attitude*
- *Coachability*
- *Mindset - resilience / response to setbacks / belief*
- *Support structure- family / friends*
- *Awareness - self / others*
- *Effort - Angela Duckworth in her excellent book Grit has a mathematical formula for achievement which sums up the main ingredient - so critical it's in there twice - effort, your best effort!*

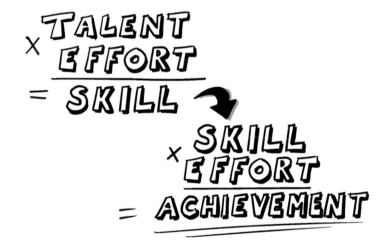

$$x\frac{TALENT}{EFFORT} = SKILL$$

$$x\frac{SKILL}{EFFORT} = ACHIEVEMENT$$

How we build the processes:
- *Doers make mistakes- it is the coach's job to ensure that the players don't continue to make the same ones. Being in an environment where a player is afraid to make a mistake is far worse than making one. We strive to build the correct environment*
- *Ask > tell. We encourage curiosity. Generation Z's want to be part of the learning process not a passive bystander.*
- *Learning happens in the mind of the learner- we haven't taught until they have learned. We check for learning and understanding and don't assume.*
- *We facilitate experiential learning: Gen Z's typically learn by doing.*

- *We prioritise 1-1 feedback individually and in-person. We aim to build reciprocal relationships with a collaborative approach to player development.*
- *We use appropriate criteria for success which is balanced and fair and also relevant to the age and development stage of the player.*
- *We are consistent in what we are looking for and understand that we get what we inspect rather than what we expect. Our attention will drive the intention.*

Common Characteristics of Successful Athletes
(influenced by the work of Wayne Goldsmith)

- *A commitment to continuous improvement recognising that success is a moving target.*
- *A belief that anything is possible. Every level of achievement is underpinned by the highest levels of belief.*
- *An understanding of where your sport has been (history of the sport), where it is now and most importantly a vision for where it is going. Most successful players are students of their game. They also tend to have a clear personal vision of their future.*
- *The confidence to be yourself – to be unique.*
- *The energy to work hard consistently.*
- *A passion for winning – a desire to be the best. Equally, this can be driven by a fear of losing.*
- *The ability and toughness needed to work through difficulties or obstacles that may arise.*

What are we Looking For?
(influenced by the work of Fergus Connolly)

1. *Character*
2. *Capacity*
3. *Capability*

Capability is the easiest component to recognise and often the most focussed upon. The ability to do one's job is naturally critical to any team's success. There are obvious physical requirements to play most sports, particularly rugby, but this is often over emphasised. We are looking at a player's technical ability here as well as their positional specific skills. In the case of capability, capacity and willingness to improve can compensate for limited capability. It is a careful balance. There are many talented people with great capability, but without a capacity and character it will be difficult for them to make it to the top.

Capacity refers to work ethic and the willingness to own your development. It is demonstrated by an eagerness to learn and improve. Not everyone is committed to being the best possible version of themselves. Often, the people with the most talent demonstrate the least capacity. Studying the pathway of previous role models can increase this capacity for players. Seeing a clear roadmap can make the commitment required more palatable. The book The Goldmine Effect by Rasmus Ankersen gives some very good examples of this in elite level performance. An appetite for hard work and training are also critical ingredients. Many of the best players also have a really clear process for getting better - they have a plan.

Character is arguably the most critical of the three and refers to the mental and moral qualities of the individual. What are your personal values and how do these impact your everyday interactions and relationships with people? There needs to be an emphasis on the development of character in young people. There are many academic definitions of culture that talk about norms, values, and beliefs, but it can be simply defined as "the way we do things around here". The players need to understand clearly the boundaries of acceptable (above the line) behaviour and unacceptable (below the line) behaviour. Having a clear personal vision and a desire to play at the highest level are key elements that become evident through a person's everyday actions and behaviours. Belief, humility, resilience and assertiveness are some of the characteristics most evident in those that progress

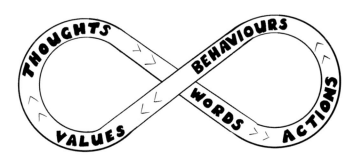

"Be more concerned with your character than your reputation,
because your character is what you really are,
while your reputation is merely what others think you are".
John Wooden

I wish you well in your endeavours,
Noel McNamara

Pat McInerney

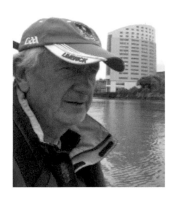

Pat McInerney is recently retired from his role as Coach Education Officer in Rowing Ireland and is also a former Junior Head National Coach and a club coach at all levels.

During Pat's time with Rowing Ireland he played a critical role in the development and delivery of their Coach Education programme. Pat is widely acknowledged as being a driving force in the creation of a Long Term Athlete Development Pathway for Rowing Ireland and in so doing making an enduring impact on generations of rowers in Ireland.

The term "Pathway" in sport describes the sequence of steps and developments along the journey from beginner all the way to elite level. This can include a guide to technical, physical and mental capacities that we would hope to find and develop in the athlete. The rowing pathway exhibits good development opportunities to all and includes competitive times and standards required at all levels of competition.

Coaches are always looking for some sign in the emerging athlete to tell them how far that person might go in the sport. Rowing is a late specialisation sport where some athletes will not start to show their capacities until after puberty or even well into their twenties. Because of this a broad base of participation is required to introduce as many as possible to the sport. We sometimes see athletes being successful early on but it's not always translated into progression to elite level. Late arrivals or late developers can do well in rowing if they are in the right setting.

The physical demands of the sport include: a Maximal Oxygen Consumption (VO2max) of > 70mL per kg per minute. An ability to perform at a high percentage of VO2max for the duration of the race (approx. 5:30 min to 7:00 mins depending on boat class and category). Good technique and an ability to utilize fat as a fuel source during exercise of longer duration at high work rates (Ref: Rowing Faster, Volker Nolte, Chapter 7).

Top international heavyweight rowers are normally tall with long levers, strong and lean with high levels of endurance and high VO2max capacity.

Rowing also has competitions for lightweights who average 70kg for men and 59kg for women. The top lightweights also show high VO2 max capacity and can be as fast as the heavyweight finalists in some events.

Development of good technique is always encouraged but particularly at the start of the pathway. Good habits learned early on will reap benefits later and it's difficult to unlearn bad habits. Rowers are constantly searching for the perfect stroke or the perfect "run" in the boat. Skill is the ability to apply technique and physical attributes efficiently, at full pressure, at top speed, in the heat of competition. To cover the 2000 meter standard racing distance can involve 220 to 250 strokes of full pressure, therefore as well as skill, we require power and endurance. Rowing is termed a power endurance sport and a large part of the training programme is devoted to building an aerobic base of fitness as well as strength and a capacity to keep top speed with high intensity interval training.

Athletes normally start rowing in the 12-14 age range which, for most, is before the growth spurt and also before many know what they want to achieve in sport. This is a time for learning the basics of how to move a boat and starting to train and learning how to train. The most important thing to remember at this stage is to ensure they develop a love of the sport and get hooked. Mid-teens is a great time for developing the aerobic engine with long distance work.

As already noted, it is difficult to know before an athlete goes through their growth spurt if they have the physical attributes required to be a top athlete. Some countries have programmes that try to find the most suited athletes at a young age and train them specifically for the sport. This requires consistent investment and resources. A more common approach, which also requires investment, has been to focus on developing the capacity of coaches and clubs to set up the right conditions to develop talent. Most athletes if coached well in a good environment will become competitive at club level, some will be competitive at national level and a small number will make it to elite. By the time rowers reach late teens or early twenties coaches will have many good indicators to help determine how successful a rower can become. Rowing is very measurable, both on the indoor rowing machine and by speed test from A to B on water as a single sculler.

Unfortunately, large numbers of athletes drop out of rowing before giving themselves a proper chance to become successful. One of the reasons for this is, as I have just stated above, that rowing is very measurable and people get to see very quickly where they stand. This can be discouraging for many and encouraging for others. Coaches must create the right environment where athletes will want to come and have fun, work hard and be given an opportunity to develop. One of the key roles of a coach is to keep young athletes in the game long enough so they can discover for themselves if they want to pursue it or not. Athletes must be open to continuously learning and development.

Apart from the technical skills and physical qualities that go into making a top rower, there are a number of other characteristics that must be developed and nurtured along the pathway. Below are some of what I believe to be the most important. It is these characteristics which allow the athlete optimise their skills and physical qualities.

Work Ethic:
The top athletes know that being on time, completing all the sessions and bringing their best effort to training are all vital factors for success. These are all a given, they are the basics and they do not require huge talent. A solid work ethic and a good attitude costs nothing but delivers a lot. Talented people who don't put in the work will not be successful. We often see athletes with less obvious sporting talent making it to the top level by sheer hard work and top class attitude.

Resilience:
The road to success is never a straight linear graph where you do something and you get results. It is often a jagged graph of ups and downs, periods of progress followed by periods of setbacks. The rowing pathway can be seen as a motorway with on and off ramps. The 'on ramps' are to enable the late arrivals to join and to allow those who may have fallen off the pathway to re-join. What is important along the road is to learn from the past and plan for success in the future. To see a continuous trend of improvement it takes time and patience. When we see an athlete on the top of the podium it is easy to forget that they were 10th, 5th or 3rd in previous years. Continuous development requires resilience, bounce-back-ability and mental toughness. There are many tools available to help in this area. A good skill to introduce early in the pathway is the ability to reflect back on a session, a block of training or a competition. All you can take from the past is lessons learned. Then plan to make changes, do the work, move on and repeat.

Focus:

Everyone will lose focus now and then. If it's at the wrong time it can cost you. There are so many things that can distract an athlete from the job in hand. Time spent learning to focus and remain calm in competition is time well invested at an early age. Regular and simple cues and triggers that get you to do basic things like listen to your breath, visualise a perfect stroke or simply look at the head of the person in front will help regain focus.

Confidence and Goal Setting:

One of the greatest things you can develop through sport is confidence. Appropriate goal setting can help build confidence. With proper goal setting comes realistic expectations and definitions of what success is for the individual. Then having some experience of success, and learning to deal with success and failure all become part of a well-managed sporting life.

Fun and Enjoyment:

Enjoying being out on the water moving boats is the most basic requirement for true success in rowing.

There is potential for development everywhere, we just need to find it. Top international rowing coach Thor Nilsen from Norway once told us, "There is a potential national champion on every street corner, and a potential Olympic champion in every county." If sport becomes too exclusive and difficult to access we run the risk of someday looking around and finding there is no one with us. The ultimate purpose of a talent pathway is to bring through the best. In order to do this, we must make the sport attractive for the rest.

Best wishes,
Pat McInerney

Mick McCarthy

Mick McCarthy is a Professional Football Manager. As a footballer he represented the Republic of Ireland on 57 occasions. Nicknamed 'Captain Fantastic', he led Ireland as captain in what was a glorious period for Irish football during Euro '88 and Italia '90. At club level he played for Barnsley, Manchester City, Celtic, Lyon and Millwall.

He went on to manage Millwall and then the Republic of Ireland where he guided Ireland to the knockout stages of the 2002 World Cup. He later managed Sunderland, Wolverhampton Wanderers and Ipswich Town. His most recent job saw him return as manager of the Republic of Ireland football team. Here, Mick shares his insights from a lifetime in football into the qualities he believes allows a player to reach their potential.

I have been involved in football for over fifty years and that's a long time! I have played and managed at both club and international level. Nobody can ever truly say they have seen it all, but it is fair to say I have seen and experienced a lot- the good times and the not so good times, the ups and the downs. The footballing landscape I grew up in is completely different to today's millionaires' club. I have worked with hundreds of footballers over the years and in this piece I will aim to give my insights into what it is I have come to believe are the most important qualities in the player.

Talent is the most obvious place to start. There must be a baseline of talent and ability there: the touch, the awareness, the vision, the speed, can they see the pass and so on. We are all looking for this talent and when watching a youth football match, the technically gifted stand out a mile… anyone can pick them out. What is not so obvious is whether or not the talented individual will be able to maximise their ability as they age and mature. The world is full of 'could have beens'.

I am always asked, 'who is your best player?' I take this question to mean, 'who is your most effective player?' The player I want is the one who can give 7 out of 10 almost every day, a half a dozen 9 out of 10s a year and I'll even allow them an odd 6. Consistency is king. To be of significant value the player must be consistently effective. Every manager wants to know: can I depend on them? For me, I really want to know what I will get when we are 1 – 0 down.

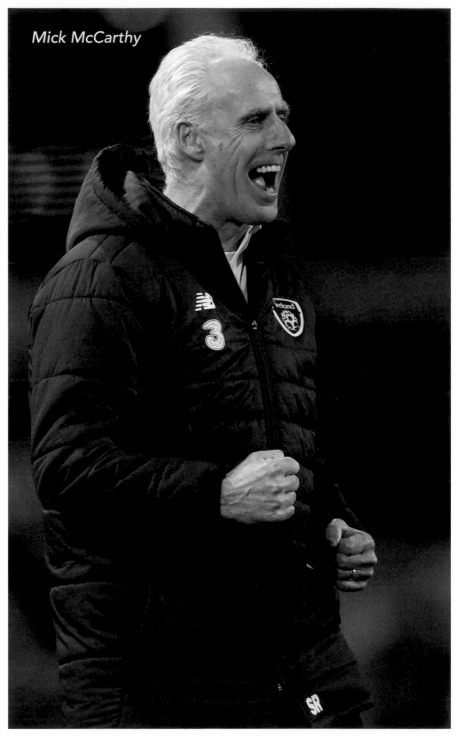

Mick McCarthy

There are a number of indicators that lead you to trust a player and their ability to be consistent. The demeanor is always one. Do I get a 'good morning gaffer' every morning or is it just when the mood takes them. This is a basic respect. For me, respect is a two-way street and it must go both ways. Respect goes a long way in sport and in life. Punctuality is another one- who is first in the door? However, it must be noted that first in the door is of little value if it simply means, first to the canteen for tea. I am looking for the players who use this time wisely and pay attention to the finer details of prehab, individual skill-based work and so on. These are things that allow you to reach your potential. These are the things that show you the player's desire and ambition.

There are so many levels in football that there is a place for almost everyone. Sometimes the most talented end up paddling along in the lower leagues. This is a shame. While everyone strives for a big contract early in their career it can be a dangerous thing if the desire, drive and ambition isn't strong. Poor decisions are there to be made. Players can easily forget why they got into football and once they lose sight of their 'why' they are in trouble. Money can make you comfortable and the comfort zone is no place for a player who wants to maximise their talents and reach their potential. It is easy to end up a relatively big fish in a very small pond. The malaise of a nice lifestyle can dampen the hunger. I find it really difficult to watch a player who with a little bit more fight and desire could really make something better of themselves. Money plays a huge part in professional football. There are many downsides to this, but give me a player who wants to strive and work towards earning a 50k a week contract over the one who is happy to coast along at 5k a week when with a little bit more ambition and drive they could aspire to better.

When managing at Championship level the players I want are the ones who want to get to the Premier League...and hopefully bring me with them through promotion. My reasoning is simple, these are the type of players who will inspire those around them, the ones who will set the standard, energise the squad and demand the best from everyone. They know why they are there and they have a fundamental belief in hard work. Their attention to detail is better, as is the focus of their life and lifestyle. The line is really so fine and many good people fall by the wayside. If you are given a chance, you have to grab it and maximise it because someone else will take it from you. The coach's job is to challenge and assist the player as best we can, but the player's job is to grab every opportunity that is given to them with both hands.

I think now of players I feel who really maximised what God gave them. Stephen Ward, who I signed at Wolves from Bohemians, is one who stands out. He has played 50 times for Ireland and spent years playing Premier League football. It is remarkable how he has made himself into a top-class player. Another one is Matt Doherty. When I signed him, he was not the fittest or the most obvious buy, but I knew I was getting something. After a couple of loan stints, he has risen to every challenge, progressing from League One, through the Championship and into the Premier League and the Europa League. He is now arguably one of the best wing-backs in the Premier League. You must remember the Premier League is the biggest and best league in the world. It is some achievement. He has absolutely maximised his potential and made 300 appearances for Wolves before recently moving to Spurs. I take my hat off to both of them. I admire them for their achievements. Other, perhaps more obvious talents, yet with that same ceaseless desire to be the best they could be were Robbie Keane and Shay Given. They stood out as teenagers and were model professionals who enjoyed the stellar careers that their talent and hard work deserved.

Application in training is an area I must address and a player who springs to mind here is Martyn Waghorn. He was a player I signed at Ipswich for 250k having been through a number of clubs. After signing him we discussed his jersey number and he said that his preference was Number 9. I explained to him that Number 9 was a 'big jersey' to fill and he assured me he was up for the challenge. After watching his first training session with the team I was really disappointed. It was as if he was afraid to stand out and was there with the mindset of being liked by the squad as opposed to being respected by them. I spoke very directly to him after the session and explained to him that that wasn't the way my Number 9 trained. From that day on he was brilliant for me. He trained with fight and fire and ignited those around him. His thought process completely changed. He trained with the intention of being as good as he could be. He went on to 16 goals that season and we sold him to Derby for 5.5 million. My kind of player!

Training is not a place to make friends, this happens away from the field. Training is a place you strive to be different and better than the rest in a positive manner. Each training session is an opportunity to maximise your talents and in order to reach your potential you must truly appreciate this. Often, you see a new or young player join training with the first-team and their mindset is that they want to blend in. I want the exact opposite. I want them to stand out but again for the correct reasons. *Flynn Downes is one such player that springs to mind. I can still remember his first training session with the Ipswich Town first team. He repeatedly demanded the ball and snapped into three tackles with no regard for names or reputations. It was instantly obvious that he meant business and was a first team player. Training and playing with focus and application is how you gain the respect of your fellow players and management.*

I view the world quite simply and this has served me well. However, I must warn you the devil is in the detail. People talk about being professional and training hard but often the pictures don't match the sound. My advice to you would be listen to your coaches, seek challenges everywhere you go, know that there is always another level and never cease to strive for it and always remember why it is you play the game. Hunger, fire and fight matched with the correct input of expertise and guidance will see you a long way. We can't all be Premier League stars but one thing we can all be is the best version of ourselves.

Good luck to you,
Mick McCarthy

References

Connolly, F. (2017). Game Changer- The Art of Sports Science. Victory Belt.
Duckworth, A. (2016). GRIT. The Power of Passion and Perseverance. Scribner
Goldsmith,W (2001), Multi disciplinary approach to performance Swimming in Australia (Lavington, N.S.W.) 17(1), Jan/Feb 2001, 6-8.
Goldsmith,W (2000), The TUF principle: technique under fatigue, Swimnews (Toronto) 27(7), Aug 2000, 10-11.
Goldsmith,W (2000), A multi disciplinary approach to performance: the Integration of the sports Sciences in smart coaching, Sports-coach-(Belconnen) 23(3), 2000, 14-15.
Kanter, R. 'Change is Hardest in the Middle', Retrieved on 3.10.2020.

CHAPTER 14: EXCELLENCE & COMMITMENT

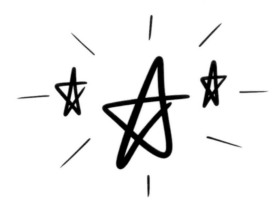

Now that we have looked at many of the skills and qualities required to maximise your talents, we will look to establish a personal understanding, or standard of excellence.

What is success? How do I know if I am 'successful'? Is it an outcome or a result? If I win does it mean I am a 'success' and alternatively if I lose does it mean I am a 'failure'? What is my best? How will I know if I am at my best? What is excellence? How do I know if I am preparing and performing with excellence? Who can tell me?

This is a short and simple chapter. At this stage in the book, you may well now appreciate that excellence and genuine success are based on the solid bedrock of character and mindset, and that a number of skills and tools must be acquired and developed to be the best you can be in sport.

Character is the foundation stone and when you are clear on who you are, who you want to be, and how you want to behave and act, answering the above list of questions will become a relatively simpler task. If 'winning' is your only measurement, and all you want to do in sport, then I suggest you drop to the lowest level of competition, find the weakest opponent or opposition, and live in the 'cage of winning'. If you wish, you can choose 'average' any day and still engineer a way to 'win'. Is this success? Is this excellence? I think not.

Learn to value and appreciate achievement through strategy and effort. Be advised that no matter what level you are at, the moment of victory is far too short to simply live for that alone. Once again, this is not a book about being the 'best', it is a book about being the 'best you can be' and seeing where that takes you in sport and in life. Excellence is being the best you can be. It is more about improving ability, rather than proving ability. Part of excellence is appreciating you are not good enough to stay the same.

Aim to avoid comparing yourself to others. Learn from them by all means, but don't simply try to be better than them. 'I'm the greatest me that has ever lived' is one of life's (not so) obvious truths. I'm sure you will be 'better' than some and 'worse' than others but the challenge will always be to be better than you would have been if you didn't do what you should have done.

Excellence is a by-product of a relentless commitment to the process of continuous improvement which is character driven. Success follows. By success, I don't necessarily mean winning. Winning is something that can often follow, but can be out of your control, especially in team sport.

Three things you can control every day are your attitude, your effort and your actions. If you strive for excellence in these three areas, you may be outscored, but you will never lose or fail (in the negative sense). The real contest that sport, and indeed life, offers us is striving to reach our personal best, and that is totally under our own control. Only one person can be the ultimate judge in this and that is you. When you achieve this, you have achieved excellence. You are a true winner- a champion!

The road to real achievement takes time, and will be full of setbacks and readjustment, but for now I want you to focus on:
(Note, an exercise like this may be best suited to the front or back of your journal. This will allow you access it easily and take a minute or two daily, or weekly, to read and review).

WHAT DOES EXCELLENCE MEAN TO YOU IN SPORT?

_____

_____

WHAT DOES EXCELLENCE LOOK LIKE TO YOU IN SPORT?

_____

'The race is long but in the end it is only with yourself'

SKILLS FOR DRAWING
ON YOUR INNER STRENGTH
SKILL NO. 7 - COMMITMENT
By Tony Óg Regan

Why is this important?

The intention and quality of your decisions, choices and actions will have a major bearing on how successful you will be in your chosen field. What you choose to believe, listen to, think, say, feel and do, can and will influence how much you improve or how well you perform. What you decide to eat and drink, how you decide to sleep and when, how you turn up to practice, what you say about yourself, your teammates, your coaches and the opposition will all impact your psychology and physiology in either a positive or negative way. When you impact people and situations with a positive energy you produce a chemical response in your biology which makes you feel more connected (oxytocin), happier (dopamine) and calmer (serotonin). The opposite is true when you bring negativity, you produce stress hormones like cortisol and over long periods of stress without recovery, this can damage your health and immune system.

"The way we do small things determines the way we do everything. If we execute minor tasks well, we will excel in our larger efforts. Mastery then becomes our way of being".
From The Secret Letters of The Monk Who Sold his Ferrari

Below is a commitment scale you can apply to any domain, including sport and can choose to adopt each day. Where do you fit on this scale right now? Where would you like to get to on it?

Level 1 - Commitment to Mediocrity

I show up to 1/3rd of my team sessions each week. I never practice outside of my set training sessions. I never watch the top players perform. I never set goals for the day, week, month, year, training or games. I never review my goals and performances. I never mentally rehearse before training and games. I never bring a positive energy to training and team gatherings. I never perform to my potential.

Level 2 - Commitment to Average

I sometimes show up for 2/3rds of my team sessions each week. I rarely practice outside of my set training sessions. I rarely watch the top players perform. I rarely set goals for the day, week, month, year, training or games. I rarely review my goals and performances. I rarely mentally rehearse before training and games. I rarely bring a positive energy to training and team gatherings. I rarely perform to my potential.

Level 3 Commitment to Train

I show up for the vast majority of my sessions each week. I sometimes practice outside of my set training sessions. I sometimes watch the top players perform. I sometimes set goals for the day, week, month, year, training and games. I sometimes review my goals and performances. I sometimes mentally rehearse before training and games. I sometimes bring a positive energy to training and team gatherings. I sometimes perform to my potential.

Level 4 Commitment to Compete

I consistently show up for all my sessions every week. I consistently practice outside of my set training sessions. I consistently watch the top players perform. I consistently set goals for the day, week, month, year, training and games. I consistently review my goals and performances. I consistently mentally rehearse before training and games. I consistently bring a positive energy to training and team gatherings. I consistently perform to my potential.

Level 5 Commitment to Extraordinary

I always aim for extraordinary levels in each session each week. I am meticulous in my preparation in terms of food, hydration, recovery and sleep. I always practice outside of my set training sessions with focus and intention on what I want to improve. I always watch the top players perform and review footage on my own game. I always set goals for the day, week, month, year, training and games. I always review my goals and performances. I always speak to my coaches on what I do well and where I can improve. I always mentally rehearse before training and games. I always bring a positive energy to training and team gatherings. I always strive to perform to my potential.

Most athletes will take a full career before they get to EXTRAORDINARY levels of performance. It can take years and years of deliberate and intentional practice and commitment to achieve this. There are a huge number of things that cost ZERO TALENT on that list. However, it does take discipline to do these things. It is very easy to take the easier option of staying up late, staying in bed, eating poorly, not doing any work on video or mental rehearsal. It is easier not to write goals and write about what you achieved and can improve. You are a collection of habits. What is the quality of the habits you have in relation to your commitment to your craft? It is only a habit if you do it almost every day.

Top Tips:
1. Identify what level of commitment you are at now (current reality)?
2. Identify the level you want to get to (ideal state).
3. Choose the areas you want to work on – for example if it is writing down goals, pick a time every week when you will write these down and when you will review them daily. Work on this consistently for one or two months until you feel it is an automatic process.
4. Build a new habit every two-three months, over the course of a year you may have changed five-six habits that will improve your performance more than your results. Habits can take 90-100 days to build in.
5. Key formula = Task/Habit + Process + Performance = Outcome + review + repeat it
6. Start with end in mind – The outcome you want is to sleep better, the task is to get 8 hours sleep a night, the process for doing this is to get off the phone by 9pm, have a hot shower and hot drink before bed, get room and light temperature correct, have your room clean and cleared of clutter, do some gentle breathing exercises to calm mind and body and the performance happens where you get good quality, and the required quantity of sleep. On waking, you feel fully rested and refreshed.

SUMMARY POINTS - Chapter 14

- Excellence and genuine success are based on the solid bedrock of character and mindset and a number of skills and tools must be acquired and developed to be the best you can be in sport.
- Excellence is being the best you can be. It is more about improving ability, rather than proving ability.
- Having a personal understanding of what excellence means to you is crucial.
- Commitment is a key component of excellence.

PART 2

This section of the book is designed to give you an overview and appreciation of many of the elements involved in physical development and preparation for sport throughout the teenage years, and beyond. It is not designed to be a comprehensive aid to help you self- program or self- coach in athletic development. Rather, it aims to offer you some appropriate information, as well as expert opinion and insight which will allow you make informed decisions with regard to your athletic development and general health

Paul Kilgannon.

CHAPTER 15: THE MATURING BODY

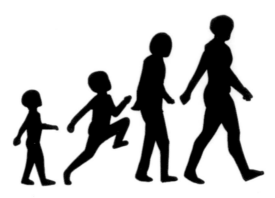

By Donie Fox

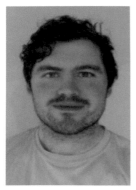

Donie Fox is a Chartered Physiotherapist and Athletic Development Coach who works with athletes across a broad range of sports, particularly GAA and Athletics. He is a frequent contributor to international coaching and physio websites, forums and podcasts. Donie contributes to two chapters in the book in the areas of Physical Maturation and Injury and Rehabilitation.

Physical Maturation
Children don't become adults overnight - that's an obvious statement. The way a young person grows and develops is a very complex journey that is never the same for two people. Scientists, doctors, psychologists, physiotherapists and many more study maturation in depth and yet what is understood about it is based on general principles and our own experience. It cannot be predicted how tall Anna will be or when Luke will grow facial hair. However, we can expect certain things at certain ages, and plan for those things. In the same way you may grow out of a pair of football boots within a short period during your early teenage years, your bones outgrow the length of your muscles during a growth spurt. This chapter aims to provide you with the knowledge of how to prepare for the whirlwind of change young bodies go through, and come through the other side a confident, competent and informed young adult.

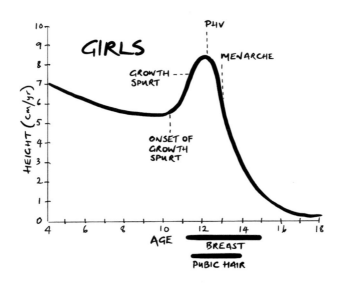

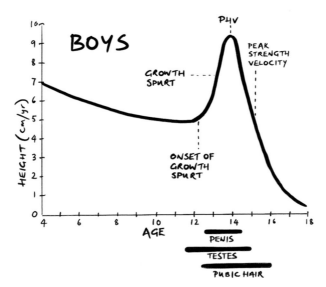

Maturity Events in Girls and Boys
(Adapted and Modified from Ross & Marfell-Jones, 1982)

It's Not Linear

One of the most important concepts to grasp is that the process of puberty and adolescence is not linear. People grow and mature at different ages, different rates and into different final products. It would be a very frustrating exercise for me to compare how I developed to other boys the same age.

I was a very early bloomer. I grew to almost 180cm by the time I went to secondary school and grew very little after that to finish up at 186cm. As you can imagine, a 6-foot first year student stands out (quite literally). It made me feel very awkward socially, but helped me a lot on the sports field. That was until everyone else caught up. While I was taking advantage of my height and physicality others were working on their speed, skills and game understanding. By the time I left school it was a level playing field, everyone had grown and I was left trying to catch up on those aspects of my development I had neglected due to my early physical advantages.

Athlete Examples
When we look at examples of some of our sporting heroes there are really important lessons to be learned about how our bodies develop at different rates. We see that where we perceive ourselves to be as adolescents often has very little to do with where we finish in terms of physical maturity as an adult. David Beckham, Henry Shefflin, Brian Fenton, Anthony Davis and Harry Kane are famous for being written off at an early age, only to develop late and go on to dominate their sports.

Biological Age
We all identify as being a certain age. It's based on the day we were born. This is our chronological age. Interestingly, across many sports those born earlier in the year tend to be selected for elite teams more often than those born later in the year. The main reason being that those born earlier in the year will tend to be, on average, more developed than those born later in the year. This seems to give those born in January, February and March an advantage over the rest. But it shouldn't. With differences in the onset of puberty, it is your biological age which is most relevant. Your biological age describes the stage of development you have reached. Though not a definite number this is a descriptor of your potential abilities based on where you are on the maturation spectrum.

Growth (Dick, 2014 & Gamble, 2019)
Growth doesn't just occur during puberty. You don't reach physical maturity until around 20 years of age. It's also important to note that it's not as simple as - taller and bigger. You need to respect growth as a complex process with a lot of give and take between different systems. The proportions of the body change massively as you grow. Imagine a 6-foot baby - that is not what an adult looks like. Each part of your body:

legs, arms, feet, head grow at different rates and at different times. It is very important that you appreciate how these proportions affect how you move and what type of training you can and should be doing.

Longer limbs are longer levers. This presents a challenge for growing bodies with regards to how you control these long levers. Muscles that were once comfortable and competent controlling your thigh bone may really struggle when that thigh bone grows 3cm in a few short months. Similarly, as your body stretches out and its limbs and trunk adopt new proportions, your centre of mass changes. What you once knew about balance and movement is now challenged by a relocated centre. This is where growth impacts upon your ability to participate and compete in sport. It affects your coordination, flexibility and ability to adapt to training.

Your skeleton is what gives you your shape and it is the focus for looking at growth, and the changes of proportion that comes with growth. The vast majority of your bones start out as cartilage and mature into bone by approximately 20 years of age. One of the important things to understand with bone growth, is that it occurs only in special parts of the bone- the growth plates. These are located between the long shaft of the bone and the end of the bone (epiphysis). These growth sites are a relatively common site of injury in adolescents.

Along with lengthening of the bones, you also have a very important process which hardens the bones. Young bones are pliable and elastic. The young skeleton has a lower ability to carry load but by progressively and consistently exposing immature bone to loading, you are encouraging and aiding the process of ossification. Ossification is the process by which your body forms solid bone and is very important for all young people. Previously it was thought that bone growth and hardening happens as a result of purely hormonal changes. What we know now is that our physical activity as children and adolescents can drastically alter how our bones adapt while growing.

As with most things in life we need to find the happy medium between too much loading and not enough loading. We have evidence that higher intensities of loading can negatively impact bone growth and healing, and conversely too little loading can lead to incomplete maturation or a lower ceiling for bone mineral density development. There is an important link here between physical activity, growth and body composition. Body composition is the relative percentage of lean nass and fat mass in our bodies. In growing bodies there is a strong link between our amount of lean muscle mass and our bone mineral density. The opposite is also true - higher fat mass is associated with lower bone mineral density.

Finding Balance

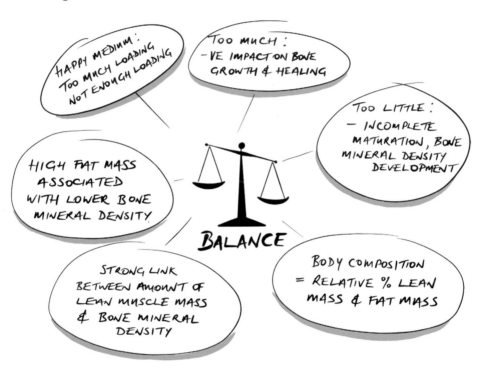

Stress + Rest = Growth

It's not just our bones (and muscles) that respond positively to the loads we place on them. Our connective tissues (tendons and ligaments particularly) respond to strain placed upon them during activity by remodelling stronger and with a greater ability to resist straining.

During this time appropriate physical activity in line with one's abilities sets up the skeleton and connective tissues for life - developing stronger bones and tissues as we expose our bodies to appropriate stress. There is a tipping point here where injury may occur. That is always a risk when it comes to vigorous physical activity but in growing bodies there are some special considerations which we will cover next.

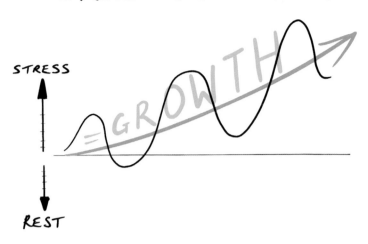

Differences between Girls and Boys

There are many differences between males and females, not least is how puberty affects their bodies. On average, females reach puberty earlier, and finish earlier than boys. The main growth spurt known scientifically as Peak Height Velocity (PHV) is reached sooner in girls than boys (~11.5 years vs ~14 years). During growth spurts there is another unique difference between the sexes. Girls, when they approach maximum height, lag behind in how strong their longer bones are versus boys. One estimation is that when a girl has reached 90% of their adult height, they only possess 60% of their maximal bone mineral density. If you seek to develop age-appropriate strength at an early age your skeleton will adapt to those stresses and become more resistant to the stresses of sport.

It is not just length of bones and how dense these bones are that summarise the differences between males and females in terms of growth. The average shape of each body begins to diverge also. In general, males will have relatively narrower pelvises and broader shoulders. Whereas females will be narrower in the shoulders and broader at the pelvis. This is significant with regards to how we move and coordinate sporting movements. The wider female pelvis can create very large demand for the control and protection of the knee joint during sporting movement. While this is sometimes described as a risk factor inherent in females the truth is a little more complicated. The difference in body shape may only be a risk factor if there isn't appropriate strength and coordination development.

There is another big difference in the development of males versus females during puberty - hormones. The higher circulating levels of testosterone that occurs naturally in males leads to significantly more natural strength development during the years of puberty (and indeed throughout life) versus females. With appropriate intervention in the guise of strength training this disparity in relative strength can be reduced. Without these interventions the relative weakness combined with the different body shapes can increase a female's risk of significant lower limb joint injury in sport.

PuBERTY	REACH LATER	FINISH EARLIER
PEAK HEIGHT VELOCITY	~14 YRS	~11.5 YRS
BONES	STRONGER & LONGER	LESS DENSE
BODY SHAPE	NARROWER PELVIS BROAD SHOULDERS	NARROW SHOULDERS BROADER PELVIS
HORMONES	GREATER LEVELS OF TESTOSTERONE LEADING TO GREATER STRENGTH.	LOWER LEVELS OF STRENGTH CAN LEAD TO INCREASED RISK OF INJURY

Technique/Skill

While we do not forget how to do a butterfly stroke, throw a left hook or do a back handspring during puberty, at times our body's changing dimensions can make the performance of these things more difficult, awkward and sometimes impossible. Your hardware (the body) has been updated but the software (motor control) has yet to be updated. During growth you need to spend a lot of time on remastering the basics in *order to ensure that you continue to improve technique throughout adolescence and into early adulthood. Your time away from structured coaching sessions should focus on making sure your body can continue to perform the basic movements, techniques and skills of your sport even as it grows and changes proportion.*

Learning to Train

One of the main issues around sports training for youths is the focus on short-term performance rather than long-term development. During the adolescent years there should be a focus on learning how to train appropriately and preparing for competition. A focus on short-term performance can negatively affect how adolescents develop as athletes. Appropriate athletic development (see Chapter 16) is a priority during these years. At different stages of growth and development your body can tolerate more, or less, training. During these times it is vitally important that you are able to identify times when you are very tired, getting sore, or struggling with technique and that this is communicated to your coach/parent. This is usually a clear sign that your training has overtaken your body's capacity to adapt/ respond positively in the short -term and that you may need to rest a little or have a different focus for a few weeks. Many of these precautions are to avoid injury to your growing, immature body. Below is some general advice for things to focus on during different stages of growth.

Each Stage - Have a Focus

Whether you are an early or late developer the key to maximizing potential is to work on various aspects of your sporting prowess during different stages of development so that you leave adolescence a well-rounded and healthy performer.

As an Early Developer

You are more likely to have a physical advantage over your opponents - faster, stronger, and bigger. This can give you a short-term performance benefit. It is imperative that you continue to hone the craft of your sport - spend extra time on skill, technique and tactical understanding. Ensuring that you are able to control your new body and train to maximise how you can utilise your physicality is bonus territory for the early developer. If you fail to do so then you can come out the other end of adolescence, when everyone else has caught up, with a small sporting toolbox.

As a Late Developer

The opposite can be true here. As late developers you tend to rely on your skills, techniques and tactical development to stay competitive against your more physically mature opponents. You may be naturally drawn to what might seem the most obvious type of training which you feel gives you an immediate advantage i.e. skills of the game. That said, by getting an early start on age appropriate athletic development you can close the gap and give yourself a springboard for when your growth kicks into gear. As we have seen earlier, physical activity prepares your tissues. If you stress your body now and develop a really good baseline of athleticism, it becomes easier to maintain that baseline and improve upon it as you grow.

Shifting Your Training Focus around a Growth Spurt

Irrespective of competition and whether you have a natural advantage or disadvantage over an opponent, you need to think about your own welfare and health. Looking after your body during this time of growth is simple but often overlooked. The duration and frequency of a growth spurt will vary greatly between individuals. You are likely to experience multiple growth spurts with some more pronounced than others. Here are some simple guidelines for how you may shift your training focus around growth spurts.

Firstly, we need to be able to tell when a growth spurt is happening. By frequently (every fortnight or so) measuring and graphing or logging your height and weight you can identify early when it is happening and behave accordingly.

- Measure your height in centimetres - barefoot, heels down, chin tucked in. You may need someone to help you.
- Measure your weight in kilograms.

Before a Growth Spurt

- Spend extra time in the week working on your athletic development sessions - speed (see Chapter 18) and strength are very important at this stage to maintain short-term performance while looking after long-term development.
- Seek out opportunities to compete with maturing teammates or opponents. This will help improve your problem solving when it comes to dealing with early developers.
- Watch sport - yours and others (see Chapter 7). You can learn a lot about tactics and styles of play which will help build your sporting knowledge. It will also help you to gain an appreciation for tactics at a time when you can't simply rely on physical advantage.

During a Growth Spurt (Once you notice a spike in your measurements you are in a period of accelerated growth)

- *Go back to basics in athletic development (see Chapter 16). You may lose the ability to effectively perform some fundamental movements during this time as your brain adapts to the growing body.*
- *Just like fundamental movement, your basic sport techniques and skills will suffer here if you do not dedicate time (see Chapter 5)*
- *Do not be afraid to take some days off if you feel very tired or start to ache. It is important that your body gets a good balance of stress and rest here. Without rest your body may not achieve its growth potential.*
- *Let your coach know that you are in the middle of a growth spurt. Coaches can lose sight of long-term development and get frustrated when previous high performers start to struggle with skills and movement. You may experience a dip in performance during this time. It is perfectly natural so try not to get frustrated. It won't last forever.*
- *If you start to experience debilitating pain or feel you might be injured, tell your parents and coach. You can experience a variety of pains associated with these growth spurts but the most common areas of pain are the knees and feet. You may need to see a physiotherapist. The therapist will assess the area and after ruling out any other conditions will prescribe a treatment usually consisting of massage and a stretching/strengthening programme for the specific area.*

After a Growth Spurt (Once you notice the spike in growth is flattening)

- *If you have continued to stay on top of the basics of athletic development then now is the time to try and build on that. With a larger frame you now need to build infrastructure for that frame. Appropriate strength training is the focus for this.*
- *If you have continued to maintain skill and technique levels during your growth spurt then it may be useful to speak to your coach and ask for advice on new skills or higher-level techniques that you can work on.*
- *If you have not maintained your fundamental movement ability or skill/technique ability then it is important to stay working on the basics until these are improved to your previous level of competency. With a level playing field, those who have continued to work on the basics and are able to progress from there will come out on top.*

Periods of Potential Accelerated Development

The principles and models of long-term athlete development are well established in the literature and are beyond the scope of this chapter. There are many models, each with its own limitations and challenges, and debate around what is the 'best way' to approach athletic development is ever-present in the industry. The periods of potential accelerated development or 'Windows of Opportunity' outlined in the timelines below, detail different stages along the maturation cycle, where there may be an accelerated adaptation to a specific focus of physical development. It must be appreciated that this model, like all others, has its limitations, however, it offers the youth athlete a simple and clear reference point. All individuals are different, so the 'best way' for one may not be the 'best way' for another and as such, chronological age can be a poor reference point for some individuals.

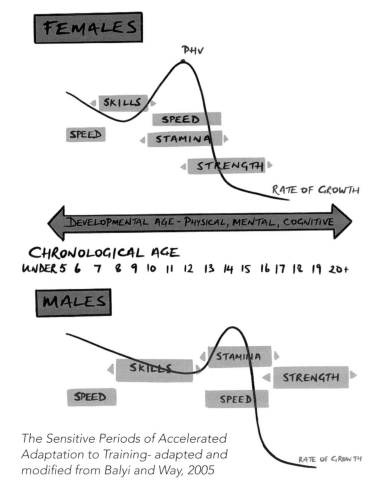

The Sensitive Periods of Accelerated Adaptation to Training- adapted and modified from Balyi and Way, 2005

Dr Katie Lydon

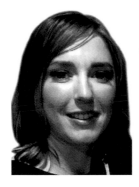

Dr Katie Lydon is currently team doctor with the Dublin Senior Ladies Football Team, having previously worked with the Irish Men's Hockey Team. She holds an honours degree in Sports and Exercise Science from Loughborough University. She is currently completing her masters in Sports and Exercise Medicine while undergoing research in the area of menstruation and performance at the Sport Ireland Institute. Below, Katie gives an overview of the menstrual cycle and how it pertains to the female athlete.

The Menstrual Cycle
The menstrual cycle reflects the changes in hormones that occur in females from menarche (when menstruation first occurs) to menopause. The cycle centres on the dynamics of the ovarian hormones, oestrogen and progesterone, which are in turn affected by the pituitary hormones, follicular-stimulating hormone and luteinising hormone. In the average female it takes approximately 28 days to complete this cycle, which begins with menstruation (Day 1 = first day of menstrual blood loss). Menstruation lasts approximately seven days (range is two to seven days). The cycle is split into two phases - the follicular phase whereby follicles mature and prepare for ovulation (release of an egg from the ovary), and the luteal phase where the uterus lining thickens in preparation for possible pregnancy.

While the average cycle is 28-days, it can range from 21 to 35 days. There are various reasons why an individual's cycle can be shorter or longer than normal (see Appendix). Once your menstruation starts, as well as bleeding, you may experience cramps, food cravings, diarrhoea and bloating. Some females also notice dry, sensitive skin during their menstruation, which generally subsides once you stop menstruating. You may notice you have more energy around ovulation–this is normal. Around this time, your skin may become oilier and you may get some spots–again this is normal. Between ovulation and menstruation, some females may experience a range of symptoms, which fall under the term, premenstrual syndrome (defined below). These symptoms can include: mood swings, food cravings, abdominal cramps, breast tenderness, headaches and you may find that you are more irritable. These symptoms generally resolve once your next cycle starts. If you find that these symptoms are impacting your everyday life it is important to speak to a medical professional.

The majority of individuals will have a normal menstrual cycle and it won't affect their ability to train and perform. However, some females express issues around their cycle and it is important to realise that this is more common than you may think. Up to 95% of the female population can experience issues, albeit mild, with their cycle at some stage in their lives. The menstrual cycle can be affected by biological, psychological and social factors. These relationships are all intertwined and if you believe your menstrual cycle is affecting you, it's important to address each of these areas with a medical professional. Likewise, it is helpful to know about some of the primary menstrual issues affecting women, which in the exercising athlete can affect her ability to train and perform (Table A).

Condition	Explanation	Prevalence
Oligomenorrhea	Infrequent menstrual periods (<nine/ year)/ a cycle >35 days in length	~14%
Primary Amenorrhea	Failure of the initiation of menstruation by the age of 14 (in the absence of secondary sexual characteristics) or 16 (in the presence of secondary sexual characteristics)	<1%
Dysmenorrhoea	Painful menstruation	Up to 90%
Hypomenorrhoea	Very light menstrual flow	<2%
Intermenstrual Bleeding	Uterine bleeding at irregular intervals, especially between expected menstrual periods	Up to 24%
Premenstrual Syndrome	A range of mood, behavioural and physical symptoms that can impact daily functioning in the period before menstruation	Up to 95%
Menorrhagia	Heavy or prolonged bleeding	Up to 30%
Secondary Amenorrhoea	The cessation of normal menstruation for three months or longer in an individual who previously had a regular menstrual cycle, or for six months or longer in an individual who previously had an irregular cycle.	Up to 8%
Polymenorrhea	Menstrual cycle < 21 days in length	~12%
Anovulation	The failure of release of an oocyte (immature egg) during the menstrual cycle.	Up to 19%

Table A. Explanation of Menstrual Irregularities.

The following are a number of tips aimed to help you manage your menstrual cycle:

- *Monitor your Cycle. A simple diary will do, or there are a variety of apps available to make this task easier. Documentation of daily symptoms, including flow and emotional state can be beneficial in identifying issues that may contribute to menstrual disturbance. In addition, the length of your cycle can inform your coach about how you are responding to training. For example, those with amenorrhoea or oligomenorrhoea may have a training regimen that is in excess of their body's tolerable limit. Furthermore, some injuries occur more commonly at certain times of the menstrual cycle (for example- anterior cruciate ligament rupture is more common in the preovulatory phase) due to the effect of oestrogen and progesterone on muscles, tendons and ligaments. Maintaining a menstrual diary can better inform coaches of the at-risk time points and training regimens can be altered accordingly if required.*

- *Talk to your Coach. Granted, this may be easier if your coach is female or you are participating in an individual sport. If you are part of a team, perhaps there is a female member of the team management you can talk to? If you are feeling out-of-sorts due to your menstruation, or even in the premenstrual phase, it may be beneficial to discuss training alterations with your coach. Additionally, providing information on your cycle to your coach may help plan future training. Tailoring training to the menstrual cycle, while currently in-vogue, has no scientific basis and is not recommended. Oftentimes there can be a breakdown in communication between the athlete and coach on this matter, however creating and maintaining an open channel of communication ensures that issues surrounding the menstrual cycle can be identified and addressed promptly.*

- *Keep a food diary. Anti-inflammatory foods (e.g. berries, fatty fish and green leafy vegetables) can assist with the treatment of some of these conditions. It is important to maintain a well-balanced diet to ensure there is no energy deficit, which could lead to a range of physical issues, including RED-S (Relative Energy Deficiency in Sport). RED-S occurs when there is a mismatch between energy availability and energy expenditure, generally because an athlete is not eating the appropriate amount of food for their activity level. Essentially, they are putting out more energy than they are taking in. This affects the hormones in the body. The result is an athlete with low energy availability, menstrual dysfunction and reduced bone mineral density, which can ultimately lead to* bone fractures (you don't need all three parts of the triad for a diagnosis). Warning signs of energy deficiency can include: not having your period by the age of 16 or missing three cycles of your period, having repeated stress fractures or shin splints and having a low body mass index. Linking in with a nutritionist and physician can help to prevent this and ensure you are getting the maximum benefit from your diet.

- Deal with stress. There is a reciprocal relationship between menstrual health and psychological wellbeing. Stress can take different forms: physical, emotional, social or cultural and can manifest as physical or psychological signs or symptoms. Stress in any form can result in adverse menstrual signs and symptoms such as dysmenorrhoea, which can in turn result in heightened levels of stress and anxiety. Speaking to a psychologist may help.

In all this, if you think you are having issues with your menstrual cycle, don't be afraid to talk to someone and seek medical assistance.

Many menstrual issues are managed using hormonal medications or implants. If you require such management it is important that you are fully informed of the potential side effects of the medication, as with any treatment plan. Seek medical assistance and discuss with your parents and coach (if applicable).

While some athletes admit that their menstrual cycle is burdensome on their ability to optimally train and perform, it is a vital sign of general wellbeing and provides clinicians and healthcare professionals with a valuable insight into the overall health status of an athlete. For instance, amenorrhoea can be a sign that the athlete has an energy deficit. Addressing this can restore energy levels, prevent possible future insufficiency fractures and reinstate optimal menstrual health, which can ultimately beneficially affect performance.

Case Study

Aoife is a 17-year-old elite boxer. She has suffered from painful periods for a number of years, relying heavily on anti-inflammatories and painkillers to get her through the start of each cycle. Due to the pain and heavy blood loss, Aoife found it difficult to commit 100% to her training schedule and because of that was slow to make meaningful gains. Her doctor prescribed hormonal medication for her, but she suffered adverse side effects (hair loss, mood swings, weight gain) and had to stop taking it. Aoife had spent a long time suffering in silence and *was slow to talk to her coach about her pain and the associated stress. Following repeated absences from training, her coach approached her to address the issue. By this time Aoife had suffered enough and disclosed her menstrual difficulties to her coach. This led to Aoife consulting with a doctor with a special interest in this area. Following evaluation, she was diagnosed with Premenstrual Syndrome (PMS), which affects up to 50% of the athletic population. Aoife was reassured and linked in with a nutritionist. She was encouraged to include more anti-inflammatory foods into her diet and was commenced on omega-3 fatty-acid supplementation, which has been shown to reduce the PMS symptoms in the general population. Over time she was able to reduce her reliance on painkillers and anti-inflammatories. She has not missed many training sessions due to her menstrual cycle and is currently reaping the benefits of improved nutrition and medical support on her physical, psychological and menstrual health, which has translated to improved performance in the ring.*

Best wishes with all your sporting endeavours,
Dr Katie Lydon

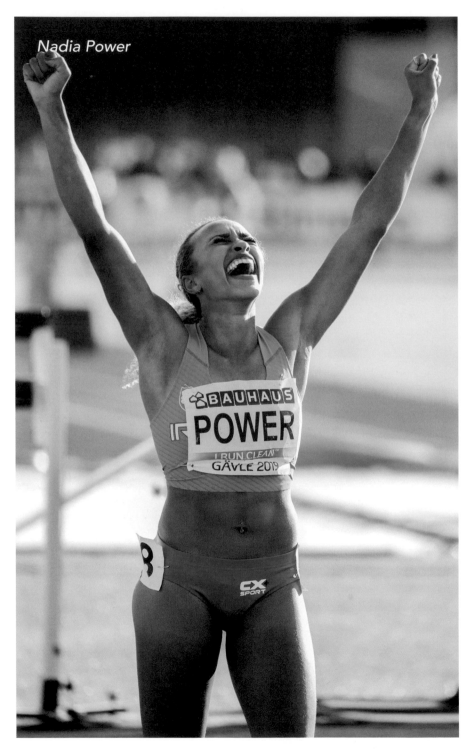

CHAPTER 15

Nadia Power

Nadia Power is a middle-distance athlete from Dublin currently studying in DCU and striving for Olympic Qualification. She is the National Senior Indoor 800m Champion 2020, European U23 800m Bronze Medallist 2019, European U20 1500m finalist 2017 & 5 Time All-Ireland Schools Champion (1500m & Cross Country). Here, she gives an insight into her experience of physical maturation through her teenage years.

I competed at a national and international level in athletics throughout my teenage years. Over this time, I had to adapt to changes in my body as I progressed as an athlete throughout secondary school. I would consider myself to have had a relatively smooth experience and was able to win national titles each year throughout this important maturation period, but not without a few frustrations.

As a teenage girl competing over 800m/1500m and cross country, it was apparent that girls were maturing and progressing at different stages and often very quickly. My own improvement stalled for a few years from around 14 to 16 despite my body getting significantly stronger throughout this time. I remember being frustrated by new competition suddenly appearing and running incredible times on the track compared to me, despite my years of consistent training. However, many athletes disappeared just as quickly, having pushed their bodies too hard during this crucial developmental stage. It has been my experience that while talent often shines brightly in teenage years, hard work and years of consistent and intelligent training comes to fruition at senior level.

Without a doubt, one of the biggest obstacles a teenage girl can face in sport is menstruation. Personally, I frequently worried about my period affecting my performance as a teenager during important competitions. This is something that still crosses my mind; however, I have learned to accept this as part of being female and know it's a challenge my competitors face also.

Sadly, an even bigger problem than getting your period as a teenage girl, is not getting it. I have witnessed a lot of my friends in endurance running struggle with this and ultimately fall out of the sport because of it. It is common for girls who are training intensively to lose their periods or never begin them in the first place. At first, this seemed to benefit performance but ultimately led to a cycle of injuries. For some of my friends, it still continued years later despite seeking medical advice and managing to regulate their periods.

As a teenage girl involved in sport, it is really important you have an open relationship with your coach. Telling your coach if your period stops or if you are finding it harder to perform well at certain times of the month will really help your coach structure your training, which will ultimately benefit your performance. I also find it useful to track my period in my training diary. That way when I am looking back, I can reflect on if performances were affected or see if it is late or irregular. If you don't feel comfortable speaking to a male coach, find a teammate or an older role model to share your feelings with. Always remember you are not alone and no athlete has a smooth or perfect journey.

Best of luck,
Nadia Power

References:
Balyi, I., Way, R., Higgs, C., Norris, S. & Cardinal, C, Canadian sport for life: Long-Term Athlete Development [Resource paper]. Vancouver, Canada: Canadian Sport Centres (2005)
Dick, F.W., Sports Training Principles: An Introduction to Sport Science. 6th edn. London, UK:
Bloomsbury (2014)
Ross, W.D. & Marfell-Jones, M.J., Physiological testing of the elite athlete. In J. D. MacDougall, H. A. Wenger & H. J. Green (Eds.), Kinanthropometry Ithica, NY: Movement Publications, (pp. 75–104), (1982)
Gamble, P., Comprehensive Strength & Conditioning: Physical Preparation for Sports Performance. Vancouver, Canada: Informed in Sport Publishing (2019)

SUMMARY POINTS - Chapter 15

- People grow and mature at different ages, different rates and into different final products.
- During periods of growth, appropriate physical activity sets up the skeleton and connective tissues for life.
- Puberty affects the male and female bodies differently.
- During growth, you need to spend time remastering basic skills and movements in order to ensure that you continue to improve throughout adolescence and into early adulthood.
- During the adolescent years there should be a focus on learning how to train appropriately and prepare for competition.
- Follow the recommendations provided for before, during and after a growth spurt.
- Menstrual symptoms generally resolve once the next cycle starts. If you find that these symptoms are impacting your everyday life or participation in sport it is important to speak to a medical professional.
- Follow the recommendations to help you manage your menstrual cycle.

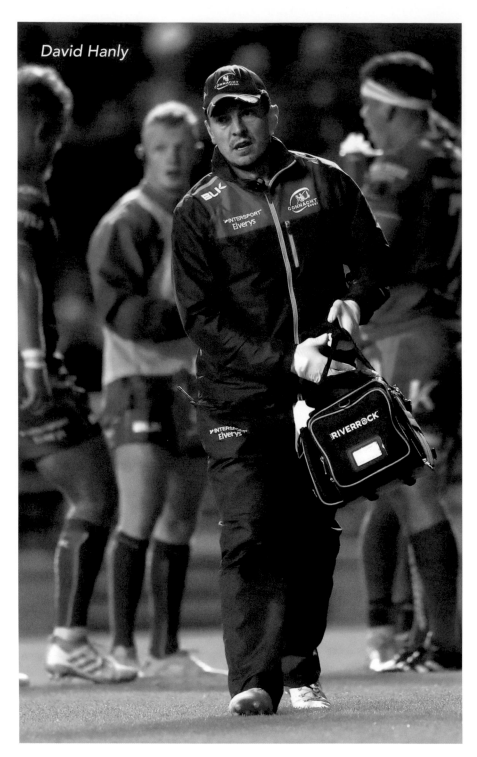

David Hanly

CHAPTER 16 : MOVEMENT EFFICIENCY

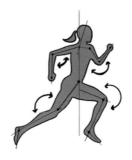

By David Hanly

David Hanly is a Chartered Physiotherapist. He is currently Senior Physiotherapist at Connacht Rugby and Physiotherapy Clinic Owner at Performance Physio Galway. He has been involved with Galway GAA intercounty teams for the past 12 years, as well as working with numerous athletes and teams across a broad range of sports at both youth and adult level. In the following chapter he gives his insights into the importance and value of developing 'movement efficiency' in the youth athlete.

My interest in 'movement efficiency' has developed as a result of frustrations in dealing with stubborn pain and injury in athletes of all abilities. It goes without saying that the older you get, the more difficult it is to stay injury-free. One way we can counteract this is by developing your athletic capabilities during your developmental years, when your body have the greatest potential to learn new movement skills. I believe that current methods of how we physically prepare our young athletes, particularly in Ireland, can be better and I will provide my opinion as to why this is the case. I hope the following text can provide you, the aspiring athlete commencing on your journey of development, with some guidance as to how to maximise your physical literacy, and set yourself up for a long and healthy sporting life.

Introduction
As time has gone by the world of medicine, for the most part, has evolved with it. Advances in diagnosis, pharmacological treatments and surgical techniques means our healthcare system is in a stronger

position now than what it was 20 years ago, with patients enjoying better outcomes. One area that has not enjoyed the same results is that of sports medicine, particularly in relation to soft tissue or muscle-tendon type injuries. Take the case of hamstring injuries in professional soccer; they are as commonplace now as they were 20 years ago. When you consider the advances in sport science made over that time period, and the resources and expertise that are poured into the care of such athletes, it is a pretty damning statistic that we have become no better in reducing the incidence of such issues.

Sport has been a huge part of my life, both personally and professionally. I played Gaelic football to a high level with my club and county. Since then, I have worked as a Chartered Physiotherapist for the best part of the last 15 years looking after athletes of all shapes and sizes with various aches and pains. Over that time period, I have been lucky enough to work with sportspeople at the very top of their game and have experienced moments that I'll always cherish. However, the curse of injury is never too far away and the disappointment of seeing one of your players "break down" has not got any easier for me as my career has gone on.

When looking for answers as to why these injuries occur, or indeed re-occur, it is my opinion that the injured tissue or structure is the 'victim' rather than the culprit. In the case of most soft tissue injuries, the injured muscle or tendon is often overworked to the point of exhaustion due to what some term an "energy leak" somewhere else in the athlete's movement system. On digging deeper into finding these leaks, it is rare that physical attributes such as strength, endurance and power are where the main deficits lie. We call such measures "quantitative" as they can be measured by number for example; how many chin-ups can you do? Most athletes will demonstrate their primary faults in the finer, more "qualitative" aspects of how they perform a movement. For example, instead of counting how many chin-ups someone can do, we instead look at how he/she performs the chin-up movement. Does it look smooth and coordinated? Are there any signs of compensation in the body? I would much rather see someone perform five good quality repetitions of an exercise than 10 sloppy reps where the movement is being performed in a manner that is not smooth and causes compensation in the system. These "bad" reps often come back to bite in the form of pain or injury further down the line.

CHAPTER 16

Quality
— OVER —
QUANTITY

Unfortunately, movement quality is not as high a priority for everyone. High performance sport is data-driven. Coaches obsess over numbers and as a result, there is a necessity to have quantitative measures on each and every athlete. How much weight can he squat? What's her Shuttle Test score? Qualitative analysis of how an athlete coordinates a landing or his/her ability to change direction quickly on the playing field is more difficult to measure and is not high on the priority list of most coaches. More importantly, the optimal period for training and developing these fundamental qualities of 'movement efficiency' has passed by the time an athlete has reached competition level. The developmental period of the athlete's life is the optimal time to train qualities such as balance, coordination, body awareness and expression of movement, i.e. the building blocks of skill acquisition. Unfortunately, the older the athlete becomes, the more difficult it can become to illicit gains in these valuable areas.

This aim of this chapter is to provide you with an introduction to the area of 'movement efficiency' and to help you develop an appreciation of its importance during this vital stage in your athletic development. In addition, I will describe 8 basic exercise streams that will serve as a starting point for you on this journey and will help form the building blocks to develop higher level movement skills related to sport. The purpose of this piece is not to act as a replacement, or a substitute, for quality athletic development coaching. The written form has limitations, which good coaching will always surpass.

Most of the content included is based on well-established principles of long-term athlete development (LTAD) and influenced by the teachings of leaders in the field of movement efficiency such as: Kelvin Giles, Steve Myrland, Vern Gambetta and Bill Knowles, amongst others. In addition, some of the material in the chapter reflects what I've experienced and learned over the years in my own practice of treating pain and injury, and how I feel we can help prepare our young athletes better in order to become robust enough to realise their sporting ambitions.

Problems

Early specialisation is a concept related to youngsters, which can be defined as an "intense and specific focus on one sport at the exclusion of others" (Myer et al, 2015). As a rule of thumb, the athlete should not complete more training hours per week, in a given sport, than their biological age. By some influence youngsters get drawn to a sport. This influence may be a parent, teacher, friend or even the media. Obviously, this can only be seen as a positive, and getting any young person involved in physical activity at an early age should be encouraged and nurtured.

The negative elements of early specialisation generally develop when an adult, not the youth, gets it wrong. This is usually as a result of placing too high a burden on the young athlete to be competitive in one sport only, when the focus during this stage should be on sampling many sports and the different movement experiences that comes with it.

So what exactly are the negatives associated with early specialisation? (See also Chapter 22) Firstly, we have an issue where if the young athlete focuses solely on one sport- he or she is tasked to perform repeated actions that demand a high degree of movement efficiency and movement resilience. In field sports, for example, there is an emphasis on such things as:

- *Acceleration/Deceleration*
- *Rapid Change of Direction*
- *Jumping/Landing*
- *Kicking*
- *Catching*
- *Striking*

The above movements place huge stresses on your body and require a proficient standard of 'movement vocabulary' to be executed efficiently, particularly when they need to be performed repeatedly and under fatigue. This highlights the need to train the fundamentals of balance, coordination and body awareness to deal with such demands. Consider the dreaded anterior cruciate ligament (ACL) injury of the knee, which has cursed some of the greatest athletes and results in a significant process of rehabilitation for the injured athlete. In the vast majority of these cases, the mechanism of injury looks innocuous. There is usually no contact involved when the injury takes place; instead, it is more likely to occur while the athlete is landing from a jump, changing direction or having to decelerate quickly. Such tasks rely on the body's ability to coordinate movement efficiently through all parts of the system, from "fingers to toes". If one part of the body's chain is not doing its job properly, another part pays the price. Unfortunately, the knee is the victim in this scenario. The second main downside to early specialisation also revolves around the issue of injury. If you are a young athlete focussing solely on playing one sport at a competitive level throughout the year (as many talented players do) the risk of 'overuse' injury, and potential player burnout, becomes a very real possibility. With this biased approach to training, areas of the body with high workload demands such as the hamstring, groin, knees and ankle can accumulate excessive stress and eventually break down. Add to that the advent of a "growth spurt" (see Chapter 15), as may occur in the early to mid-teens, and these tissues are under even greater load again.

A real-life example that highlights the importance of multi-sport participation is Ajax Amsterdam FC in the Netherlands, who have been one of the top football clubs in Europe for a number of decades. Their academy system is regarded by many as the best in world football and has produced superstars such as Wesley Sneijder, Christian Eriksen, Frenkie de Jong and Matthijs de Ligt, the youngest ever Champions League captain at 19 years old. When young players enter the Ajax Youth Academy, 40% of their training is non-football related for the first couple of years. Judo and gymnastics feature heavily in the programme, with the goal of developing whole-body strength and coordination. Their training centre "De Toekomst", which translates as "The Future", is equipped with mini basketball and badminton courts, as well as track and field facilities where the young athletes get to sample the various movement challenges of a wide variety of sports. Focus on a player's football ability only becomes a priority later in the development cycle, at which point they will have attained a strong level of athleticism to deal with the high demands of the professional game.

The main message I'd like you to take home is that this period of your development offers the best potential to build a foundation of 'movement vocabulary' that will serve you long into your career. Focusing only on playing one sport during these important development years can have its drawbacks. Instead using this period to sample many different activities, organised or otherwise, where your body can experience many types of movement challenges, will only serve to maximise your athletic potential as you progress. My experience to date is that I invariably see athletes in their mid-teens who are "adapted", yet we should have athletes that are "adaptable" (Myrland, 2007) to the challenges that present themselves over the course of the athletic development journey.

Athlete Development Overview

As noted in Chapter 15, the principles of long-term athlete development are well established in the literature. It cannot be denied that there are limitations and challenges to every model and debate is ever-present in the athletic development industry as to what is the 'best way'. The stages of training outlined below have been defined by Balyi & Hamilton (2001). This is just one athletic developmental model but for the purposes of this piece, it offers a simple and clear point of reference. It must be qualified and appreciated that there are limitations to this model and all individuals are by their very nature different. Chronological age (related to your date of birth) may be a poor reference point for some.

STAGE	AGE
FUNdamental	6-10yrs
Training to Train	11-14yrs
Training to Compete	15-20yrs
Training to Win	20+yrs

For many of you reading this book, you will be in what can be referred to as the "Training to Train" phase of your development as an athlete. Your nervous system is almost fully developed at this stage, therefore it is wise to make the most of this 'window of opportunity' in how you train during this period. There should be a focus on developing qualities such as balance, coordination and agility. In general terms, the focus should be to improve both Mobility and Stability through your system in different movement patterns, in all directions or dimensions of motion. As a rule of thumb, we are striving for QUALITY rather than QUANTITY in everything we do during this stage of athletic development. "Strength and Conditioning", as it relates to adding Load or Weight to your exercises, may only come later in the process, under the guidance of a qualified professional, after you have established a level of 'movement efficiency' that is sufficient to progress to such activities (see Chapter 17). In essence, you need to "Earn the Right" to put extra load on your body by achieving satisfactory control of your own bodyweight first. I need to stress that this development of 'movement vocabulary' is very much an ongoing process that should continue well beyond this development stage. On entering the "Train to Compete" stage where formal strength training is often introduced, the emphasis on further developing our movement qualities should be even greater, to match the demands of a progressive strength programme and greater game intensity. In truth, the journey of maximising you movement competencies never ends.

Movement Efficiency

So, what exactly is 'movement efficiency'? For me, the best definition for it comes from Kelvin Giles who describes it as the:

> *"process that puts the body in the right position, at the right time, all the time so that it can effectively produce, reduce and stabilise force. In relation to athletes who play field sport, we need to consider this process in a multi-joint, multi-plane and multi-directional setting"*
> *Giles, 2012*

In trying to achieve this, you may need to think differently about how you prepare. In my experience, traditional strength and conditioning programmes for this crucial phase of development do not place sufficient focus on the areas highlighted above. For me the opportunity to develop these qualities must be ceased by the youth athlete. As you progress, your ability to improve the attributes of balance, coordination and agility diminishes.

Mobility and Stability

It goes without saying that the human body is an amazing piece of machinery. For it to work efficiently, you want to achieve the right balance of 2 key attributes: Mobility and Stability. Without going into too much detail, certain joints are designed for certain actions, just as certain muscles are designed for certain tasks. For example, the hip joint is a ball-and-socket joint. Due to its anatomical make-up, it is designed to travel through a wide range of movement in all 3 dimensions of movement, i.e. it is built for mobility. The knee, on the other hand, has a completely different shape and structure, and it is generally seen that its primary responsibility is to provide stability. However, if you have a hip that becomes too mobile or a knee that develops to be too stable, this can lead to problems in the future, such as pain or injury. If your brain senses a movement problem or "energy leak" at one body part or joint, it will react by driving that stress to another joint. This increased burden often results in pain if these faulty movement patterns persist.

A common example of this issue would be where an athlete develops knee pain due to excessive movement at the hip. In this scenario, if the muscles that control the movement of the hip are not working efficiently, it leads to excessive stress developing at the knee. As a result, we have an already mobile joint becoming more mobile, and an already stable joint becoming more stable. This causes a big imbalance in the system and, more often than not, pain and potential injury will result. Therefore, to avoid the scenario above, we want to use exercises in training according to the "Goldilocks principle". That is, for a movement to be efficient, the load is spread evenly through the system. Once this is achieved, we can be satisfied that movement at each body part or joint will be "not too little, not too much, but just right".

Assessing Movement Efficiency

Below I will outline eight exercises which can help to build a foundation of basic athletic movement competency. However, I want to stress that performing a battery of tests, or screens, is not the agenda here. The idea behind these exercise streams is that they will form a foundation for your 'movement efficiency' training programme, and can be progressed in complexity and demand over time under the guidance of a professional athletic development coach (see Chapter 17). Once again, there is no substitute for on-site coaching and feedback.

Below you can gain an understanding of why each movement is important for you and an appreciation of what proper execution of each movement looks like. In the absence of a qualified and knowledgeable coach you can practice these exercises at home or in the gym in an unloaded manner with quality of movement being your primary focus.

The movements we will focus on are as follows:
1) Squat: Double Leg
2) Hip Hinge
3) Split Lunge
4) Squat: Single Leg
5) Trunk Stability
6) Hip Stability (Hip Lock)
7) Lower Limb Stability
8) Hop + Stick

Your ability to execute the eight movements will provide a foundation upon which to develop your 'Movement Efficiency' and will enable you to recognise any potential weaknesses or imbalances that may be present. More importantly, these movements will form the building blocks of your future training programme and your capacity to perform and progress these different exercise streams will have a carryover in realising your potential in sporting endeavours.

See Appendix for more information on how to correctly preform each exercise

Also see Appendix for QR Codes for all video links shared here, and in the chapters that follow.

Exercise 1: Double-Leg Squat
Why is it important?
The squat is a hugely important movement pattern in relation to athletic performance. It has a strong carryover into training proper jumping and landing mechanics and teaches you how to lower your centre of mass efficiently for deceleration and change of direction manoeuvres on the field of play. It is also one of the fundamental gym exercises to develop strength in key lower body muscle groups such as the quadriceps and gluteal area. In executing the squat, you need to pay close attention to positioning of your trunk and pelvis during the movement to ensure you are moving efficiently and not putting excess stress on certain structures, in particular the spine and the groin/front of the hip.
See Video: https://www.youtube.com/watch?v=n4roa3-TGVg (QR Code 1)

Exercise 2: Hip Hinge
Why is it important?
The hip hinge is another fundamental athletic movement that should be developed from an early age. It involves being able to bend at your hips by shifting your weight backwards, while keeping the rest of your system in a relatively neutral position. An effective hip hinge is important in sport to allow the athlete to "load and explode" in order to change direction or accelerate. In addition, it is an excellent gym exercise to build strength and capacity through the gluteal and hamstring muscle groups, as well as developing control and stability through the trunk and pelvis.
See Video: https://www.youtube.com/watch?v=B0gum_dwoSw (QR Code 2)

Exercise 3: Split Lunge
Why is it important?
This exercise looks at your ability to flex one hip while simultaneously extending the opposite hip. This reflects the position the body needs to achieve for efficient high-speed running and acceleration actions on the field of play. It is also an excellent gym exercise to build lower body strength and is an excellent transition drill from double to single-leg strength training.
See Video: https://www.youtube.com/watch?v=PXHA9aPjv9k (QR Code 3)

Exercise 4: Squat (Single-Leg)
Why is it important?
The ability to perform a single-leg squat movement with satisfactory control is of huge importance for optimal athletic function. This exercise forms the foundation for a number of high-intensity sporting movements

such as acceleration, deceleration and change of direction tasks. It is also a brilliant exercise to develop single leg strength and control in the gym and should be a staple in any athletic development programme.
See Video: https://www.youtube.com/watch?v=zCDi8Md-000 (QR Code 4A)
See also Single Leg Skater Squat: https://www.youtube.com/watch?v=eGhfzYHTKOM (QR Code 4B)

Exercise 5: Trunk Stability Drill
Why is it important?
The abdominal muscle group has a major role to play in athletic movement and must be trained to meet the necessary demands. The abdominals, or "core" musculature, refers to the muscles of the trunk and pelvis that are responsible for the maintenance of stability of the spine, pelvis and rib cage, and also help to transfer energy from large to small body parts during sporting actions. In essence, this region of the body is built for work and cannot be too strong in my opinion. Weakness of the abdominals generally means other body tissues have to withstand excessive stresses, which can result in pain or injury. For the purpose of this chapter, we will focus on the stability role of the abdominal/core muscle group.
See Video: https://www.youtube.com/watch?v=opR2TUJfBL0 (QR Code 5)

Exercise 6: Hip Lock
Why is it important?
The hip lock movement involves placing the hip and pelvis in a position from where they can be most efficient during running. Essentially, it is the position where maximum recruitment of the hip musculature is achieved, helping you meet the force demands of high-speed running and change of direction movements. The ability to achieve and reproduce this position under increasing levels of difficulty enhances movement efficiency of the region to both increase running performance and reduce injury risk.
See Video: https://www.youtube.com/watch?v=g8tNEGqUp_M (QR Code 6)

Exercise 7: Lower Limb Stability Drill
Why is it important?
When we look at the common lower limb injuries that occur in sport, such as hamstring pulls, knee ligament injuries and ankle sprains, these injuries usually occur when there is a "system failure" when the foot contacts the ground. Sprinting, changing direction rapidly and landing from a height can all put the athlete at risk of injury due to the nature of the forces transmitted from the ground into our body during such

actions. Inability to tolerate these stresses due to lack of muscle control over your lower limb joints can predispose these structures to overload and potential damage. Therefore, it is really important that you train your ability to adopt the right joint positions from the ground up in preparation for such high-intensity tasks.
See Video: https://www.youtube.com/watch?v=k6oL9jHVJZM (QR Code 7)

Exercise 8: Hop and Stick

Why is it important?
The previous lower body stability exercise provides the foundation movement pattern for the hop and skip. The hip, knee and ankle joint angles achieved in the last exercise are exactly what you are looking to reproduce in the hop and stick drill. The aim of this exercise is to be able to demonstrate these stable joint positions both in your starting position (as we prepare to hop), and your finishing position (as we land or stick).
See Video: https://www.youtube.com/watch?v=GF7GmUFVI7A (QR Code 8)

Summary
Not many people realise that LeBron James, probably the greatest basketball player of this generation who is currently in his 18th season in the NBA, was once touted to play in the NFL as a wide-receiver on the back of the talent he showed while in high-school. Wayne Rooney was a top-level boxer in his youth before being persuaded by an Everton FC coach to choose football. He is now enjoying his 17th season as a professional football player. The great Zlatan Ibrahimovic, who has played for some of the world's most famous football clubs over the last 20 years, earned his black belt in Taekwondo at the age of 17. Former Manchester United and England centre-half Rio Ferdinand won a scholarship to the London Central School of Ballet at age 11, and remained there for four years while he was a youth player at the West Ham United Academy. His professional career spanned over 20 years. Closer to home, our own Katie Taylor showed talent across many sports, including GAA, athletics and soccer (where she played internationally), before going on to become the top female boxer on the planet.

While Katie is still at a relatively early stage of her professional career, the other three athletes have not only managed to play to the highest level of their respective sport, they have done so well into their 30's. Part of the reason for this has been their ability to stay healthy and injury-free by developing astonishing levels of movement resilience during their youth that served them into their professional careers.

Sporting organisations around the world spend billions of euros every year in trying to keep their players fit. It is common nowadays to see professional field sport athletes engaging in alternative programmes such as gymnastics, calisthenics, martial arts and track and field in an attempt to improve some of the movement competencies I have described earlier, with the ultimate aim of improving performance and reducing risk of injury. However, in my opinion, the time to maximise development of these qualities has passed and needs to be addressed much earlier in their sporting journey.

The key to training good movement habits is to start early and practice regularly. Renowned movement specialist Bill Knowles, who has helped some of the biggest stars in world sport recover from injury, calls it the "Dollar-a-Day" approach. Set aside 10 minutes every day to let your body explore its vast movement potential and watch this develop over time. The cumulative effect will be huge and it will help you realise your long-term sporting ambitions. The challenge for you is to capitalise on your body's capacity to build strong movement efficiency and resilience. I urge you to embrace the great opportunity you have at this stage of your development.

Enjoy the journey!
David Hanly

References:

Balyi I, and Hamilton, A.E. Key to success - Long-term athlete development: The FUNdamental stage - Part two. Sports Coach, 23, 23–25. 2001.
Gambetta V, Athletic Development: The Art & Science of Functional Sports Conditioning. Champaign, IL: Human Kinetics, 2007.
Giles K., Penfold L., Giorgi A., A Guide to Developing Physical Qualities in Young Athletes. Queensland, Australia. Movement Dynamics Pty Ltd. 2005.

SUMMARY POINTS - Chapter 16

- Injured tissues and structures are often the 'victim' rather than the culprit.
- *With regards to exercise execution, quality is more important than quantity.*
- *Your youth offers you the best potential to build a foundation of 'movement vocabulary' that will serve you long into your career.*
- *Sampling many different sports and activities, organised or otherwise, where your body can experience many types of movement challenges, will serve to maximise your athletic potential as you progress.*
- *The journey of maximising your movement competencies never ends and should continue throughout your sporting career.*
- *For a movement or exercise to be efficient, the load should spread evenly through the system (body).*
- *The eight movements provided will form the building blocks of your future training programme and your capacity to perform and progress these different exercise streams will have a carryover in realising your potential in future sporting endeavours.*

CHAPTER 17: THE INDIVIDUAL NATURE OF STRENGTH TRAINING

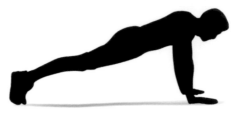

By Niall O'Toole

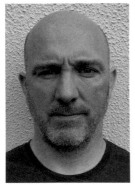

Niall O'Toole is a professional athletic development coach who has worked across a number of sports, at both youth and adult level. He excels in the area of coaching the individual and catering for their specific needs in strength training. He has an expert eye when it comes to exercise selection and execution. In this short piece I have asked Niall to leave you with an appreciation that strength training is much more than merely 'lifting weights'. My hope is that this understanding will allow you to approach strength training in a mature and intelligent manner, when the time is right for you.

'Pick it up and leave it down', 'Lift weights to get bigger and stronger', 'Squats, deadlifts and bench press (The Big Three) are great strength exercises'... It all sounds very simple, and in essence, it is. However, in order to reach this place of simplicity, there are many factors to consider. Ultimately, our job as athletic development coaches is to choose exercises which will make you 'better' at your chosen sport. This should be achieved by appreciating the fact that you are not a 'weight lifter' and strength training is only 'part' of the bigger picture.

As an athletic development coach, I strive to make athletes 'strong'. Strength creates a solid foundation from which you can develop all other athletic qualities i.e. speed, power, change of direction. Strength is the ability of the muscles to create tension across a spectrum, from absolute maximal force at one end, to extreme endurance at the other. Each is an exhibition of strength but must be trained for using different approaches.

Marathon runners, for example, must develop high levels of strength endurance and so the training focus should be primarily concerned with low levels of force development over long periods of time. This is markedly different from a rugby player, who must generate large amounts of maximal force at high velocity, in order to break a tackle or out-sprint an opponent to the try line. This is not to say that an endurance athlete cannot gain any benefit from developing some maximal strength (this has been shown to improve running economy) or the rugby player cannot gain any benefit from the ability to maintain a constant output of strength, over the duration of a game. It merely highlights the broad nature of strength and how we must match it appropriately to each individual and the tasks they engage in.

I have worked in strength training all my adult life. In many ways I feel it is a very misunderstood and undervalued profession. To the layperson the athlete is merely 'doing an exercise', 'working out' or 'pumping iron', but to the professional coach, with an expert 'coaching eye', there is so much to look for and so much to take into consideration.

'Lifting weights leads to injury', 'weights make you bulky and slow you down', 'exercise X is bad for you'.... Such half- truths and mistruths are widespread when it comes to strength training. This is understandable, as strength training can be poorly performed. The truth is that strength training is a skill and every strength exercise is a skill in itself. Like all skills, strength exercises can be performed well, and performed poorly. Certain skills come easier to some than others. For optimal execution, most skills require coaching. This is most certainly the case in strength training. Strength exercises are only as good as the athlete's ability to execute them properly. In my opinion, how we do things is far more important than what we do.

The knowledge application, and understanding, of strength training has increased exponentially in recent times. Much time and resources have been spent on scientific research which has helped shape how we program for you. In pursuit of the most effective programming, the evidence clearly tells us that if we manipulate the acute training variables (training loads, rest times, lifting velocity or exercise order) we can alter the specific outputs of our programmes. In other words, we can achieve the desired muscular adaptations (strength, power, hypertrophy etc.), whilst reducing unnecessary loads on the athlete. The prudent coach must stay current with the literature and intelligently apply this knowledge in their programme design. However, this is only half of the *picture. The other half is how we match this scientific knowledge with an equal understanding of you, the individual, and your specific exercise requirements.*

In this short piece I will seek to give you an appreciation of the complex nature of strength training. While we may not uncover what exact exercises work best for you, or what is the best way for you to execute them, I hope I will leave you with an appreciation that individualised exercise selection and coaching is important, and that there are various factors which may affect your ability to execute an exercise properly. My aim is not to equip you with the information required to design your own strength programme. This is beyond the scope of this piece. I am seeking to give you a broad overview of certain elements you may not have considered heretofore, and so develop your understanding in the area of strength training.

It is my contention that strength training is often over-simplified, misunderstood and poorly utilised. Strength training, and particularly youth strength training, must always be performed under the guidance of a qualified and experienced coach. Complex loaded exercises require expert coaching.

Individualising the Strength Programme

The concept of individualising a strength programme is simply not a case of using a percentage of maximum lifts for athletes, adjusting exercises based on athlete injury or adding exercises to programmes based on individual sports. These aspects should be considered more of a given in an athlete's programme.

True Individualised strength training takes into account many elements such as: chronological age, biological age (see Chapter 15), athlete training age and athlete assessment encompassing all their physical qualities – strength, power, aerobic endurance, injury history, movement quality and physical limitations. An in-depth discussion on each of these elements is beyond this piece. However, we will look at 'movement quality', an area I feel is critical for athletes and coaches. I hope this insight will give you an appreciation into the many variables that must be considered by the coach and that strength training is far from a 'one size fits all' activity.

Movement Quality Assessment

The mastery of movement quality assessment requires the coach to have some understanding of physics, biomechanics, musculoskeletal mobility and anthropometrics. This provides the coach with a knowledge of torque, levers, forces on the body etc. However, it is ultimately our 'coaching eye' that will determine our ability to put this knowledge into practice.

For each exercise I like to form a general image of the most effective way of executing it and cross reference this with scientific acumen. This allows me to place the athlete in the optimal position to apply force in the right direction, with the most appropriate mechanical advantage, without compromising joint integrity. Finally, I aim to fit you (the individual athlete) around this picture and adjust your position, if necessary, to meet the unique characteristics of your body's levers (e.g. length of arms/ legs).

The Straight Bar Deadlift

To provide an example of this process I will highlight how I take a specific exercise and adapt it, where possible, to suit the individual. I have chosen the Straight Bar Deadlift. Executed well, the straight bar deadlift is a great exercise to develop lower limb musculature and total body strength and coordination.
The purpose of the deadlift is to pull the bar from the floor, to a standing position. This must be performed by keeping the bar close to the body, while moving it through the shortest distance possible. This will dictate how we set up the athlete in relation to the bar.

Although it is a complex exercise and may not necessarily be a go-to exercise for the novice, I have selected it for a number of reasons:
- It is popularly seen as one of the 'Big Three' strength exercises and as such is used by many athletes, often without the aid of a professional and knowledgeable coach.
- It is an advanced strength exercise which is more often than not, performed poorly.
- It is an exercise that elicits fear in many quarters largely, in my opinion, due to it being poorly executed and poorly tailored to the athlete's needs.
- It is an exercise that does not suit a large percentage of the population for a number of reasons which we will look at.
- It is an exercise that the youth athlete often rushes into, without mastering the required foundational work.

Indeed, many strength coaches no longer use the straight bar deadlift because they feel it takes too long to coach and as a result, is a poor large-group, or team appropriate, exercise.

The Journey to the Exercise

I like to look at the deadlift as a journey of movement mastery, with the execution of the straight bar deadlift as the final destination. The same is true of many other complex lifts. A mistake that is often made by the novice athlete is to start the journey at the end point instead of at the beginning. We should never encourage the 'just lift' mentality. It is prudent to establish a sequence of steps for the athlete to master before attempting the straight bar. Every coach may form their own, but I have found the following extremely helpful.

- Quadruped Hip Extension – Helps teach the strong neutral spine position, whilst extending at the hip.
- Romanian Deadlift - Teaches standing bi-lateral hip extension with a minimal knee bend.
- Trap Bar Deadlift – Teaches us to pick something off the floor with some hip extension and a strong spine.
- Kettlebell Elevated Deadlift – teaches the same as above but with the hands in the specific pronated grip position required in the deadlift.
- Straight Bar Deadlift.

Coaching the Straight Bar Deadlift

The purpose of this example is not to detail the perfect straight bar deadlift technique or indeed suggest it as an exercise you should include in your programme. I am neither saying you must, or should, use the straight bar deadlift. I must also highlight that there are many less complex alternatives which can render similar outputs.

My purpose here is to highlight how an exercise can consist of many layers of complexity and how the coach must have the skill to alter it to suit the individual requirements of the athlete.

The Set Up

To help the athlete achieve their best 'form' I like to visualise the perfect deadlift and use this as a guide. I checklist this throughout the set-up phase.

The Feet	In general, I like to begin with a narrow stance with the feet inside the shoulder width and the toes pointing ahead. There will be degrees of freedom here; for example, some athletes may benefit from a more toes out position if their hips lack the necessary mobility to maintain the toes straight ahead. Poor hip mobility is a deadlift red flag for me. There is sufficient evidence at present to show the negative outcomes of long term lifting on immobile joints.
Grip Position	This is an area for debate. The traditional approach is for the athlete to have an alternate grip, i.e. one hand on top (pronated) - often the dominant hand and one hand underneath (supinated)-often the non-dominant or weaker hand. I feel there is value in alternating this grip position to avoid any lifting asymmetry, which can be caused by having a protracted or rounded shoulder on the pronated grip side and having a retracted shoulder on the supinated side. The double overhand grip is also another option.
The Shins	I feel this is the most important area of set up. The deadlift is best performed with a hinging pattern to allow the torque at the stronger hip musculature as opposed to it being at the weaker muscles surrounding the knee. This requires a vertical shin position; which in turn allows you to create a vertical line of force into the ground which has been shown to be preferential in execution of the lift.
Bar Position Relative to Shin	Close to if not at the shins. The further the bar is away from the shins the further it travels from the centre of mass of the athlete and consequently the more work it can potentially place on the spine, which can be troublesome for some.
Hip Position	In general terms, we are trying to find the hips optimal pulling height. A common mistake made by novices to the deadlift is starting with the hips too low. This turns the movement into a squat-type movement which is not an advantageous pulling position. Finding the optimal starting position will be highly dependent on your body type and limb lengths (see sample case below).
Spinal Position	Biomechanical analysis has taught us that the spine should be held in a neutral position throughout the lift. This is particularly true for beginners, where safety is paramount. We can see some rounding of the thoracic (upper spine) in advanced lifters as the weight exceeds the grip strength and spinal control of the athletes. This is the reality of lifting heavy and should only be seen in advanced athletes whose sport absolutely requires it.
Shoulders	At the start of the movement, the shoulders should be in line with the bar or slightly in front. This allows the athlete to bias the hip, countering the weaker squat position mentioned earlier.
Head	The head should be in a neutral position, like the spine. We can see a variety of neck positions, but excessive extension (head ack) sould be avoided. I prefer a more 'packed' chin tuck position.

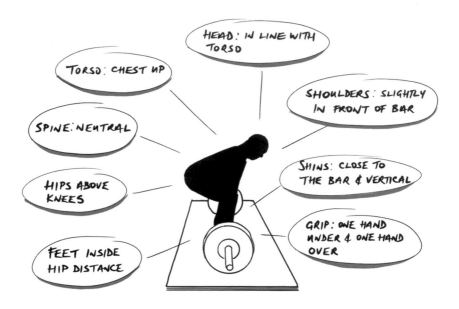

The next step is to tailor the exercise to meet the individual's body shape without compromising the integrity of the checklist above.

Sample Case

If I take myself for example, I have relatively short arms and a longer torso. This requires me to lower my body height or fold my joints through a greater range of motion. This, in turn, leaves me with a narrow hip angle at the bottom, and with my hips extremely far from the weight, which is certainly not optimal if seeking to apply high levels of force. It is widely accepted that the greater the hip joint is open, the greater torque that can be applied by the joint. A simple solution for me is to elevate the height of the bar with plates or boxes to simulate longer arms. This will mean I will not have to compress my joints as much, and I will achieve a more powerful open hip angle, which should allow me to load my body more safely. See video for contrast: https://www.youtube. com/watch?v=bsc3naDyDsw (QR Code 9)

Others may need to alter grip or stance width, while some may need to go with a different version of the lift for example:
- Wide Sumo Deadlift
- Modified Sumo Deadlift
- Rack Pulls
- Trap Bar Deadlift

Demonstrating and Cuing

What remains is the actual coaching element. Our ability as coaches, to successfully instruct, is critical to your long-term retention and transfer of movement skills into future sporting practice. It is commonly accepted that one can instruct in two ways:

- *The first is visually. This could involve showing you the said skill performed perfectly, i.e. providing a demonstration.*
- *The second way is verbal instruction. This may involve providing you with one or two cues that can attune your focus to the task at hand. This verbal information can either have an external (e.g. push the floor away from you) or internal focus (e.g. squeeze the glutes). Appropriate cuing can be extremely beneficial to help you to optimally execute an exercise*

In order to refine your movement patterns, it is then necessary to give feedback. This can come in various forms. Every athlete is unique, hence the importance of the coach being able to adapt to suit the individual. This is where the coach excels.

Summary

Although highlighting only a singular exercise I hope I have demonstrated the relative complexity of strength training. Certain individuals are suited to some exercises and others are not. The ability of the coach to spot this is a crucial skill for long-term athlete, and indeed coaching, success. Performing weighted lifts with poor form is simply not what strength training for athletic development is about. This is what has given strength training a bad name. It often leads to poor movement patterns, which can lead to muscular imbalances, which could cause future injury. This can, and must be, avoided.

Applying external load to the body requires a significant amount of emotional maturity on the athlete's behalf and expertise on that of the coach. Strength training, when performed properly, is an excellent training modality for you. However, strength training, when performed poorly for whatever reason, is both dangerous and counter-productive. My advice would be to find a knowledgeable professional coach and use their expertise to allow you to get to know your body and what works well for you. It is your body, so ultimately it is your responsibility as to how you nurture and develop it. I hope I have given you an understanding that strength training is not as straightforward as it may appear.

Best wishes,
Niall O'Toole

SUMMARY POINTS - Chapter 17

- *Strength creates a solid foundation from which you can develop all other athletic qualities i.e. speed, power, change of direction.*
- *Strength exercises are only as good as the athlete's ability to execute them properly.*
- *Strength training, when performed properly, is an excellent training modality for you.*
- *The coach must apply scientific knowledge with an equal understanding of the individual, and their specific exercise requirements.*
- *Complex unloaded and loaded strength exercises require expert coaching.*
- *Complex strength exercises are to be viewed as a journey of movement mastery, with the execution of the exercise as the final destination. A mistake that is often made by the novice athlete is to start the journey at the end point instead of at the beginning.*

CHAPTER 18: SPORT SPECIFIC SPEED

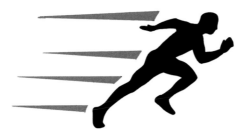

By John Duggan

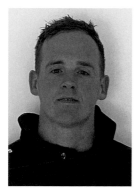

John Duggan is an accredited UKSCA S&C Coach with experience teaching and coaching across a multitude of sports throughout the world. He is currently lecturing in Strength & Conditioning/Sports & Exercise Sciences in Galway Mayo Institute of Technology, Galway. He is also a PhD candidate in Cardiff Metropolitan University researching training load monitoring in female GAA players. This chapter serves to provide you with general guidelines for sport specific speed (acceleration, upright sprinting and agility) and hopefully help increase your awareness of your sport specific speed technique. Practical recommendations are included, but again, it will never replace a good coach's eye.

Sports specific speed is a highly desirable quality frequently associated with successful sporting performance. It can be broken into three components: acceleration, upright sprinting and agility. Generally speed in sport is a game-changer. For example, straight linear sprinting is the most frequent action before goals are scored (for both the scoring and assisting player) in professional football (Haugen et al., 2019). Indeed, the Premier League Goal of the Season 2019/2020 saw Heung-Min Son gather the ball for Tottenham in his own defensive third and sprint the length of the pitch to score against Burnley FC. In a sporting context... speed kills!

To work on improving sport specific speed, we must break it down and build it back up again piece-by-piece. Speed can be broken into two phases: acceleration (take-off and build up) and maximum velocity (high speed running and maintenance). Acceleration is important to enable you to move quickly from a stationary position, moving/rolling start or getting off the ground (horizontal force application). Maximal running velocity (upright sprinting) enables you to transition quickly into attacking or defensive situations. In short, improving acceleration and upright sprinting technique will improve individual performance and reduce the potential risk of injuries.

In speed development, it is useful to have a technical model to work from. A technical model can help you determine where you need to work on and what you need to do to improve. In acceleration and upright sprinting, PAL (Gambetta, 2007) is a useful framework for both the athlete and the coach. PAL stands for Posture, Arm action, Leg action. Sport specific speed development is all about the position of the body or body shapes, and the PAL framework can help you optimise body shapes to improve sports specific speed. PAL can assist you during sport specific speed activities to develop good sprinting technique and become a faster athlete. See Figure 1 & 2 for positional cues on PAL for acceleration and upright sprinting.

Acceleration

During the acceleration phase, you need to increase the forward lean of your body to initiate movement, which helps increase horizontal force production (see Figure 1). Your posture should look like a straight line from foot to head on the take-off foot (back foot) and your front foot should be used to push hard into the ground to propel yourself forward. Optimal acceleration mechanics (see Figure 1) for athletes include:

- Starting Position- split stance, feet parallel, push down onto front foot (like a coiled spring), opposite elbow in line with front knee.
- Parallel shin and torso angle (front shin and torso should be parallel- they should look like a hashtag tilted at 45o).
- Forward trunk lean.
- Full extension of the back leg.
- Rapid and short step with the front foot so it contacts the ground immediately when the back leg is at fully extended.
- Powerful arm drive.

Figure 1: Optimal Acceleration Shapes for a Team Sport Athlete

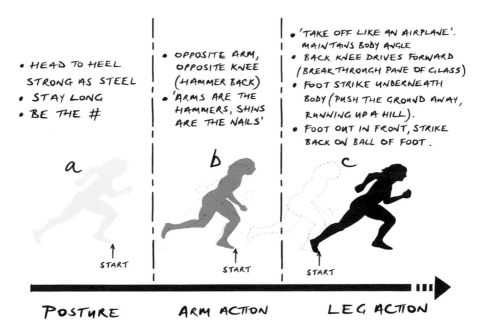

- HEAD TO HEEL STRONG AS STEEL
- STAY LONG
- BE THE #

a

↑ START

- OPPOSITE ARM, OPPOSITE KNEE (HAMMER BACK)
- 'ARMS ARE THE HAMMERS, SHINS ARE THE NAILS'

b

↑ START

- 'TAKE OFF LIKE AN AIRPLANE'. MAINTAINS BODY ANGLE
- BACK KNEE DRIVES FORWARD (BREAK THROUGH PANE OF GLASS)
- FOOT STRIKE UNDERNEATH BODY (PUSH THE GROUND AWAY, RUNNING UP A HILL).
- FOOT OUT IN FRONT, STRIKE BACK ON BALL OF FOOT.

c

↑ START

POSTURE   ARM ACTION   LEG ACTION

Acceleration Task
To check whether you are completing all the steps correctly, ask a coach or a friend to give feedback using the following checklist (Table 1).

You can also get feedback yourself by recording your technique with the video on your phone. Use the slow-motion app. to compare your positions against Figure 1 above and the checklist which follows:

Table 1: Acceleration Checklist

No.	Acceleration Coaching Checklist	Correct	Incorrect	What do I need to do better next time?
1	Toe Off - triple extension (45°), positive shin angle, torso and shin angle should be parallel (Figure 1a)			
2	Mid Flight - Back foot comes through- Piston like action (Figure 1b)			
3	Ankle Cross – back foot crosses over ankle (Figure 1b)			
4	Ground contact – Foot slightly in front or below (Figure 1c)			

Table 2: Suggested Progressions for Acceleration Development

You can include some of the following activities in warm-ups and training sessions that will improve your acceleration technique:

Level	
1	Wall Drill Posture Holds https://www.youtube.com/watch?v=-OEZybvQ3-0 (QR Code 10)
2	Wall Drill Acceleration Posture Switches https://www.youtube.com/watch?v=Kpkj9SmPKlI (QR Code 11)
3	Resisted Band Acceleration Marches https://www.youtube.com/watch?v=4M9vnnPtO9o (QR Code 12)
4	Resisted Band Acceleration Skips https://www.youtube.com/watch?v=Kc3-49wlQc8 (QR Code 13)
5	Partner Assisted Tall and Fall into Acceleration https://www.youtube.com/watch?v=Uo1lVZ0tgBU (QR Code 14)
6	Two-Point Acceleration Starts/False Step Start https://www.youtube.com/watch?v=WjN4m9MAnGM (QR Code 15)

Upright Sprinting

Optimal upright sprinting mechanics for field-based athletes include:

- *An upright body position where your hips are high to ensure you are travelling across the ground vertically (Figure 2a- imagine there is a piece of string attached to your head, pulling you up towards the sky).*
- *On your supporting leg (leg on the ground) the ankle, knee and hip should be fairly straight (Figure 2b). Torso and leg out in front of you should look like a hashtag # (Figure 2c).*
- *When your front foot is about to contact the ground (Figure 2c), it should be pointed towards the sky to take advantage of the elastic energy created by the muscle and tendons (like a rubber band).*
- *Your foot should hit the ground in line or very slightly in front of your hips (Figure 2a).*
- *Your opposite knee (in the air) should cross the knee on your standing leg as this the quickest and most efficient movement of the limb (Figure 2 b & c).*

You can practice efficient running mechanics in your warm-ups through: different types of skips (A, B, C skips), ankling, dribbles, pogos, low level plyometric type activities and rolling sprints type activities (see link to videos below). This is especially the case in-season when your primary focus is on sports specific skill development.

For an example of field-based athletes with good upright sprinting mechanics, see Gareth Bale https://www.youtube.com/watch?v=EK63Tpa1fZQ (QR Code 16) or Christen Press https://www.youtube.com/watch?v=R0JAMY2m2vl (QR Code 17) in action.

For upright sprinting positional cues, coaching checklist and progressions, see Figure 2 and Tables 3 and 4.

Figure 2: Optimal Upright Sprinting Shapes

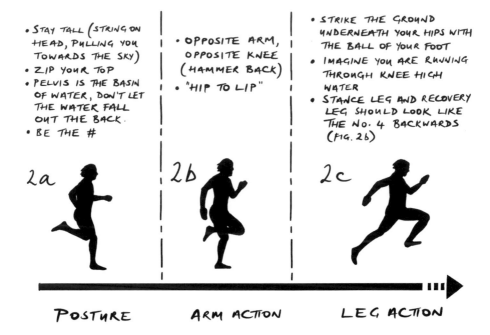

- STAY TALL (STRING ON HEAD, PULLING YOU TOWARDS THE SKY)
- ZIP YOUR TOP
- PELVIS IS THE BASIN OF WATER, DON'T LET THE WATER FALL OUT THE BACK.
- BE THE #

- OPPOSITE ARM, OPPOSITE KNEE (HAMMER BACK)
- "HIP TO LIP"

- STRIKE THE GROUND UNDERNEATH YOUR HIPS WITH THE BALL OF YOUR FOOT
- IMAGINE YOU ARE RUNNING THROUGH KNEE HIGH WATER
- STANCE LEG AND RECOVERY LEG SHOULD LOOK LIKE THE NO. 4 BACKWARDS (FIG. 2b)

2a   2b   2c

POSTURE   ARM ACTION   LEG ACTION

Upright Sprinting Task

To check whether you are completing the steps correctly, ask a coach or a friend to give feedback using the following checklist. You can also get feedback yourself by recording your technique with the video on your phone. Use the slow-motion app to compare your positions against Figure 2 above and the checklist below:

Table 3: Upright Sprinting Checklist

No.	Upright Sprinting Coaching Checklist	Correct	Incorrect	What do I need to do better next time?
1	Posture upright (Figure 2a)			
2	Pelvis neutral (Figure 2a)			
3	Powerful arm action (Figure 2b)			
4	Heel recovery is close to glute, knee crosses the standing leg, which needs to be driven up and forward, foot should be pointed up ready to hit the ground (Figure 2a & b)			
5	Foot contact on the balls of feet (Figure 2b)			
6	Foot contact underneath centre of mass (Figure 2b)			
7	Rapid cycle of recovery leg recovery (knee crosses knee of stance leg) (Figure 2b) with emphasis on positive front side mechanics (Figure 2c)			
8	Head up			

Table 4: Suggested Progressions for Upright Sprinting Development

You can include some of the following activities in warm-ups and training sessions that will improve your acceleration technique:

Level	
1	Ankling https://www.youtube.com/watch?v=Klm8mD1OizY (QR Code 18)
2	A skip https://www.youtube.com/watch?v=Da11WEU2ke8 (QR Code 19)
3	B skip https://www.youtube.com/watch?v=2DplrYCTpbY (QR Code 20)
4	Dribbles Bleeds https://www.youtube.com/watch?v=_5F70l3-lOo (QR Code 21)
5	Wickets https://www.youtube.com/watch?v=9Voi-QjkARE (QR Code 22)
6	Flying 60s (20m jog, 20m stride, 20m sprint)

Sport Specific Speed Development during Growth and Maturation

Pre-puberty is a time when the central nervous system is primed for physical and neurological development. This is a time when learning new skills should be prioritised (i.e. emphasise acceleration and sprint skill acquisition) (see Figure 3 in Chapter 15). Your brain during this period is essentially like a sponge, and this is considered a heightened window for learning new skills. In post-puberty, when your brain has stored the information (coordinated skill movement), this is a time when both males and females can take advantage of an increase in anabolic hormones. If you think about your body as an F1 car, in pre-puberty, you have started to develop the suspension, installed new tires and on-board technology (speed and agility motor skills stored in the brain). The test driving with the new specifications occurs during the growth spurt. This takes time to synchronise and get used to the new specifications. In post puberty it is time to build the engine- strengthening muscles, tendons, ligaments and skeleton. By the time you have reached adulthood, you have the complete F1 car with a fast engine, excellent breaks, solid suspension and the best on-board computer running all the systems in the car in synchronicity (coordinated movement).

From a training perspective, it is advised to focus on speed-strength (ability to execute movement against a small load i.e. bodyweight, medicine ball, resistance band etc.), strength-speed (ability to execute movement against a large load i.e. barbell jump squats, Olympic lifts, sleds etc.) and resisted modalities (e.g. sled marches, sled accelerations). Once technical proficiency has been mastered in post puberty, a combined/complex training (combining resistance training with similar plyometric movement, i.e. a weight squat with a standing long jump) may be used to obtain further transfer to speed and agility. Other advanced training methods can be utilised such as resisted/ assisted methods, once technical proficiency isn't directly affected by the training modality itself. Finally, exposure to maximal acceleration and sprints in sports specific environments i.e. skill and game-based scenarios is imperative once the fundamentals have been mastered.

Agility
Agility is the ability to change direction quickly in reaction to what you see in front of you. For example: when Virgil Van Dijk adjusts his feet to intercept the ball and start the attack, or Dean Rock uses a dummy solo to deceive a defender in Gaelic football, or when Serena Williams aggressively cuts and accelerates across the service line to return a shot from the opposite side of the court. These are all examples of agility related movements in sport specific environments.

Agility has two main components: change of direction (COD) speed and a perceptual/decision-making component. The COD speed is the physical component of agility, this requires strength and coordination to enable you to stop, change direction and re-accelerate into the specific movement based on what is in front of you in the game context. The decision-making element is often overlooked, as athletes must make rapid decisions in a split second. In youth male football, effective agility was one of the determining factors in predicting successful future performance (Mirkov et al. 2010).

If an individual lacks the ability to move effectively in an open, chaotic environment, they will be unable to apply their technical skills to the tactical requirements of the game. A good example of this is Johnny Sexton, the Irish rugby player, who is arguably not the fastest physically but has exceptional decision-making abilities and an innate skill for reading the game, to break the game line using his agility and deception.

A SAQ ladder should never be used to develop agility, as it lacks the specificity of decision making and encourages the athlete to look down. A ladder should only be used for DIY related tasks!

The development of both reactive agility and COD speed components are important. With the invasive nature of team sports, the ability to create space and penetrate through the defensive/offensive line is important to create scoring opportunities. This is where agility-based movements come into play. For a practical example of Cristiano Ronaldo using his exceptional agility (COD and decision making) skills see https://www.youtube.com/watch?v=hZqEj-Qyg6U (QR Code 23).

In youth, there are three components to agility development. These include Movement Efficiency (see Chapter 16), COD speed (deceleration ability, shuffle, side-step etc. in a closed environment), and Reactive Agility Training skills (previously mentioned skills in a sports specific environment, i.e. mirror drills, cat & mouse, tagging and chasing games, 1v1 situations etc.) (Lloyd et al. 2013). These specific qualities should be developed and mastered throughout growth and maturation.

An often-overlooked aspect of agility is deceleration. The athlete who decelerates the fastest allows themselves to make a better decision. Essentially, good deceleration allows your brain time to select the appropriate action for the next decision. A high proportion of severe sporting injuries (i.e. ACL) happen when an athlete is decelerating, so improvement here will protect your muscles, joints and limbs from serious injuries (F1 car, strengthening the suspension and quality tires). A rapid and efficient deceleration allows you to transition quickly into an attacking or defensive situation, side-step/deceive a defender to create a scoring opportunity or jockey an attacker with a good defensive stance to push them out towards the sideline and away from the scoring area. Learning how to correctly decelerate in order to make your movement qualities more efficient and prevent injuries is important.

The key components of deceleration are stopping as quickly as you can with the following optimal technique:
- *Feet should be shoulder width apart or slightly wider.*
- *Heel to toe like action to apply the brakes.*
- *Chest comes over knees at a 45° angle.*
- *Head is up scanning for the next movement.*

See video:
https://www.youtube.com/watch?v=36KWbuqN1jU (QR Code 24)

The beauty of this position (the athletic stance) is that it enables you to transition into the next movement like re-acceleration, turn shuffle etc. and so it puts you in the best position possible to make the first and hopefully the most decisive decision. A structured, integrated speed and agility program will enhance your ability to handle the high forces produced during COD and agility.

Training Prescription
Overall, development of sport specific speed tasks need to be short in duration (ranging from 20-60m depending on the speed or agility task). Maximal intent (between 85-95% intensity) needs to be encouraged throughout repetition. Therefore, the intensities of the tasks should be high, volume should be low and work to rest ratios should be relatively long (for every 10m sprinted = 60 seconds recovery). Furthermore, sets and reps recorded as meters covered per repetition can be progressively overloaded on a weekly basis. A good rule of thumb is to increase training load by 10% from the previous week with a week of reduced training load every four weeks. This will ensure appropriate physiological, psychological and technical improvement in the sports specific speed (See Table 5 for practical applications).

Case Study: Female Camogie Player
Mia is a 15-year-old corner forward playing camogie with her club. She is passionate about her game and is keen to become a better player. Mia feels she is not as fast or as agile as she used to be. She has noticed in games that she is lacking the ability to solo at speed and feels she lacks the ability to beat her marker in 1v1 situations. Following a positive discussion with her coach, they decided to implement the program below (Table 5) and to work on her speed and agility for 15 minutes before each training session for the next 6 weeks. The program will progressively overload the volume, intensity and reps in the coming weeks.

After a 6-week review, Mia feels lighter on her feet, faster, and has improved her ability to beat her marker in those 1v1 situations. In the next six weeks, they have decided to continue to implement the sports specific speed training before her main sessions as her technical proficiency has improved significantly. They will also continue to work on PAL shapes and mechanics for all components of sports specific speed.

Best wishes,
John Duggan.

Table 5: Sport Specific Speed Training Prescription for Mia

Session 1: Upright Sprinting	Session 2: Agility
Warm Up	*Warm Up*
• Work Time: <5secs • Distance Run: 10-60m max • Reps per set: 2-4 • Total sets per session: 2-4 • Total distance per rep 20m-60m • Total distance per set 60m -300m • Intra set recovery 45-60 secs per 10m run of maximum upright sprinting • Inter set recovery 1.5 – 2x intra-set recovery	• Work Time: <5secs • Distance Run: 10-40m max • Reps per set: 2-4 • Total sets per session: 2-4 • Total distance per set 10m-40m • Total distance per 60m -200m max • Intra set work: recovery ratio: 1:6

Adapted from Duggan et al. 2020

References:

Duggan JD, Moody JA, Byrne P, Ryan L. Strength & Conditioning Recommendations for Female GAA athletes: The Camogie Player. Strength Cond J 42: 105-124, 2020.

Gambetta V, Athletic Development: The Art & Science of Functional Sports Conditioning. Champaign, IL: Human Kinetics, 2007.

Haugen T, Seiler S, Sandbakk O, and Tonnessen E. The training and development of elite sprint performance: an integration of scientific and best practice literature. Sports Med 5: 1-16, 2019.

Jeffreys I. Gamespeed: Movement Training for Superior Sports Performance. 2nd ed. Monterey, CA: Coaches Choice, 2017.

Mirkov DM, Kukolj M, Ugarkovic D, Koprivica VJ Jaric S. Development of anthropometric and physical performance profiles in young elite male soccer players: a longitudinal study. J Strength Con Res 23: 2677-2682, 2010.

Lloyd RS, Read P, Oliver JL, Meyers RW, Nimphius S, Jeffreys I. Considerations for the development of agility during childhood and adolescence. Strength Cond J 35:2-11, 2013.

SUMMARY POINTS - Chapter 18

- *Remember PAL.*
- *Technical proficiency is King!*
- *The best way to run fast is to run fast!*
- *Acceleration = horizontal force production.*
- *Max velocity = vertical force production.*
- *Be the hashtag (#)*
- *For every 10m run = 60 seconds rest to ensure optimal velocity.*
- *Agility = COD speed and decision-making skills.*
- *For agility development, context is god- practice in environments that replicate your sport.*

CHAPTER 19 : INJURY & REHABILITATION

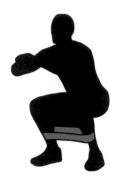

By Donie Fox

Injury is part of sport. In certain circumstances there is nothing you can do to prevent it, but there are many times you can certainly protect against it. Understanding and rationalising pain is the first step in learning about your body and injury. One of the struggles I frequently see with younger athletes is learning the difference between injury and pain. Pain is subjective and fully individual. Injury is quantifiable, we can test it and measure it.

Pain does not always mean damage; it is simply a sensation and a signal. It is highly complex but in simple terms pain starts off as a warning signal - a response to a perceived threat. In this way, pain can be a sign of imminent injury or a protective mechanism against further injury. The longer pain goes on, however, the more complex it becomes. The relationship between threat and pain becomes cloudy and sometimes disconnected. It is important for us all to remember that pain is always real, though it may not always be reliable in terms of assessing injury.

In order to rationalise and understand your body and how it reacts to training and stress it is important to define a few things:
- *Soreness from training is not an injury. It usually does not prevent you from training or playing. Yes, it is painful but there is no particular structure that is torn/fractured/bruised/inflamed. Soreness from training is feedback. It tells you how prepared your body was for the session you did. If there is excess soreness then either the body was underprepared or the coach/ athlete overestimated the body's ability.*
- *Sometimes you will get local soreness in a particular area; what most people would describe as 'a niggle'. In these instances, pain*

is telling you that some structure here is getting irritated. I like to refer to these niggles as 'hot spots'. For the most part, in these cases, continuing to play and train will aggravate the issue and can lead to an outright injury. It is important that you don't decide whether you play or not yourself. You should seek out advice from a physiotherapist or doctor and get the issue sorted before it becomes more serious.

- *'Time loss injuries' occur out of the blue or result from 'hot spots' for the most part. This is when it is next to impossible for you to train or play without obvious and major compensation to how you move or play/perform. How serious this injury is or seems dictates how you proceed. Particularly during the developmental periods of your life it is of utmost importance to follow the most appropriate plan of care laid down by a health professional.*

Why an Injury Occurs

Injuries occur for different reasons and at different times. There are certain hallmarks we look for when trying to diagnose an injury or figure out why it occurred in the first place. A simple classification of injury we use is acute or chronic/overuse. Acute injuries are those which occur all of a sudden, usually with a clear mechanism of injury. These include: bone fractures, bone bruises, muscle strains, ligament strains, contusions, tendon strains. Chronic or overuse injuries are those which occur over time, usually with a protracted history. These include: stress fractures, tendinopathies, apophysitis injuries, nerve irritations. Sometimes there will be a crossover where a chronic issue may undergo an acute loading and present like an acute injury.

<u>*See Appendix for a more comprehensive breakdown of injuries.*</u>

With any injury we look into why it happened. It is rarely ever just a case of bad luck.

- *Intrinsic risk factors (those things which are part of your own body and how it functions) include: bone density, strength, range of motion, previous injury, skeletal development, illness, lifestyle, physical literacy*
- *Extrinsic risk factors (those things which are not part of your body, as well as the things you do to your body) include: equipment, training errors, weather, surface, opponents, refereeing.*

Some sports come with a higher risk of injury and with different injury profiles: Contact versus non-contact sports. Speed versus endurance sports. Tactical versus technical sports. It is important we accept the risk within our chosen sports and prepare appropriately for that risk.

The majority of our intrinsic risk factors are modifiable and thus trainable. It is usually the role of the coaches to ensure that the extrinsic injury risk is minimised for each athlete they are responsible for.

I Think I'm Injured

If you think you may be injured then it is important to figure out what the most appropriate next step is. Usually this comes down to the severity of pain or how obvious an injury may seem. With more painful and obvious injuries such as fractures, dislocations and complete muscle or tendon ruptures, then the most appropriate path to follow is to attend the Accident & Emergency unit. For the less obvious, but still painful issues, it may be less clear.

The POLICE Principle is something you can use to treat the initial stage of acute soft tissue or structural injuries. The steps involved are: Protection, Optimal Loading, Rest, Ice, Compression, and Elevation and should be applied within the first 24 to 72 hours immediately after an injury. This should control the amount of swelling to the injured area, prevent further injury, reduce pain and quicken your recovery and rehabilitation.

Protection	Prevent further injury through use of crutches, a sling or a boot etc.
Optimal Loading	The right amount of activity can help manage swelling and quicken recovery while in some cases complete rest would prevent this.
Rest	Rest is important to allow for healing. You should avoid activities that stress the injured area to the point of pain or that may slow or prevent healing. However, as with the above, some movement is often beneficial.
Ice	The most common way to do this is a simple plastic bag of peas or ice placed over a towel on the affected area. Limit the cold exposure to 15 minutes. Cycles of 15 minutes on and 1 to 2 hours off are generally more effective than longer periods of continuous ice application.
Compression	Use a compression wrap, such as an elastic bandage, to apply external force to the injured tissue helps minimise swelling and provides mild support.
Elevation	Helps reduce the pooling of fluid in the injured limb or joint.

If you are struggling to perform basic tasks at home such as walking or dressing then you should attend your GP or chartered physiotherapist for an examination.

In other cases, unless there is obvious worsening with time alone, then a few days rest from strenuous activity is usually best. Gradually reintroducing some basic athletic development work (see Chapter 16) will give you an indication whether you may be ready to resume training or need professional advice. Regardless, it is important to continue to move frequently rather than fully resting. Do what you can pain-free and make note of what you are struggling with. These notes will inform both you and the physiotherapist/doctor about what structures are affected and how best to proceed.

During a physiotherapy assessment you will be asked questions about your activity prior to the injury, the injury itself and what you've been doing since. It can be very helpful to make note of these things prior to the session so that all of the relevant information is shared. The physical part of the assessment will usually involve some movement tests followed by some testing of the injured area. Based on this information the physio will devise a plan of care for you to return to activity and sport. This plan will dictate what you can't do for the short term but more importantly will describe what you can do to get back to sport.

I am Injured
This is when the work begins. You've been given a diagnosis and a plan of care. It is important to be diligent here - contact your physiotherapist if you have any questions.
You may not be allowed to sprint or butterfly or hit drives but:
- *Can you strike a ball off a wall?*
- *Can you swim backstroke?*
- *Can you practice putting?*

Now is the opportunity to work on and master something you may have neglected.

You should still attend scheduled training sessions if feasible. You can help out your teammates and learn a lot by simply watching practice and chatting to coaches and players. There are things we cannot see when we are taking part ourselves and this may be the perfect opportunity to get a different perspective on your sport. It may even be a great time to catch up on study, piano practice or visiting your grandmother. Take some time away from sport if you feel you might benefit from it. A break can be very important to realise how important, or not, your sport is to you.

I Think I'm OK

Staying in regular contact with your physiotherapist and reviewing with them when you begin to feel better is very important in successfully returning to sport. Your physiotherapist may have things for you that can bridge the gap to return to full training. At this point you should now be taking part in some portions of team or coached practice. It is vital at this stage that you continue to follow the physiotherapist's guidelines and not jump in at the deep end. Many injuries can recur if too much is done too soon. Be patient, be diligent and wait until you are given the green light.

I Am OK

Now you are back training and playing. It is always prudent to continue some of the physiotherapist's rehabilitation exercises in your athletic development sessions. This will ensure that you are continuing to build support for the old injury so that it doesn't recur sooner or later. Any risk factors that the physio highlighted in your assessment should be addressed in some degree by now. Be sure not to slip into bad habits and neglect what your body needs to stay healthy.

The Gift of Injury

While painful and irritating for the most part, injury can be a nice time to reflect on our sport. It can be a gift whereby we get some time to iron out kinks, address issues in our lifestyle or gain some perspective. While easy to become frustrated with not being allowed to play or train, you must stay positive and look for the little wins.

Best wishes,
Donie Fox

Michael Fennelly

Michael Fennelly is a highly decorated former Kilkenny and Ballyhale Shamrocks hurler. Throughout his playing career, he won eight Senior All-Irelands with his county and five All-Ireland Club titles with Ballyhale Shamrocks. He is a former Hurler of the Year, as well as a three time All-Star. He is currently the Offaly Senior Hurling Manager. Injury is a very personal experience and not purely a physical one. Michael paints a very real picture of his struggles with injury and how he made the best of the situations he encountered.

Unfortunately, injuries played a big part in my hurling career. Here, I will give you an insight into some of the more serious ones that shortened my playing time with club and county. Ankle injuries came first in my early twenties, two of them costing me three months each. I then went on to break the scaphoid bone in both of my wrists; twice in my right one and I had a screw implanted in my left. I also broke a metacarpal bone in my right hand during the 2011 season when I won 'Player of the Year'. In terms of soft tissue injuries, reoccurring hamstring tears and strains plagued me throughout my career. Serious back issues began to surface in my mid-twenties with bulging discs, and a protrusion in two of the discs. There was other issues with my back, which mystified specialists at times, and caused me a lot of doubt and frustration. It was something I learned, with great difficulty, to manage. A ruptured Achilles in my left leg in 2016 was a major blow, especially as by then I was in my early thirties. It brought a prolonged and challenging rehab period, over the course of seven to eight months. A micro fracturing procedure of my right knee was one of my final big ones in 2019, which needed approximately six to seven months rehab.

Sometimes, you are more predisposed to injury due to your mechanical make up, and sometimes your playing style and position, can leave you more prone to contact injuries and bone breaks. On reflection, I believe I fell into both categories. With regard to injury: some of it is bad luck, some of it can be avoided and some of it can only be managed.

Injury can be frustrating with thoughts of blame, negativity and emptiness. I missed numerous games with my club and county. I found it very difficult. I always felt I was letting my teammates down. In 2016, I missed an All-Ireland final for Kilkenny, followed 6 weeks later by a

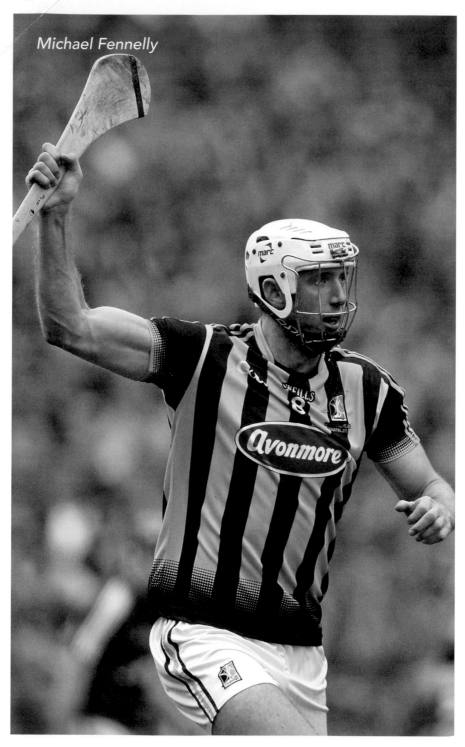

Michael Fennelly

county final with Ballyhale Shamrocks. We came out on the wrong side on both occasions. Being on crutches for those games was devastating. There is nothing you can do to help, only encourage your teammates and not let your disappointment be seen. I was lucky I didn't miss many more finals through injury. In my misfortune with injuries, I was fortunate in that they mostly came early in the year. Always be grateful for small mercies.

Prehabilitation work became central to my training and gym work as I strove to reduce the incidence of injury. My aim was go the extra mile, attention to detail, thorough preparation. I leaned on expertise, and sought and listened to those who I felt could help me. A comprehensive strengthening, activation and mobility warm-up became central to keeping my body as healthy as possible and reducing my chances of injury. I can't emphasise enough the importance of doing your prehab/ activation work before your training and gym sessions. It is often not until athletes get older that they realise this, and in many cases, it can be too little too late.

Any time I received a major injury, I would have initially been very 'down on myself' and withdrawn from friends and family. I never blamed anyone for my injuries and even though I felt heartache and misery, my focus would quickly move to what I needed to do to get back to full health and fitness. I never looked for excuses, or blame, even though you might want to at times. These negative thoughts are like weeds that strangle your self-belief. I looked at injury as a challenge where I would have to prove my worthiness to get back on the team, and become even better and stronger. This perspective was crucial.

During the rehab phase of any injury I would focus on other elements of my game that would need improving. You may be restricted in terms of what you can do due to your injury, but you can always improve in some component whether its skill, nutrition, strength or flexibility for example.

As time would tick by, my appetite to get back playing would grow and grow. Being at matches, where I couldn't play due to injury, would make me reflect on the privileged position I had as a hurler. Being able to play for both my club and county was a gift, and injury made me realise it was a gift that should be cherished and that it wouldn't last forever. Every game became more and more important to me as I grew older, and I would play each one as if it were my last.

Please don't take it all for granted, there will be setbacks in your playing career, but how you respond to them will determine your future. Becoming a stronger and more resilient teenager both physically and mentally, will support your transition to adulthood later in life. Enjoy the journey and prepare yourself as best you can.

'You never see a crowd on the extra mile'

Best wishes,
Michael Fennelly.

Joe Carbery

Joey Carbery is an Irish and Munster rugby player. He had been a European Champions Cup and Pro14 winner with Leinster before moving to Munster to actively seek a new challenge. He also won a Six Nations Championship with Ireland in 2018. He is seen by many as a prodigious talent and noted for bravery in play. Unfortunately, at the time of writing, he is a player who has struggled with injury for an extended period. Here Joey tells his story of how he has dealt with his injuries and looks forward to returning to play a better player and person.

I play rugby, a sport where injury is common and can sometimes define a career. If you pick up a serious injury, or a series of injuries for example, around contract negotiation time, it can have a significant effect on whether you are kept on or let go. This can add a huge amount of stress and anxiety at a period when you are already struggling.

Up until a little over a year ago, I was fortunate enough to get away with only a couple of minor injuries. Then, in the middle of the 2019 Six Nations campaign, I tore my hamstring. Eight weeks later I re-tore the same hamstring 30 minutes into my first game back. This led me to miss most of the business end of the year. I returned to fitness to play the last game of the season. Our annual summer break followed and I returned to Ireland training in preparation for the Rugby World Cup 2019. Training went well that summer and I was feeling great coming into the warm-up games. I broke my ankle in the first warm-up game against Italy and it required surgery. After much painstaking work, I managed to still make the World Cup squad, but then returned home to face another two months rehab on the same ankle. In my second club game back against Ulster, I damaged ligaments in my wrist that required surgery. During the recovery from surgery, I was advised by an ankle specialist that I needed another procedure on my ankle.

Looking back on this year, it has been a whirlwind of emotions. The main and most obvious emotion has been disappointment. Every time I have suffered an injury, it has been in the middle of or just before very important games. The hardest part of being injured for me is missing out on big games and not having the opportunity to do my thing on the biggest stage. It has been heartbreaking. Not being able to go out with my teammates and best friends and help them out. The best I can do is cheer them on from the sidelines. The days are a lot longer and drawn

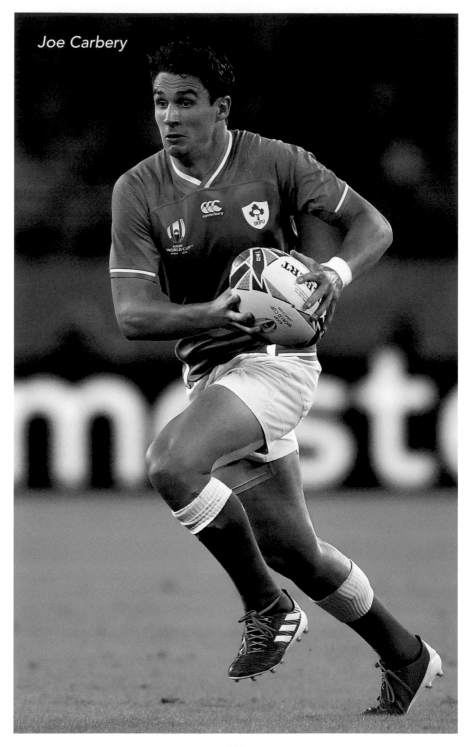

Joe Carbery

out when you're injured. I start earlier, have tough sessions alone, and cannot play the game I love.

From being injured a lot over the last year, I've had some time to think about how I can get the most out of this situation and how I will come back a better player and a better person. I have tried to create a mindset whereby my aim is to get better each day. Every gym session, every wattbike work-out, every rehab session; my goal is to improve. I think of it as like building a brick wall. Each session I am adding another brick. I'm motivated to come back stronger and faster, so I can hopefully avoid another injury setback.

I'm very fortunate to have great physios and coaches around me to help me during these times. They help me with rehab, strength and rugby specific skill sessions I can do without irritating the injury. Without them, it would be so much harder. They also help a huge amount with the mental side of the injury. Being able to chat to them daily about worries or concerns is a massive benefit. They can reassure me that I am on the right path and doing absolutely everything to return as soon as possible, while also being able to have a bit of fun and make it somewhat enjoyable. Small games in between sessions, or simply changing up the regular routine into a more stimulating day; little things like this go a long way to help me stay positive and mentally engaged.

A major skill I have learned from being injured is the ability to listen to my body and to then be able to relay this back to the medical staff. Sometimes I have said I was good to go, when deep down I knew that I wasn't 100 percent. This is because I'm so eager to get back out on the grass. This is not a good thing, and I'm lucky to have learnt this lesson at an early age. Usually, your body knows more than any test or scan. Scans are incredibly important and can give great clarity surrounding the nature of the injury; however, when it comes to rehab and returning to training and games, you've got to listen to your body and make sure that it feels as good as possible. It's something I am now fully committed to and is going to be the main indicator as to when I return. A huge component of this is being able to trust your doctor and physio that they will not look past how you actually feel. They must listen and sometimes put their egos to the side and allow the player to speak their mind.

While being injured, I have tried to improve my rugby knowledge. I spend time watching games and training clips to keep my rugby stimulus sharp. Chatting to the relevant coaches about rugby and ways in which we can do things better, helps a lot as well. It presents an opportunity to grow my rugby brain and see things differently. By doing this, I will not have to catch up on as much, when I do return to training and games.

Being injured sucks, but it is a part of the game I love. It is a time where you have a lot of time away from your team, often rehabbing and going to the gym alone, without getting to play. Remaining positive, focused and trying to learn and improve are so important. I fully believe that you can return a better player after an injury. Working and training hard, along with a combination of rest, spending time with friends and family and having a good team around you enable this.

Best of luck,
Joey Carbery
September 2020

Reference:
Brukner, P. & Khan, K., Brukner & Khan's Clinical Sport's Medicine. 4th edn. Syndney, Australia: McGraw-Hill Australia (2012)

SUMMARY POINTS - Chapter 19

- Pain is subjective and fully individual. Injury is quantifiable and can be tested and measured.
- Injuries occur for different reasons and at different times.
- The POLICE Principle is something you can use to treat the initial stage of acute soft tissue, or structural injuries.
- If you feel you are injured you should attend your GP or chartered physiotherapist for an examination.
- Occasionally, injury can be more psychologically challenging than physically challenging.
- Commit to your rehabilitation under the direction and guidance of a quality physiotherapist. Go the extra mile!
- Injury can be an opportunity to focus on other elements of your game, or parts of your life.
- Stay in regular contact with your physiotherapist and review your progress with them.
- The aim should to return from injury a better athlete than the one who left.
- On your return from injury, continue some of the physiotherapist's rehabilitation exercises in your warm ups and athletic development sessions.

CHAPTER 20: NUTRITION

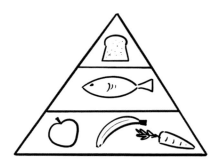

By Michael Day

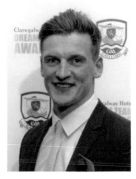

Michael Day is a Performance Nutritionist and Sports Scientist. He provides nutrition education and support to athletes of all ages at club and intercounty level, along with high performance athletes at 3rd level colleges.

I have asked Michael to share with you the Fundamentals of a 'Food first' Approach to Performance Nutrition.

Introduction

Achieving your nutritional requirements is not only essential in order for you to reach peak performance, it will allow for your healthy growth and development, reducing the chances of injury and sickness. This will allow you to have greater participation in sport which is the overall aim. Furthermore, the timing of nutritional intake before and after activity is critical in order for you to maximise performance adaptations. Over the course of this section, appropriate nutrition required for health and athletic performance, along with timing of intake will be discussed and practical recommendations provided to help achieve these goals.

Youth athletes that follow appropriate nutrition guidelines for their sport will have adequate energy to sustain high performance, prevent muscle breakdown, accelerate recovery, and reduce symptoms of hunger and sickness. While there is a greater energy requirement for youth athletes compared to their sedentary counterparts, the food sources recommended for optimizing athletic performance are very similar to those recommended for optimal health. When guiding the youth athlete to attain adequate calories, I would recommend a diet rich in whole grain carbohydrates, fruit, vegetables, lean animal and vegetable protein. Following a diet rich in these nutrients will allow you to be adequately fuelled for performance, along with reaching vitamin and mineral requirements, essential for your physical growth and repair[1].

What to eat and where to get it?

The Eatwell Guide displayed in Figure 1 is a good resource for you to see what sources you can get your food from[2]. The three macronutrients you will be in taking are carbohydrates, protein and fats. These three macronutrients all play a vital role in your sporting performance and overall development. Each of these make up a percentage of your daily calorie needs and should be met to improve performance.

Due to the high volume of training undertaken by youth athletes, having enough energy is crucial so you don't fatigue early, impacting performance. Carbohydrates are the fuel that will provide this energy so 55-65% of daily intake of calories should come from healthy carbohydrate sources shown in the Eatwell Guide i.e. whole grains, fruit, vegetables, milk and yoghurts. Protein is an essential part of the young athlete's diet, and the role of protein for you includes building, maintaining, and repairing muscle and other body tissues. Between 15-25% of a youth athletes' diet should come from good quality protein sources i.e. lean meat and poultry, fish, eggs, dairy products, beans and nuts. Finally, 20-30% of your daily calorie intake should come from healthy fats i.e. olive oils, oily fish, nuts, seeds, avocados. Healthy fats are important for the absorption of fat-soluble vitamins (A, D, E and K) allowing immune function to work at its optimum, which is important to help prevent fatigue and illness. This will help reduce sessions missed and chances of injuries occurring[4].

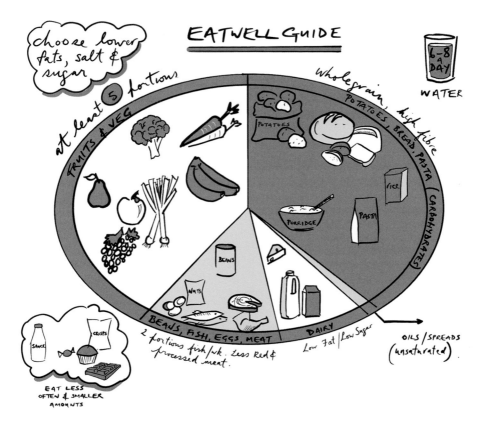

Figure 1. Adapted from Eatwell Guide from Public Health England

Carbohydrates – What are they and what do they do?

Adequate consumption of carbohydrates supports usual training intensity along with promoting recovery. If the intensity or duration of the session is high, then the carbohydrate requirements increase. So, depending on your sport, level and weight, carbohydrate requirements will differ. Those playing and training regularly in high intensity sports i.e. GAA, soccer, rugby, boxing, swimming etc. require approximately 4-6g of carbohydrates per kg of body weight daily, i.e. 70kg athlete will need to take in 280-420g of carbohydrates daily to be adequately fuelled for performance and to promote adequate recovery, reducing injury prevalence. As for athletes who regularly compete and train for longer duration sports which can last 90 minutes i.e. cross country running, long distance running, road cyclists etc. the requirements are higher. These athletes need to be consuming eight to 10g per kg of body weight daily i.e. 70kg athlete requires between 560-700g of carbohydrates daily to be adequately fuelled for performance and to promote adequate recovery, reducing injury prevalence. Therefore, it is essential that each day you are getting in enough healthy carbohydrates from the sources listed in Table 1.

Table 1. Sources of Carbohydrates and what ones to choose

Choose More	**Choose Less**
Potatoes with skin – Normal or Sweet baked with olive oil boiled in unsalted water	Skinless potatoes made with high amounts of butter, salt. Butter fried/ baked
Rice – wholegrain or basmati	Rice – low fibre white. Highly sweetened versions
Cereals – Normal porridge oats, Weetabix	Cereals – High sugar cereals
Fruit – All types of fruit, honey, dried fruit	Fruit juices, sports drinks
Pasta – whole grain options	Low fibre white versions. Carbonaras
Bread – brown breads, brown pitta	Bread – White or fruit breads. Cakes
Grains – Quinoa, lentils, bulgur wheat, couscous	Grains – Highly sweetened versions
Snacks – wholegrain rice cakes, corn cakes	Snacks – jellies, highly sweetened snacks
Vegetables – All types	Vegetables with high sugar, salt, butter additives

Once consumed in the diet, carbohydrates are stored as glycogen in the muscles and liver. Pre-exercise consumption of carbohydrates in the hours and days leading up to exercise has been found to increase the glycogen stores in the muscle, leading to reductions in fatigue. If exercise is lasting longer than 60 minutes, consuming some fast-acting carbohydrates can help reduce fatigue onset. It has been reported that the body only needs approximately 30g per hour, so not a huge amount. Many sports gels contain these. Even one to two mouthfuls of sports drinks with a cereal bar can do the trick, but trialling this in training is highly recommended as is keeping these types of foods to training and competition days[3].

Figure 2 gives a visual of how much carbohydrates should be consumed during exercise depending on duration. Following exercise, it is extremely important to consume a meal within 30-60 minutes to maximise recovery, in order to get the most out of each session[3]. If adequate post exercise nutrition is not ingested fast enough, even if a delay by only a couple of hours, there is a decrease in muscle glycogen storage and protein replenishment. So, make sure not to miss this window of opportunity. This meal must contain a mixture of carbohydrates and protein. Both complement each other well, to maximise recovery.

A quick and easy recovery meal that you can have with you can be 500ml of milk, 1-2 pieces of fruit and 1-2 handfuls of trail mix. This will provide you with what you need along with helping rehydrate the body

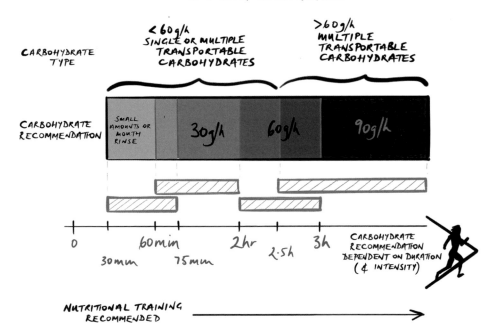

FIGURE 2: RECOMMENDATIONS FOR CARBOHYDRATE INTAKE DURING EXERCISE

Carbohydrate Sources – What is best?

Table 1 shows where carbohydrates should be sourced from the majority of the time i.e. fruits, vegetables, wholegrains. There are many reasons why these should be consumed. They are nutrient dense, contain high amounts of vitamins and allow for a slow release of energy, maintaining a steady blood sugar level. Consistent long-term consumption leads to healthier lives and increased performance. A wide variety of colour should be taken in through the diet to get the greatest number of vitamins, minerals and fibre in the diet. This can be achieved through *increasing fruit and vegetable content of meals. Immune function and body composition are highly likely to improve from implementing this policy.*

In addition to nutrient density, glycaemic index or load should be considered. Glycaemic index or load of an individual food or meal is a measure of how quickly it causes blood sugar levels to rise and fall. Foods high in glycaemic index/load usually contain highly added or refined sugars that can be seen in Table 1 i.e. sweets, white bread, cereal bars, sugary drinks etc. These foods will cause blood sugar to spike and dip rapidly, not providing sustained energy and should be avoided in most situations. They can play a role during exercise as fast acting sources of energy but other than that should be avoided. Alternatively, foods low in glycaemic index/load can maintain steady blood sugar levels throughout the day and during exercise, which not only influences physical performance positively, but also aids in maintaining mental performance and reduction in excess calorie intake later in the day[3].

Protein – What is it and what does it do?

Protein plays a critical role in an athlete's diet and should be consumed through a variety of sources daily. It promotes growth and repair of muscle, hair, nails and skin. While it is not a primary fuel source during high intensity exercise like carbohydrates, protein can aid the recovery of muscle glycogen, delaying onset of fatigue. Furthermore, it strengthens the immune system through growth and repair of the cells within the body.

There are varying recommendations for protein intake, with a lot of this coming down to the level of activity of the individual. As a general recommendation for maintaining health in the non-active population, protein intake should be between 0.8 and 1.2 grams of protein per kg of body mass daily i.e. 70kg individuals will need to take in 56-84g of protein daily. This recommendation has been found to be adequate to meet the bodily demands of 97.5% of the population[7]. The American College of Sports Medicine recommends the active youth and adult athletes should be consuming between 1.2 and 1.8g/kg of body mass to sufficiently deal with the load of their activity by promoting muscle growth and repair. Regularly doing this will also help the body adapt to the training load, improving performance.

Table 2. Sources of Proteins and what ones to choose

Choose More	Choose Less
Skinless Chicken and Turkey with no added sauce	Breaded or marinated turkey/chicken
Skinless Fish with no added sauce	Breaded or marinated Fish
>90% Lean Meats	<90% Meat Versions
Butcher Meats (Less salt and additives)	Packaged and cured meats
Tuna in Springwater	Tuna in brine or sunflower oil
Low fat dairy products with no added sugar	Full fat dairy products with added sugars
Grains – Beans, Quinoa, lentils	Grains – Highly sweetened versions
Eggs	Eggs with excessive butter and salt added
Nuts, seeds and 100% nut butters	High added sugar versions (Chocolate/Yoghurt)

Protein – What is best?

Table 2 gives a good guide where to source protein from the majority of the time i.e. lean meats, breadless meat and fish and grains. In most developed countries, youth athletes appear to meet protein requirements[8]. This shows that there is no need to use protein supplements as a youth athlete if the diet contains rich amounts of protein daily. The main thing is to get protein intake from the good sources highlighted in Table 2.

Fats – What are they and what do they do?

Fat is the major fuel source for low and moderate intensity exercise. Fat is necessary to absorb fat-soluble vitamins (A, D, E, K), to provide essential fatty acids, aiding immune function, which is crucial to reduce onset of illnesses and fatigue[3]. Fat, like protein, also provides the feeling of fullness. However, it is the most calorie-dense source of energy (one gram provides nine calories) and is more difficult to use during exercise. Daily intake of fat should be 1 gram per kg of body weight i.e. 70kg individual requires 70g of fat. Daily consumption of saturated fats should exceed no more than 20g with the remainder coming from polyunsaturated and monounsaturated, heart healthy, fats.

Fat Sources – What is best?

Good sources of fat are polyunsaturated and monounsaturated (Omega 3 and 6) as seen in Table 3, and they include lean meat, oily fish, nuts, seeds, low fat dairy products, olive and seed oils. Deep fat fried foods, creams, butters, highly processed meats and baked goods should be minimized. Consuming high amounts of these types of foods are not good for health or youth athlete's performance goals. Substituting the good sources of fat for the bad sources will aid in healthy bodily function and possible performance improvement. As such, youth athletes will benefit from focusing on foods containing healthy, rather than unhealthy, fat sources for long term health.

Table 3. Sources of Fat and what ones to choose

Choose More	Choose Less
Olive, vegetable and seed oils for frying	Coconut oils and butters for frying
Oily Fish (Mackerel and Salmon)	Breaded or deep fried
>90% Lean Meats	<90% Meat Versions
Butcher Meats (Less salt and additives)	Packaged and cured meats
Nuts, seeds and 100% nut butters	High added sugar versions (Chocolate/ Yoghurt)
Low fat dairy products	Full fat dairy products
Freshly baked foods from home	Store bought baked goods

Fluids

Fluids, especially water, play an important role in all athlete's diets. The amount, timing and type of fluid that is ingested can play a significant role in your performance. Water is the best source of hydration for your performance. Drinking adequate water before, during and after exercise can help you perform more effectively and for a longer duration, along with aiding the recovery process through replenishment of fluids lost in sweat. Sports drinks can play a role to, but only in long distance or high intensity competitions to provide energy and hydration. During normal training and daily activity, they are not needed and may have negative health and/or performance implications if taken excessively[4]. Hydrate through water instead and make sure to do this daily. The better the hydration, the better your body will work.

When hydration levels are poor, your physical and mental performance can decline especially in hot, humid conditions or longer duration activities. Figure 3 gives a good breakdown of the side effects linked with a poor hydration status during exercise[9].

A good guideline on how much water to consume daily is to multiply 35ml by body weight i.e. 70kg individual must consume 2450ml minimum daily and an extra one litre for every hour of exercise completed in the day. Recent research on how dehydration affects performance found that athletes who lost 2% of body weight during exercise i.e. 1.4kg for a 70kg athlete, resulted in a 20% decrease in performance during normal temperatures and up to 40% in hotter climates[10]. It is vital that water is consumed throughout activity to minimise the fluids lost, improving performance.

A good method of monitoring changes in hydration levels daily, and following exercise, is to check the colour of your urine. It should be a light, pale yellow colour and if it is darker, more fluid intake is required. Another method is to take your weight before and after exercise in shorts and socks. The amount you have reduced in weight you must replace with fluids. The two best methods of replenishing what has been lost is to drink water and approximately 500ml of milk. The milk contains electrolytes, proteins and carbohydrates needed to improve recovery while also replenishing the fluids lost in sweat.

The majority of daily hydration should come from water. However, other good sources that can be included daily are low fat/skimmed milk, no added sugar cordials, teas/coffees with no sugars and fruit juice but only one small glass daily.

Figure 3. Side effects of dehydration.
Adapted from Maughan et al. (2007)[9]

SIDE EFFECTS OF DEHYDRATION

⌃	RISK OF HEAT ILLNESS
⌃	HEART RATE
⌃	FEELINGS OF EFFORT
⌄	PERFORMANCE
⌄	MENTAL FUNCTION
⌄	ABILITY TO REGULATE BODY TEMPERATURE
⌄	DEVELOPMENT OF HEADACHES, NAUSEA

What and When to Eat – Fuelling for Exercise

Within sport, the timings and compositions of meals/snacks play a crucial role in maximising performance and recovery in athletes. In order to reduce the chances of being in an energy deficit and negatively impacting performance, it is advised that athletes consume at regular intervals daily (approximately every two to three hours) eating five to six times daily through three main meals and two to three snacks. In general, energy intake should match the energy usage, with consumption of foods at times when the body can benefit most from them to maximise performance and recovery.

Pre-Exercise Timing and Composition

The purpose of pre exercise meals and snacks is to increase the energy stores (glycogen), before competition or training, so to minimise chances of fatigue, improving performance. All athletes have different requirements and foods they like, so it is important that they trial foods in training to see how it affects performance and if they could use it in competition. Never trial new food on the day of competition[4].

It is generally recommended that athletes should eat the last main meal approximately three to four hours, and last snack one to two hours before exercise to avoid feeling tired or hungry, and to keep the body energized for activity. Typically, a high carbohydrate, moderate protein and low-fat meal or snack that is easily digested should be consumed. Minimise high fat meals or snacks so as to avoid delayed stomach emptying and resulting cramps[4]. This is easily achievable with afternoon and evening events but for early morning events where it can be difficult to achieve. It is recommended that youth athletes should consume a high carbohydrate meal and snack the night before and a light carbohydrate snack with proper hydration that morning. Avoid consumption of simple and refined sugars (sweets, soft drinks etc.) as these foods result in a rapid increase and decline in blood sugar, which can negatively impact energy levels during sports[3].

As the athlete gets closer to their competition or training, the lighter the meal or snack should be in order to allow appropriate digestion and to avoid stomach upset. It is recommended not to eat within 30 minutes of exercise, as foods will have less time to be digested. Blood will also flow to the stomach, away from the exercising muscles, upsetting the stomach and reducing performance. There are some easy and effective pre exercise meals and snacks displayed in Table 4 below.

Table 4. Pre-Exercise Meal and Snack options

Pre-Exercise Meals 3-4 hours	Pre-Exercise Snacks 1-2 hours
Bowl (2+ servings) of Porridge with fruit, nuts, seeds and a tablespoon of honey	Smoothie made with water, mixed berries, honey and 100ml of natural yoghurt
1-2 eggs with 2 slices of brown toast, 150ml of yoghurt with honey/granola	1-2 handfuls of dried fruit and 100ml yoghurt
2+ serving of brown rice/pasta or normal/sweet potato with 1 serving of breadless chicken/fish/turkey and mixed vegetables in a homemade tomato sauce	2-3 wholegrain rice cake/oatcake/ crackers with hummus
2 brown bread/pittas with ham, tomato and light mayonnaise	1 Cereal bar or 2 servings of fruit

Guide to Serving Sizes
- One serving of Protein- Palm of hand size
- One serving of Carbohydrate- Cupped hand.
- One serving of Fats- Thumb size
- One serving of Vegetables- Fist size

During Exercise

For events lasting longer than 60 minutes, consuming fuel during competition can improve performance through sustained energy levels. However, for those lasting less than 60 minutes, the food and fluids consumed the day of and before will be enough to fuel you. The same applies to trainings that are not high in intensity or long in duration i.e. greater than 90 minutes.

Coaches should encourage youth athletes to drink fluids at regular intervals beginning early in a training or game, and throughout the duration of activity. Every 5 to 10 minutes players should consume two to three mouthfuls of water to reduce the onset of fatigue. Only in events lasting longer than 60 minutes should sports drinks be used, as their mixture of electrolytes and carbohydrates can reduce fatigue onset. Sports drinks are designed with 6 to 8% sugar, which is quickly absorbed and used for energy[3]. However, fluids higher in sugar like soft drinks and fruit juices should be avoided during exercise, as they may cause stomach distress and negatively impact performance[3].

Post-Exercise/Recovery

The purpose of post-exercise nutrition is to aid the repair and recovery of the youth athletes' body while also replenishing the glycogen stores in the liver and muscles used during exercise. Follow the 3 R's of recovery after any activity: Rehydrate with fluids (milk, water, sports drinks), Replenish energy with carbohydrates and Repair the muscle with a protein source. (The 30-60 minutes following exercise is when the muscles are at their most receptive to energy uptake and youth athletes should be prepared so not to miss this window. Muscles store more glycogen immediately after exercise than in later hours. However, another similar meal one and a half to two hours post exercise will further aid recovery. The post-exercise meal or snack should contain a mixture of high carbohydrates, moderate protein, and sufficient fluids to replace sweat loss.

Table 5 gives a list of simple and effective ideas that will hit these targets.

Post-Exercise Meals 30-60 Minutes
Dinner with 2+ servings of Carbohydrates, 1 serving of protein and 1-2 serving of vegetables
500ml of low-fat milk, 1 banana and a handful of mixed nuts or trail mix
A Smoothie made with a cup of mixed berries, 1 banana, 300ml of low-fat milk with a handful of mixed nuts
1 brown pitta bread sandwich with ham/chicken and 500ml of low-fat milk
1 cereal bar, 1 banana and 500ml of low-fat milk

Putting it All Together

Match at 2pm on Sunday	
Saturday Morning – Breakfast	1-2 eggs with 2 slices of brown toast
Saturday Mid-Morning – Snack	150ml of yoghurt with honey/granola
Saturday Afternoon – Lunch	1-2 brown bread/pittas with ham, tomato and light mayo
Saturday Early Evening – Snack	1-2 pieces of fruit with 100% Peanut Butter
Saturday Evening – Dinner	Homemade dinner with 2+ serving of potato/pasta/rice, 1 serving of meat/fish and 1 serving of vegetables
Saturday Night - Late Night Snack	A Smoothie made with a cup of mixed berries, 1 banana, honey, 300-500ml of low-fat milk
All Day Saturday	Drink 2-3L of Water

Sunday - Pre-Game	
Wake up	Begin hydrating with water
Breakfast 8-9am	Bowl (2+ servings) of Porridge with fruit, nuts, seeds and 1-2 tablespoons of honey
Last Main Meal 10-11am	1-2 brown bread/pittas with ham, tomato and light mayo
Last Snack 12.30-1pm	Smoothie made with water, mixed berries, banana, honey and 100ml of natural yoghurt

Sunday - During Game	
1st half	Take 2-3 mouthfuls of water every 5-10 minutes - Especially in warm weather
Half Time	Sip on water and sports drink at half time
2nd half	Take 2-3 mouthfuls of water every 5-10 minutes - Especially in warm weather

Sunday - Post Game	
Immediately after game	Begin sipping on water to replace sweat loss
Within 60 minutes	500ml of low-fat milk, 1 banana and a handful of mixed nuts or trail mix
Within 1-3 hours	Dinner with 2+ servings of pasta/potato/rice, 1 serving of meat/fish and 1-2 servings of vegetables
Remainder of Day - Fluids	Keep Hydrating until urine is a light, pale yellow colour
Remainder of Day - Food	Keep consuming a mixture of Carbohydrates, Protein and good fats to further recovery

Conclusion

It is vital that you get a healthy, well-balanced diet from a variety of sources in order to maintain proper growth while simultaneously maximising athletic performance. Ideally, a youth athletes' diet should be made up of 55-65% carbohydrates coming from sources like whole grains, fruits, vegetables and low-fat dairy products. With a higher percentage focused on training and days before competition. Protein intake should be 15-25%[4] of daily intake and sourced from lean meat and poultry, fish, eggs, low-fat dairy products, beans and nuts. With a higher percentage focused on rest and recovery days. For fats, 20-30%[4] of daily intake in youth athletes should come from healthy fats i.e. olive oils, oily fish, nuts, seeds, avocados. Hydration is hugely important for health and performance. The majority of your fluids should come from water and be increased on days of high exercise activity and temperature. Minimising the amount of water lost during exercise will reduce chances of fatigue.

Finally, timing food consumption is another important method to optimise your performance. Your main meal should be eaten a minimum of three to four hours before exercise and light snacks should be eaten one to two hours before activity. Recovery foods should be consumed within 30-60 minutes of exercise finishing and again within one to two hours of activity to allow your muscles to rebuild and ensure proper recovery. Doing the above and getting the energy from these foods will not only fuel you during your sporting endeavours but will also optimise your performance and provide you with the necessary nutrition for proper growth and development.

Best Wishes,
Michael Day
See Appendix for Sample Recipes

SKILLS FOR DRAWING ON YOUR INNER STRENGTH
SKILL NO. 8 OPTIMISING RECOVERY AND HEALTH
By Tony Óg Regan

Why is this important?

One of the often-overlooked factors in relation to performance is recovery. Most athlete's sports performance is dependent on a short window of time. They may have 70 minutes to perform in a game. In hurling for example, you might be on the ball somewhere between 10-20 times in a game depending on your position. This equates to 20-40 seconds in which you will have the ball in your hand; a short time frame to make an impression on the ball. Your decision-making and movement must be clear and fast in those moments. Therefore, every aspect of your lifestyle, preparation and practice must be at an extraordinary high level if you want to produce an extraordinary performance. What you eat will affect what you think and feel and how you move; what you drink will do the same. How you sleep will affect your mood, energy levels and movements like anticipation, reaction times, decision making. It is all connected!

Pillar One: Sleep

Sleep is measured by the quality and quantity we get. The recommended number of hours for youths is a quantity of 10 hours and, for adults, between 7-8 hours. How do you gauge the quality of sleep? On waking do you feel rested, relaxed and excited by the day ahead? Here are some important things to look at regarding sleep.

- Do I go to bed consistently at the same time each night and wake at same time each morning?
- Do I get off all devices at least an hour before sleep? As we can see from the graph below, we start to produce a hormone called melatonin at 9pm. This is the hormone that makes us drowsy and sleepy. When we are on devices, we are exposing ourselves to blue light which stops us producing melatonin.
- Building in a warm up routine before a game gets our bodies and minds ready to perform. It is crucial to our performance that we do this consistently and properly. You should have a similar routine before bed. You should start to wind down mentally and physically.

- *Some Key Tips to Promote Better Sleep: Have a shower or bath to wash off the day, drink a hot water and lemon, ensure right temperature (approximately 16 to 19 degrees Celsius) and darkness in your room. Have clean bed clothes and a tidy room. Read a book or do some writing/ journaling. Do a light meditation or breathing routine to relax the central nervous system.*

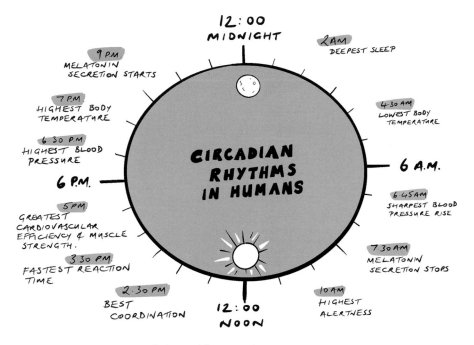

Adapted from praisemoves.com

Pillar Two: Nutrition
A vital pillar- See Previous

Pillar Three: Hydration
A vital pillar- See Previous

Pillar Four: Movement
The benefits of exercise and movement has many great health rewards. When we exercise, at a neurological level, we create new connections between brain cells, higher levels of thinking, improve concentration and memory, and prevent degeneration of brain cells. We release a hormone called BDNF which helps our processing speed and recall. At a physiological level, we release endorphins like serotonin and dopamine which give our system a strong mental boost, a greater appreciation for

nature and a stronger sense of well-being. At a psychosomatic level, we release tension and stress from the muscles, this gives us a mental boost as well as allowing us to sleep better and reduce anxiety. At a psychological level, when we exercise our perception of ourselves improves increasing our self-confidence and self-image.

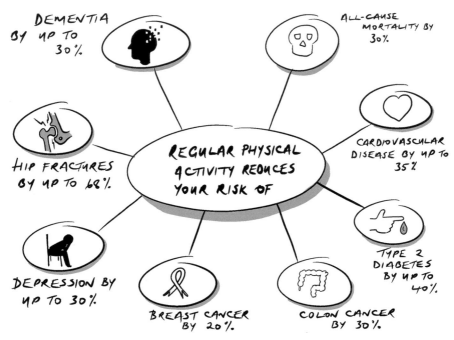

Adapted from publichealthmatters.blog.gov.uk

Top Tips

As part of your recovery from the stress of training, it is important you look at the variety of your movement each week. Activities like walking, swimming and yoga can promote great healing in the mind and body. As athletes, we produce a lot of chemicals such as adrenaline and cortisol during exercise and under stress. Cortisol is a stress hormone that weakens our central nervous system, which, in turn, can make us prone to illness and injury. You must strengthen your immune system by incorporating new ways to promote more relaxation in your mind and bodies. What you listen to (media, other opinions, podcasts, TV/Radio), who you spend time with, where you go and what you do can all have an impact on how you heal, regenerate and recover. Find activities, people and environments that put you at ease, grow your energy and confidence and promote more calmness in your life.

References:

1. Gidding SS, Dennison BA, Birch LL, et al. Dietary recommendations for children and adolescents: a guide for practitioners: consensus statement from the American Heart Association. Circulation 2005; 112:2061-75.

2. Public Health England, 2016. The Eatwell guide.

3. Sacheck, J. and Schultz, N., Optimal Nutrition for Youth Athletes: Food Sources and Fuel Timing.

4. Purcell, L.K., Canadian Paediatric Society and Paediatric Sports and Exercise Medicine Section, 2013. Sport nutrition for young athletes. Paediatrics & child health, 18(4), pp.200-202.

5. Baechle, T.R. and Earle, R.W. eds., 2008. Essentials of strength training and conditioning. Human kinetics.

6. Jeukendrup, A., 2014. A step towards personalized sports nutrition: carbohydrate intake during exercise. Sports Medicine, 44(1), pp.25-33.

7. Smith, J.W., Holmes, M.E. and McAllister, M.J., 2015. Nutritional considerations for performance in young athletes. Journal of sports medicine, 2015.

8. Meyer, F., O'Connor, H. and Shirreffs, S.M., 2007. Nutrition for the young athlete. Journal of sports sciences, 25(S1), pp. S73-S82.

9. Maughan, R.J. and Shirreffs, S.M., 2010. Dehydration and rehydration in competitive sport. Scandinavian journal of medicine & science in sports, 20, pp.40-47.

10. Péronnet, F., 2010. Healthy Hydration for Physical Activity. Nutrition Today, 45(6), pp. S41-S44.

* References have been left as authour intended.

SUMMARY POINTS - Chapter 20

- *Always take a 'food first' approach. Supplements are not required for youth athletes.*
- *Eat and drink for optimum health to reduce chances of illnesses and injuries. This leads to greater participation in sport which is the overall aim for youth athletes.*
- *Aim to consume meals and snacks, which contain good sources of carbohydrates, protein, and fat so there is no deficiency in any nutrient.*
- *Consume at regular intervals daily (approximately every two to three hours) - eating five to six times daily through three main meals and two to three snacks to reduce chance of energy deficiency, impacting immune system and performance*
- *Fuel for the work required i.e. the higher the energy used, the greater the energy required - increase carbohydrates. The lower the activity, the less energy required and more emphasis on recovery - increase intake of lean protein and healthy fats.*
- *Monitor your urine colour throughout the day along with weight before and after training to reduce chance of dehydration.*
- *Have as much variety as possible in your diet with a mixture of colours to keep your immune function at its optimum.*
- *Follow the three Rs of recovery after exercise.*
- *Enjoy your food and never feel guilty for having a treat every now and again.*
- *Develop a solid sleep routine to ensure the adequate amount of quality sleep.*
- *As part of your recovery from the stress of training, look at the variety of your movement each week. Activities like walking, swimming and yoga can promote great healing in the mind and body.*

PART 3

This section of the book deals with lifestyle, as well as pastoral and self-care issues. It is my wish that this book is as comprehensive as possible, and helps many people in many ways. Sport can and must be a source of good for everyone. Sport can and must enrich both life and society.

Paul Kilgannon.

CHAPTER 21: TIME & ENERGY MANAGEMENT

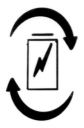

One of the few things we all have in common in this world is that we all have 24 hours in any given day. We all work from the same clock and we all have limited amounts of energy to give each day. Time is an asset; one you should learn both to manage and spend wisely. Time well spent is something we cherish and benefit from.

It is important you know how, and where, you want to put your time and energy to use. As with almost everything, being proactive and intentional is key. A certain amount of self-discipline is necessary in order to avoid putting short term desires ahead of long-term values and goals. It is vital you learn to respect time and consciously prioritise what is important in your life. The world will get out of the way for someone who knows where they're going. The aim is to focus on energy management, time management, and indeed where possible, environmental management (where and who you surround yourself with). Productivity is a by-product of these three skills. How you manage your energy, time, and environment provides structure, and structure delivers function. Yes of course there will be 'lazy' or 'off days' (perhaps even weeks and months) and these are vital and need to be factored in. Life, especially your youth, isn't all about productivity and planning. Indeed some would flippantly suggest, it should have nothing to do with it, but I think deep down everyone knows this is foolhardy. Real freedom comes from not being ruled by your unconscious habits and patterns. Real freedom arises when these habits and patterns are put to rest and you have control and clarity to make decisions on your own. Occasionally you will lose your way and maybe that too is part of the process of finding your way.

"The chains of habit are too light to be felt
until they are too heavy to be broken".
Warren Buffett

The modern world is full of distraction and what can be termed 'time and energy zappers ' such as: phones, email, social media, computer games, YouTube, television, the internet and, indeed, people who may want to pull you in a certain direction and distract you from what is important. Many devices and applications are purposely designed to be addictive and all-too-many people become addicted to 'the scroll'. Learning how to manage distractions is important. Leave your phone out of sight when your goal is productivity, no matter the domain. Out of sight, out of mind. Go one further, switch it off from time to time, once you get over the initial anxiety it is truly liberating. The message is simple; control your smartphone and other such devices, or they will end up controlling you.

Limit notifications on your smartphone and laptop. Keep the most important things the most important things. I am confident you understand that you don't need to be instantaneously alerted every time the most trivial of 'events' happen on social media or in your friendship circle. Reacting to numerous notifications can literally devour your time and energy and pull you away from living in the real world.

Take control of how you consume social media and use your devices. Social media, with its ability to devour your time, can negatively impact your mood and perspective and can lead you into negative mental states. Consciously choose who, and what, you follow. Imagine the content you consume to be books. Now ask yourself, what does your library currently look like? What are you consuming? What are you filling your head with? Appreciate that what you consume profoundly affects and influences your values. Now ask yourself, how can you improve the quality of the content in your library? Who or what is draining your time and energy and isn't enriching your life at any level? Who or what do you need to unfollow? Who, or what, can you follow that will improve the quality and value of what you are consuming on social media?

Do a social media and devices time-audit by utilising tools that track how and where you are spending your time online. Tools you can use to actively audit and limit your time spent on social media, devices or online include: Social Fever, My Addictiometer, OFFTIME and App Usage. Actively and consciously control your relationship with social media or it will control you.

Email is an important part of modern life but again, you can also learn to manage it optimally. Like social media, it can be a serious time zapper. Simple tips include: finding maybe two times in the day where you can check your emails, deleting content once you've read it, and responding straight away where appropriate. Aim to touch each email once. Manage the content you receive. Unsubscribe from promotional emails that, by and large, are trying to sell you something you don't need. When buying online, untick the box to receive further promotional information from these suppliers. Build good habits. As these and hundreds of other small improvements accumulate, positive results can come quicker than you imagined. Success is the by-product of the accumulation of a series of positive daily habits.

The Habit Poem
I am your constant companion.
I am your greatest helper or your heaviest burden.
I will push you onward or drag you down to failure.
I am completely at your command.
Half the things you do, you might just as well turn over to me,
and I will be able to do them quickly and correctly.
I am easily managed; you must merely be firm with me.
Show me exactly how you want something done, and after a few
lessons I will do it automatically.
I am the servant of all great men.
And, alas, of all failures as well.
Those who are great, I have made great.
Those who are failures, I have made failures.
I am not a machine, though I work with all the precision of a machine.
Plus, the intelligence of a man.
You may run me for profit, or run me for ruin;
it makes no difference to me.
Take me, train me, be firm with me
and I will put the world at your feet.
Who am I?

I AM A HABIT
Author Unknown

When you are clear on your priorities, you can make daily or weekly commitments to them. You can begin to actively and consciously build your identity as the person you want to be, and your credibility will begin to grow in the fields and areas you prioritise, as the quality of the time and effort you put into them improves.

There is a short mantra I love around choices:

*"There is a choice you have to make in everything you do.
So keep in mind that in the end the choice you make makes you".*

You must understand and appreciate there is a price to be paid for achieving anything of significance no matter the domain. You can strive to have anything you want, but you can't have everything. Things exist in contrast and conflict. Being intentional with your time is key.

Occasionally, you must be willing to pay the price of dedication and sacrifice. It cannot be denied that having a strong 'athletic identity' is a necessary requirement for an elite athlete. There are no secret training methods or quick fixes. To achieve excellence at any level you must do the work and do it consistently well. There will be times you will have to ask yourself; what am I willing to sacrifice for the things I want in life? However, you must appreciate that having too strong an 'athletic identity' (see Chapter 3) may result in over-commitment, which can lead to extreme and dysfunctional practices culminating in overtraining, anxiety when not training, and often burnout. You will hear stories which glorify the extreme, but I certainly don't want this book to be about that. This is not to say that self-discipline is not a critical quality in all areas of high performance. To live an extraordinary life, there are many occasions in which you will have to resist an ordinary approach.

Having a balanced life can be challenging depending on your level of commitment to your sporting endeavours and studies (see Chapter 23). However, be advised that more isn't necessarily better- better is better. Quality is key. You can't continue to empty the proverbial cup and expect to be able to keep drinking from it; you must fill it too. Downtime, recreation and friendships inside and outside of sport are key. Consciously make time for friendships and relationships, don't go it alone. Your peer group is a huge influence, and old and dear friends should always be cherished. I must warn you to be aware of the wrong company because it's the first step that leads to a bad way. When it comes to fostering relationships, spend less time with people who deplete your energy and more time with people who inspire you.

*"Walk with the wise and become wise,
for a companion of fools suffers harm".*
Proverbs 13:20 NIV

You will need to be able to switch off and you will need to consciously make time for this. Being constantly emotionally involved in your sport is neither helpful, nor healthy. Having a broad range of hobbies and interests is important. While you actively engage, and thrive in your athletic role, don't relinquish the adequate exploration of alternative skills and interests. You want and need a balanced lifestyle. You want to be a balanced person. You can't invest all your time into your 'athletic identity'. There are numerous stories of athletes in their prime, getting injured, being dropped from teams and squads, or simply falling out of love with their sport. What do these athletes do then if all they ever knew was being an athlete and identifying solely with that role? Other options or future decisions can become limited. Make time for fun and play. Explore other hobbies, identities and interests. This is a marathon not a sprint.

WHAT'S IMPORTANT TO YOU?

EXAMPLES INCLUDE: HEALTH, FAMILY, FRIENDS, SCHOOL/STUDY, SPORT, HOBBIES & RECREATION, DOWNTIME.

_____

_____

Audit and examine where, and how, you spend your time. Be clinical but don't overcomplicate it:
1. List all your weekly activities including free time; be thorough, list everything.
2. Spend a week tracking your behaviours and time spent in each weekly activity.
3. Once finished break them up in to categories with descriptors e.g. School, sport, health, down time.
4. Assign each category a percentage based on how much time you spend on it per week.
5. Draw a simple pie chart based on these percentages.
6. Do your values and priorities match how you are allocating your time? Is there alignment? If not, what changes need to be made in order to align your priorities with how you spend your time?

Identify your key priorities this week. Each week will vary priorities wise, however your health should always come first as it is key to being at your best in the other areas. Sleep is vital, especially for a maturing and changing body.

WHAT ARE YOUR KEY PRIORITIES IN YOUR LIFE THIS WEEK?

WHAT ARE THE MOST IMPORTANT AREAS FOR YOU?

WHEN WE WRITE THESE DOWN & REVIEW THEM WE

ARE 80% MORE LIKELY TO COMMIT TO DOING THEM.

YOUR JOURNAL COMES IN HANDY HERE.

_____

_____

'To do lists' or 'daily priority lists' are excellent life skills tools to utilise rather than relying on your brain to remember everything that has to be done. Make a list- prioritise 3 or 4 of the most important things. You may not get to everything, every day, but ticking things off the list will highlight your progress and drive motivation. Break large tasks down into smaller parts. You can break your list into short tasks and longer ones. Prioritise what needs to be done and then look at what would be nice to do. Learn to schedule effectively. Some tasks are easier in the morning when you are fresh and motivated. Others can be left until the evening. Again, such practices can be incorporated into your journal.

Morning and evening routines are great ways to begin and end your day. Your journal can be used here to set out your priorities and consciously explore how you wish to attack the day. As part of your evening journal reflections you could write down 5 things you are grateful for that day or answer a simple set of questions (see Chapter 2). Such a practice promotes feelings of happiness and contentment. When you reinforce what you have in your life you feel a greater sense of emotional wellbeing and energy. You can measure your success each day based on your own standards and priorities not anyone else's. Again, learning how to ask yourself 'empowering questions' for example; 'How can I…', 'What can I ….', is key.

As I have mentioned in Chapter 2, I believe it can be a good idea to have both a journal and a diary. The journal for ideas, thoughts and reflection and the diary for scheduling. Your diary should have day, monthly and yearly planners that can help you navigate how you spend your time.

My 168 hours- Setting out your Week

24 hours x 7 days leaves us with a total of 168 hours in a week. It really is your choice what you get out of these hours. Once again, it is critical you plan and schedule time for practices that renew and expand your energy such as: movement, friends, family, hobbies and down time.

An example of key daily practices to prioritise health would be:

1. Bed each night before 10pm and phone off by 9pm.
2. Ensure a minimum 30 minutes of movement each day – walk, run, cycle, gym, etc.
3. Eat a balanced and nutritious meal every 2-3 hours.
4. Meditation or mindfulness practice for 10 minutes every morning.
5. Spend time in nature for mental clarity and to reset your central nervous system.

WHAT WOULD BE YOUR TOP 5 PRACTICES EACH DAY THAT MAKE YOU THINK, FEEL & MOVE AT YOUR BEST?

_____

_____

We have limited amounts of time and energy each day and week. It is important you don't get caught up being reactive to everyone and everything. Learning to say 'no' can be an important skill, but I hasten to advise that you don't get so self-absorbed that you end up saying 'no' too often. Overuse of the word 'no' can become a crutch that merely leaves you in your own little cage, in your own little world.

When we prioritise our time and energy and build good habits we find we are more productive, happier and achievement follows. Never forget that how you chose to spend your time is, either consciously or unconsciously, how you choose to spend your life.

Sample Week Planner (see next page)

(Note the planner starts at 6:00 and ends at 24:00 to allow for up to 10 hours of sleep. Some of you will be morning type, while others will be more night type people).

PRIORITIES	TIME	MON	TuE	WED	THUR	FRI	SAT	SuN
	6.00							
	6.30							
	7.00							
	7.30							
	8.00							
	8.30							
	9.00							
	9.30							
	10.00							
	10.30							
	11.00							
	11.30							
	12.00							
TO DO	12.30							
LIST	13.00							
	13.30							
	14.00							
	14.30							
	15.00							
	15.30							
	16.00							
	16.30							
	17.00							
	17.30							
	18.00							
	18.30							
	19.00							
	19.30							
	20.00							
	20.30							
	21.00							
	21.30							
	22.00							
	22.30							
	23.00							
	23.30							

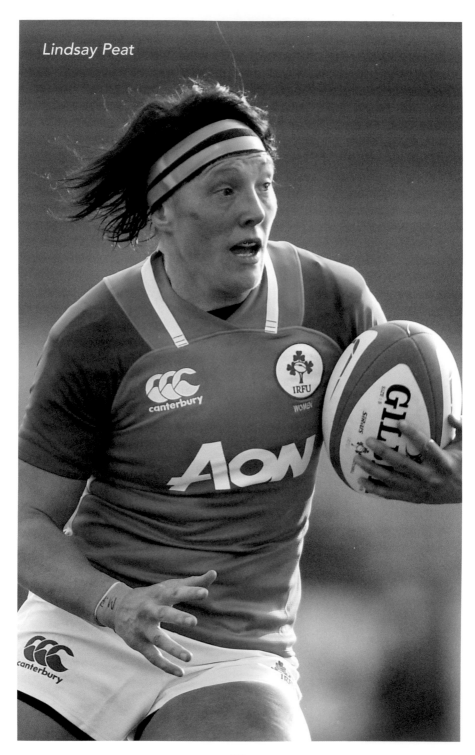

Lindsay Peat

CHAPTER 21

Lindsay Peat

Lindsay Peat is an all-round sportswoman who has managed a full and broad sporting life in which she has served many masters. She is a highly decorated athlete across numerous sporting codes and was Ireland Rugby Women's Player of the Year in 2017. Here, she shares with you some hard learned lessons on time and energy management and making priorities.

Where do I begin? I suppose introducing myself might be the best place to start. My name is Lindsay Peat and I am an athlete who has played across four different codes at the highest level for over 15 years now. I have represented Ireland in soccer, basketball and rugby. I have also had the honour of representing my beloved Dublin in Ladies Gaelic Football, winning an All-Ireland in 2010 and playing in two other All-Ireland Finals in 2009 and 2014. I've played in the European qualifiers for the U18 Irish soccer team, numerous 6 Nations Rugby Championships, a Rugby World Cup in 2017, co-captained the Irish Senior Women's Basketball Team and won many club and personal honours throughout my career. While juggling these various sporting commitments I also managed to go back to college as a mature student, get married and have a beautiful son.

After giving you a basic and broad outline of the commitments I have had over the past number of years, hopefully it will instil confidence in you that I might be somewhat 'qualified' to lend some advice on the subject of 'time, energy, choices and priorities'.

Miles Davis the great jazz musician once wrote that, "Time isn't the main thing, it's the only thing". We all have the same amount of time available to us: 24 hours in a day, 168 hours in a week, 730 hours in a month and 8,760 hours in one calendar year. If we were to place a monetary value on time would it change our thinking, would we be more cautious about how we spend it; how we invest it?

Looking back, I think if I had applied such an analogy to my time I may have spent or invested it a little more wisely in some areas of my life, other than sport. I am extremely proud of my sporting accomplishments but I must be honest and truthful when I look back at the time and energy I invested in sport. As you can see, I certainly reaped the rewards and have a clear and identifiable "athletic identity"; but what about the other areas that make up my life: family, friends, career? Did I allocate the time and energy needed here? If I am honest then, no, I didn't. Could I have been more efficient, organised and intentional with my time? Yes, I could have.

There have been extensive periods in my life where I simply lived in the moment and rode the crest of whatever wave I was on, which was, let's be honest, a sporting wave. I simply did not have the tools to take a step back and look at what I wanted to achieve in all areas of my life, not just sport. Life is for living and my journey on life's highway has helped shape me into the person I am today; however, if I could go back and give my young self some advice I would be saying to sit down and take stock of all that I want to achieve in life. To take 'a call to action' so I could list, sort and prioritise what were the areas of my life that were important to me and what I wanted from life. I think this would have been a great tool to help me stay focused, ensuring I was sticking to the plan that I had set out for my time or if necessary write a new plan. After all, it is my life.

With this said, I cannot deny that my life's journey has taught me strict lessons regarding my time and my energy. I feel I am more of an accomplished master of my time now rather than the apprentice I most certainly once was.

Here is my advice and what tools have worked for me. I love lists. I always make a to-do list. They are modest, informal ways of keeping you focused and provide huge fulfilment as you tick off each part that you have accomplished for that day, week, month or year. Lists take very little time and energy to complete, thus allowing you to use your full complement of time and energy more productively.

Be realistic when allocating time to tasks. If I think a gym session will take me an hour, I at least add half an hour on. I've miscalculated on so many occasions my time, as I tried to cram too many things into one day, leaving me stressed, void of energy and not enjoying that part of my day I should've been enjoying.

Most notably over the years, the one area of my life that I let slip were friendships, simply because I didn't allocate the required time to them. Make the time, relationships are a priority and need to be treated as such. Proper scheduling will help here. I have learned its value. As regards to your phone, use it to maintain relationships. Use it as a means of communication not as a means to scroll through how everyone else is living their lives. Limit your time on it and go and live your life.

Time is such a valuable asset and learning to manage it properly can add great value to your life. Your sporting career will no doubt take up much of your time but it certainly shouldn't take up all of your time. Make time for the things in your life that are important. Making living life important.

Best wishes,
Lindsay

SUMMARY POINTS - Chapter 21

* *Time is an asset and one you should learn both to manage and spend wisely.*
* *Consciously prioritise what is important in your life.*
* *Actively and consciously control your relationship with social media.*
* *Success is the by-product of the accumulation of a series of positive daily habits.*
* *Occasionally, you must be willing to pay the price of dedication and sacrifice.*
* *'To do lists' or 'daily priority lists' are excellent life skills tools to utilise.*
* *Schedule time for practices that renew and expand your energy such as: movement, friends, family, hobbies and down time.*
* *How you chose to spend your time is, either consciously or unconsciously, how you choose to spend your life.*

CHAPTER 22 : MULTI-SPORT ACTIVITY

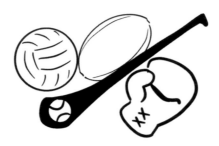

By Dr. Damien Young

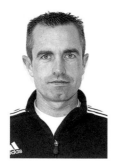

Dr. Damien Young is a lecturer in Sports Strength and Conditioning at Limerick Institute of Technology. He has represented both his club, Drom & Inch and County, Tipperary at every level on the field of play. He has served as Performance Analyst with the Tipperary Senior Hurlers since 2008. Damien is also a GAA Coach and Coach Educator. He has published a number of research papers in International Sports Journals. Here he gives an overview of the research around multi- sport activity for the youth athlete which may help inform your choices as you age and develop.

Over the last number of years, there have been increased opportunities to participate in a wide variety of sports. Depending on your access to these sports, you may have participated competitively or recreationally with your friends in more than one sport to-date. Now, as you progress through your adolescent years, you may be considering reducing your involvement in other sports to concentrate on your "main" sport. Before you make up your mind, let us consider what the research suggests.

The opinion of focusing on one sport was of great interest a number of years ago when research carried out by Ericsson and colleagues (1993) suggested that those who accumulated hours of deliberate practice would have a major advantage over those who did not. This intensive practice method was also known as the "10 year/10,000 hour rule" (Ericsson, Krampe and Tesch-Römer, 1993). This concept was developed from studies that focused on a small number of chess players and musicians who had been termed "experts" as a direct result of very high volumes of training hours. However, studies which involve sportspeople that focus only on one sport in their childhood and perform high amounts of training is not a guarantee for success (Myer et al., 2016). There are negatives associated with early specialisation, such as overuse injuries (see Chapter 16), a lack of time spent with friends, and burnout (Malina, 2010). However, if the sport requires a peak performance before puberty, for example, gymnastics, there are benefits of focusing just on one sport provided that proper programmes are put in place (Myer et al., 2016). However, these sports are in the minority. The same authors suggested that those involved in team sports and some individual sports should wait until middle adolescence to specialise.

What if you play multi-sports? Research was carried out to identify whether focusing on one sport (early specialisation) or playing multiple sports (sporting diversification) throughout childhood and adolescence can influence performance levels before adulthood (Bridge & Toms, 2013). One thousand and six subjects (46% males, 54% female) participated in a study. The sport that the subjects were playing the highest standard at between 16-18 years was considered their "main" sport. Of the sports identified, 362 people were involved in individual sports, and 549 played a team sport. Each participant in the study was asked to provide information about the number of organised competitive sports that they had participated in each year between the ages of 7 and 18 years. The results showed that those who were competing in three sports when they were aged 11, 13, and 15 years were more likely to play at National level when they were between 16-18 years compared to those who only reached club level (Bridge & Toms, 2013). A further study showed that adult world-class athletes from different Olympic and International sports reported a moderate amount of training in their main sport at an early age but had extensive involvement in various other types of sports (including non-organised sports) at the same time (Güllich, 2014). It is suggested that, while organised sport-specific practice is important to sport success, it must also be recognised that early specialisation is unnecessary and may even be detrimental to long-term success, while multi-sport practice and peer-led play experience facilitates the effectiveness of later specific practice (i.e., late specialisation) and long-term achievement (Di Fiori et al., 2017).

The role of multi-sports does not hinder elite sports participation, it provides a wider range of experiences and an opportunity to develop fundamental movement skills and cognitive skills (Strachan, Côté and Deakin, 2009). Some research suggests that there is a transfer of skills between sports (Collins et al., 2014). One such case is that, in developing golfers, participation in sports such as table tennis, pool/snooker, and *racket sports such as squash and badminton were helpful (Toms, 2014). Participation in other sports may also help develop decision-making skills. It was suggested that practicing in other sports, especially those, which have common decision-making experiences, may reduce the hours of sport-specific practice needed to become an expert in team ball sports (Baker, Côté and Abernethy, 2003). The research suggests that sports specialisation would begin in late adolescence. In particular, for sports assessed in centimeters (e.g. track & field), grams (e.g. weightlifting) or seconds (e.g. swimming), research showed that those who reached the elite level specialised at a later age, trained less in childhood but intensified their training in late adolescents more so than those who were near elite (Moesch et al., 2011).*

The Benefits of Participating in Multi-Sports:
- *Greater overall athleticism.*
- *Improved foundational motor skills and transferable skills.*
- *Lower chance of drop-out.*
- *Increased fun and enjoyment.*
- *Wider circle of social relationships.*
- *Reduced chance of overuse injuries.*
- *Longer sport career and involvement.*
- *Promotion of lifelong physical activity skills.*
- *Greater intrinsic motivation.*
- *Opportunity to learn new sports.*

(Roetert, Woods and Jayanthi, 2018)

In summary, for those who are currently playing multi-sports, the research supports your choice to maintain your participation in these sports, especially until mid-adolescence. Your performance in your main sport will benefit from the technical skills, physical movements, and decision making experiences that you practice in these other sports. In addition, playing multi-sports allows you to participate with a wider circle of friends, learn from different coaches, travel to different places and provides you with an all-round sport experience. It may be difficult to maintain your participation in multi-sports from a time and cost point of view. However, even if you play a range of sports in your recreational time, they will benefit you.

Best wishes,
Damien Young.

Billy Walsh

Billy Walsh is a world renowned boxing coach. He was Head Coach of the Irish High Performance Boxing Team from 2003 to 2015, a period of unprecedented success for Irish Boxing. His current role is as Head Coach at USA Boxing. Billy is a former Olympic Boxer and also played hurling and Gaelic football for Wexford in his youth. Here, he tells of his long and varied sports career and the virtues of participating in multiple sports

Billy the Kid

As an overactive, aggressive young lad, little did I think or even dream that I was going to become an Olympian. As for my late father, Liam, he may have dreamt a little, but I don't think the Olympics were in his sights. The facts were clear, nobody in my family had ever been close to an Olympian, and nobody from Wexford town, where we came from, had ever been to the Olympic Games. Did my father foresee the end journey as he brought his first born of six (five boys and one girl) to play hurling, to play Gaelic football, to play soccer, and join the local boxing club.

Whether it was to burn off my energy and aggression, to teach me discipline, respect, confidence and self-belief, or indeed to become an Olympian, only my father can say. If he was still with us he would tell you he planned it all, every minute of it. As it happened, he started me on an unbelievable journey not only in sport, but also in life. Some of those guys I played football, hurling, and soccer with as a child, are my best friends to this day. As I grew older I gained more friends playing through the underage systems and into the adult teams for all those sports. As my love for sports grew, so did my discipline. Sport kept me on the straight and narrow. I knew if I got into trouble outside the boxing club I would be thrown out. I loved the game of boxing so much I couldn't take the risk of being excluded. By the time I reached my 14th birthday I was playing soccer, Gaelic football, had won a Leinster hurling medal for Wexford and also my first National Boxing Title.

I continued to participate in all four sports through my teens. We were competing well at club level, winning a few county medals, losing a few county medals, but always learning. By the age of 18 I was captain of the

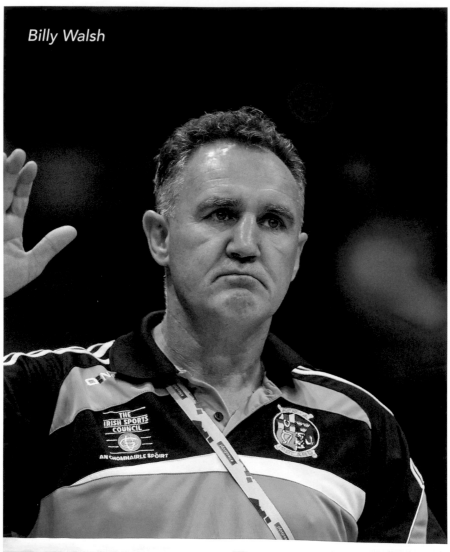

Billy Walsh

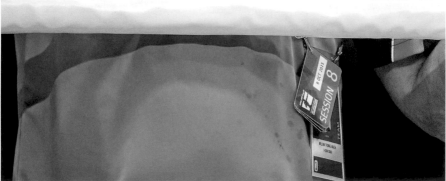

Wexford Minor Football team, wing back on the Wexford Minor Hurling team and four times National Boxing Champion. By this stage, soccer had been removed from my sporting schedule; something had to give.

After a one-point loss to our closest rival, Kilkenny, in the Leinster Final in Croke Park in 1981, I decided to focus on the sport where I had only myself to rely on. I set out in pursuit of my Olympic dream. I achieved that dream competing in the 1988 Olympic Games in Seoul. As soon as I returned home, I went back to playing my other sports, winning county senior championships for hurling and Gaelic football and a cup winners medal with soccer. I played both Gaelic games, hurling and Gaelic football, competitively until I was 40 years old.

I'm not sure about my father's vision; was it by chance and was he simply trying to tame this wild kid of his or had he studied Istvan Balyi's Long Term Athletic Development Model? Whichever one it was, he equipped me with a broad range of skills and tools that gave me a full and enjoyable life on the playing fields of this country and in the boxing rings of this world. I lived a sporting dream.

Billy the Coach

Having spent the last 20 years as a Professional Boxing Coach, and having studied and presented with Istvan Balyi on Long Term Athlete Development, I often wonder had my father read his findings? I have witnessed many athletes grow and develop. Undoubtedly the most rounded and developed are those athletes who played multiple sports while young, focusing solely on their chosen sport in their mid to late teens. Katie Taylor has multiple caps playing underage soccer for Ireland. She went on to be Ireland's greatest ever boxer as a 5 times World Champion and Olympic Champion. Darren O Neill played minor and u-21 hurling for Kilkenny before becoming an Olympian and a European Boxing Silver Medallist. There are endless examples of world class athletes who played multiple sports in their youth.

My advice to all you future Athletes is that in order to give yourself a chance of reaching your full potential in sport, and indeed in life, you should play as many sports as you can when you are young; narrow it down in your mid to late teens and then focus on your best or favourite sport thereafter. Finally, be sure to enjoy the friendships that will last you a lifetime.

All the best,
Billy Walsh

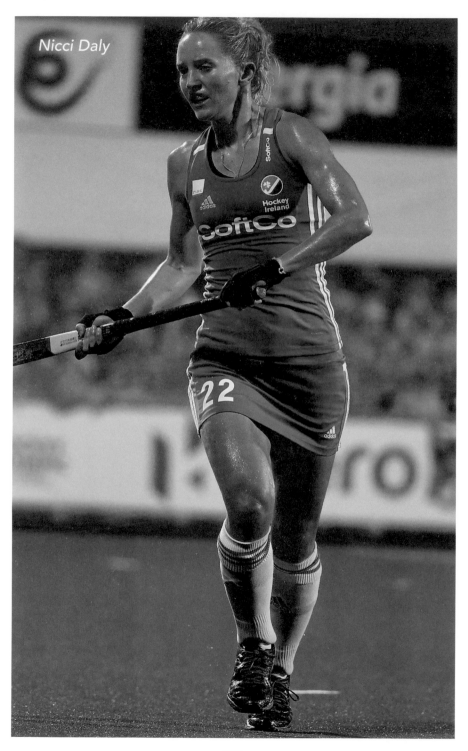

Nicci Daly

Nicci Daly

Nicci Daly is an Irish Women's Field Hockey International. She was a member of the Irish team that played in the 2018 Women's Hockey World Cup Final and is currently looking forward to the Tokyo 2020 Olympic Games. She has also played Senior Ladies' Gaelic football for Dublin. Her family is steeped in sport. Her late father, Vivion, was the most successful racing driver in Ireland in the 1980s and 90s. Her uncle, Derek Daly, raced in Formula 1 and IndyCar and her cousin Conor Daly, currently races in the IndyCar Series. Her grandfather Pascal Burke, was a professional snooker player and her mother's first cousin, Paddy Mulligan, played soccer for Chelsea.

Nicci runs a schools initiative called Go Girls Karting & STEM (Science Technology Engineering & Maths) which aims to encourage more girls to get involved in motorsport and highlights the different career opportunities available in the motor industry. Below she outlines the central role sport played in her youth and the value of taking a multi-sport approach before going on to specialise in a chosen sport.

Growing up, I was always looking to be outside, kicking a ball or swinging a tennis racket. I grew up in a motorsport family and racing was always my dream, but it was too difficult at the time with my father already involved in the sport. I took to most sports quite naturally and through primary school I tried a bit of everything- swimming, karate, athletics, Irish dancing, basketball, cricket and Gaelic football in the yard with the boys. I loved swimming and completed my primary level lifesaving course as a youngster. I continue to swim to this day for both leisure and recovery. Sport is so much more than merely the competitive based activities we often pigeon hole it to be. Although today, I am only involved competitively in one sport, I still partake in many sports such as golf, swimming and soccer recreationally.

Sports day was always my favourite day at school. I loved all the different disciplines involved. I represented the school in athletics before joining the school Gaelic football team in 5th class. We had a mixed team, but in reality I was one of the only girls that played. Gaelic would be the sport that would take me into my teenage years. I developed a love for the fast flowing nature of the sport. Two days a week training just wasn't enough for me; I spent my days kicking balls and soloing up and down the garden as fast as I could. Sport was a cornerstone of my youth.

I began secondary school just as I was beginning to really develop my Gaelic skills and knowledge of the game. Unfortunately, there was no

Gaelic football team in the school. I was really disappointed. "You'll play hockey instead" I was told, as the school was primarily a hockey school. I wasn't overly impressed. I had no idea how to play the game and knew nobody who played it. Being honest, I had never even heard of this game before. Little did I know that it was a game that would come to play a huge part in my life.

Reluctantly, I started hockey in secondary school. I began to enjoy it, the more I played. I was still playing Gaelic football and went on to represent Dublin at Under 14. Unfortunately, shortly after this the club I was playing Gaelic with, Ballyboden Wanderers, disbanded and as a result I began to focus on hockey. While in school, I played hockey for Leinster at Under 16 and Under 18 level and grew to love the game. However, on leaving secondary school I parked the hockey for a period and returned to Gaelic football. Before I knew it, I had been invited to join the Dublin Ladies B team. I did well there and was named in the Dublin Senior panel for the 2009 National League. Around the same time, an old hockey coach of mine, Joe Brennan, approached me to return to the sport. After a three-year hiatus from hockey, I returned to play with Glenanne Hockey Club and the Leinster U21 panel. Shortly after this, I joined the Irish Senior hockey panel.

I remember talking to both my Gaelic and hockey coaches at the time, to discuss their training and competition schedules for the summer ahead. I soon realised it would be almost impossible for me to balance both at an elite level. This is a situation many athletes find themselves in; having to choose between two sports they love. While in discussion with my hockey coach, he mentioned the words 'Olympic Games' and my mind was made up. Up until that point, I hadn't even realised that hockey was an Olympic sport. I decided to focus my talent and attention on hockey and to this day I am happy with my decision. The Dublin Ladies Gaelic team have gone on to have fabulous success and I am delighted for them. Occasionally I wonder 'what if….', but again, I am happy with my decision to prioritise hockey.

The more I began to focus on elite level hockey, the more I began to appreciate the value of a youth spent playing and sampling many different sports. There are many skills that crossover from Gaelic to hockey. As a forward in both sports, 'leading' and 'timing of the lead' is very important. Having learned this in Gaelic has allowed me to make the same 'leads' for hockey. The 'give and go', is another skill I learned in Gaelic which transfers to hockey, just expressed differently as a 2v1.

Making the defender commit before eliminating them is yet another. Although the object is different, a stick and a ball compared to just a ball, it is the movement of the feet and body that forces the decision of the defender. The same is true of tackling technique; the qualities required to perform the skill in both sports are similar. I also try to attack in hockey very much the same as I did in Gaelic; by running hard and cutting on the inside. I think if you were to watch me play Gaelic and then hockey, you would see many of the same movement patterns.

I think in every sport there are players who: 'look like' or 'play like' a typical player for that sport, some who look unorthodox but extremely effective and others that sometimes look like they are carrying a skillset from a previous sport. I think the latter is true of me. I feel I don't display all the typical characteristics, or have the complete skillset, of a traditional hockey player, but rather a hockey player with some skills that have been transferred from a previous sport. This is also easily spotted for those on our hockey team who have played camogie. They will often have a different technique of hitting the ball on their reverse side than your 'typical hockey player' and it is usually pretty effective. Another example are those who have previously competed in athletics. The athletic ability of these players is evident, and their strong running technique is very much representative of their athletic training.

For a team like the Irish hockey team, having a wide range of skills outside of the traditional hockey skillset, has proven to be an asset. Most hockey teams will never have defended against a camogie player or a Gaelic footballer, and so for this reason, we can be unpredictable to them and harder to read and defend against.

My advice to any youngster setting out on their sporting journey would be to sample as many sports as possible. This will provide you with a broad base of athletic qualities, skills and experiences that can be adapted to many sporting arenas. I would also advise that your sporting journey may take many twists and turns, and it may lead you to places you never imagined. Doors can open and close, and then open again. There may be tough choices to make along the way and at some point sacrifices will have to be made. Find your passion, follow your heart, commit to what you do and never give up on your dreams.

Best wishes,
Nicci Daly.

References:

Baker, J., Côté, J. and Abernethy, B. (2003) 'Sport-specific practice and the development of expert decision-making in team ball sports', Journal of Applied Sport Psychology, 15(1), pp. 12–25.

(Bridge & Toms, 2013)

Bridge, M. W. and Toms, M. R. (2013) 'The specialising or sampling debate: A retrospective analysis of adolescent sports participation in the UK', Journal of Sports Sciences, 31(1), pp. 87–96.

Collins, R. et al. (2014) 'Change of plans: An evaluation of the effectiveness and underlying mechanisms of successful talent transfer', Journal of Sports Sciences, 32(17), pp. 1621–1630.

Ericsson, K. A., Krampe, R. T. and Tesch-Römer, C. (1993) 'The role of deliberate practice in the acquisition of expert performance.', Psychological Review, 100(3), pp. 363–406.

Di Fiori, J. P. et al. (2017) 'Debunking early single sport specialisation and reshaping the youth sport experience: An NBA perspective', British Journal of Sports Medicine, 51(3), pp. 142–143.

Güllich, A. (2014) 'Many roads lead to Rome – Developmental paths to Olympic gold in men's field hockey', European Journal of Sport Science. Taylor & Francis, 14(8), pp. 763–771.

Malina, R. (2010) Early Sport Specialisation: Roots, Effectiveness, Risks, Current Sports Medicine Reports. doi: 10.1080/07303084.2010.10598525.

Moesch, K. et al. (2011) 'Late specialisation: the key to success in centimeters, grams, or seconds (cgs) sports', Scandinavian Journal of Medicine and Science in Sports, 21(6), pp. 1–9.

Myer, G. D. et al. (2016) 'Sports Specialization, Part II: Alternative Solutions to Early Sport Specialisation in Youth Athletes', Sports Health, 8(1), pp. 65–73.

Roetert, E. P., Woods, R. B. and Jayanthi, N. A. (2018) 'The benefits of multi-sport participation for youth tennis players.', Coaching & Sport Science Review, (75), pp. 14–17.

Strachan, L., Côté, J. and Deakin, J. (2009) '"Specialises" versus "samplers" in youth sport: Comparing experiences and outcomes', Sport Psychologist, 23(1), pp. 77–92.

Toms, M. (2014) 'Early Developmental Experiences Of Elite Golfers- A Case Study From The UK", World Scientific Congress of Golf', in World Scientific Congress of Golf.

SUMMARY POINTS - Chapter 22

- Sport participation can be with a club or played recreationally with friends.
- A minority of sports requires a peak performance before puberty, for example, gymnastics. In these instances, there are performance benefits to focusing on one sport.
- There are negatives associated with early specialization, such as overuse injuries, a lack of time spent with friends, and burnout.
- There are numerous benefits of participating in multiple sports in your youth.
- From mid-adolescence onwards, you may wish to limit your participation in some sports and specialise in your favored one(s). This is an individual choice.

CHAPTER 23: THE STUDENT ATHLETE

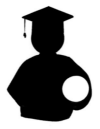

By Colm Flynn

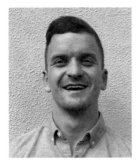

Colm Flynn is a guidance counsellor and secondary school teacher. His literary work includes a dissertation on the role of the guidance counsellor in supporting the student athlete. Colm holds a keen interest in the athlete creating a blend between their education, sporting life and other important elements in their personal development. Here he advises how to balance the demands of study and sport.

In combining school and study, with your sport you will inevitably encounter challenging scenarios. You may be entering a crucial year of study, such as your Junior Certificate or Leaving Certificate, and this coincides with an important competitive sporting year. You want to navigate both successfully. Sometimes your competition or training schedules mean that you will miss significant days of school, study or school assignments. You will need to catch up during, or after, your competition or training. Having a solid friend in each class that will share notes, or explain homework, is a great advantage. A common, but very effective, tool that all student-athletes should create and follow is a study and training schedule. Planning and scheduling are key (see Chapter 21). Be realistic, factor in the times you train and plan to work your homework and study around them.

It is possible that you may pick up an injury, be deselected from a team or panel, or experience worry about how well you are playing. This can result in low mood or self-doubt and impact on your studies. If demands become too much at certain times, it is important to notify teachers, your year head or your guidance counsellor about the extra challenges you may be facing.

Due to the individual nature of scenarios and circumstances involving different sports or school structures, there's no blueprint or 'right way' to overcome the challenges and difficulties that balancing study and sport presents. However, the common theme in helping and guiding students, lies in their own personal development. It is simply the further development of disciplines, habits and rituals that drive performance, which hold the key to both excelling in and balancing education and sport.

Competencies You Need to Develop

A wealth of research focuses on combining a sporting career with education. This simultaneous endeavour of educational and sporting achievement is referred to as a 'dual career' in sport psychology literature (Stambulova et. al, 2015). Recognising its prevalence, the European Parliament's (2016) policy department outlines key recommendations in relation to the standards of dual career programmes and services in their publication of EU Guidelines on Dual Careers of Athletes. The challenges and scenarios you are likely to face are recognised on a global level. While it may often feel that nobody realises the commitment it takes to combine education and sport, remember, many great athletes who have achieved at the top of their game have been through the same struggles.

An interesting European study, that surveyed 4,196 'dual career' athletes across various countries and fields of sport, may give you an insight into how the top performers manage it. When asked what they believed to be the most important attributes which helped them overcome different scenarios and challenging times in their careers, they outlined a range of different competencies that they felt were crucial. Below are the top 10 competencies the athletes felt were most important. These competencies, or principles, are applicable to all performance domains.

Adapted from the Gold in Education and Elite Sport Handbook for Dual Career Support Providers (2016).

Top 10 Competence Profile for Perceived Importance in Rank Order
1. Perseverance during challenging times and in the face of setbacks.
2. Understanding the importance of rest and recuperation.
3. Ability to cope with stress in sport and study.
4. Dedication to succeed in both sport and study.
5. Belief in your own ability to overcome the challenges in sport and study.

6. Willingness to make sacrifices and choices to succeed in sport and study.
7. Ability to use your time efficiently.
8. Ability to collaborate with support staff in study and sport (e.g. coach, teachers).
9. Self- discipline to manage the demands of your study and sport combination (e.g. work independently without the supervision of others).
10. Assertiveness- being self- assured and acting with confidence.

LIST THE COMPETENCIES YOU FEEL YOU HAVE WELL DEVELOPED & EXAMPLES OF WHY YOU FEEL SO.

_____

_____

LIST THE COMPETENCIES YOU FEEL YOU NEED TO DEVELOP IN THE MONTHS & YEARS AHEAD.

_____

_____

Ultimately, being a student athlete and competing in sport requires a large degree of self-focus. Challenging scenarios will often present themselves, be it your performance in school or sport, or relationships with your parents, friends or coaches. Know that your success lies with your ability to be aware of, and develop, the appropriate competencies needed to navigate the challenges of a dual career. It's also important to remember that the disciplines and skills developed through sport will complement your application to your study. Dedication, self-discipline, assertiveness, organisational and time management skills (see Chapter 21) and work ethic are all skills that are transferable to your studies if you so choose.

Future Study Plans

Selecting the best study plan and making the best choices in order to integrate both your sport and study is hugely important. Remember, sport is something you do as opposed to who you are (see Chapter 3). It is important you keep all things in context. It can be very challenging to strike a balance between your sporting career and studies.

An important time for recognising this need for balance is when you start to consider your future career path. As you progress through secondary school your curiosity will heighten around what options are available to you after you finish school and how your sport can complement those plans. Whether you hope to pursue a sports-related career, or something away from the sporting arena, the important questions remain the same.

- *What institutes offer the post Leaving Cert course, apprenticeship or college course you are interested in?*
- *Does the location and offerings of these institutes impact the possible balance between study and training or competition you wish to strike?*

Diligent research is your friend here. In addition to meeting your guidance counsellor in school, ensure you use available websites, prospectus and open days to gather all the information you need. As well as researching your course of study, which is paramount, perhaps you can consider the sporting facilities that the various institutes offer and the level at which they play, or regard, your sport.

Consideration may also need to be given to the possibility of scholarships being offered by different institutes. Again, research is crucial here. It is important not to choose a certain course of study, or a particular college, based on their scholarships. Applicant success in your sport is usually low and spaces are held for elite athletes only. However, the majority of third-level institutes offer sports scholarships to incoming students every year. Some colleges also offer additional CAO points to successful scholarship applicants. Other important questions may need consideration:

- *What sports scholarship options do the various institutes offer?*
- *What does the scholarship application involve?*

Some application processes can be detailed, so make sure you ask for help from your parents, coach or guidance counsellor to ensure you have a strong application complete before the deadline.

Plan B

There are numerous stories of athletes getting injured, being dropped from teams and squads or simply falling out of love with their sport. What do these athletes do now if all they have ever known is being an athlete and identifying solely with that role? Other options or future decisions can become limited. As a guidance counsellor, I urge students to always consider their Plan B.

I've seen the other side as well- athletes that progress to the highest level of their sport, but also work hard and plan out their education and future. This is the ideal scenario and usually results in a life where they work in a job they enjoy and get to play the sport they love.

I have also seen students make future decisions based entirely on their sporting goals. They repeat a Leaving Cert year or choose a certain college solely based on playing for a specific team. Don't be the athlete that forgets about their education. When performance and competition has ended, these athletes can be left on their own without a plan. Be wise, have a future focus.

Ultimately, you don't want to run the risk of neglecting your future career development or career decisions. While you actively engage, and thrive in your athletic role, don't relinquish the adequate exploration of alternative skills or interests. Whether it is work shadowing on certain jobs you think you might like, signing up to some online workshops of interest or simply reading material that is outside the sporting domain. You just don't know what interest or passion can be uncovered that could work hand in hand with your sporting career or even offer you an alternative avenue from your sporting life.

As your sporting career progresses, tough decisions will inevitably have to be made. The awareness and development of your skills and competencies will ensure that you can create the balance needed between your sport and education. Occasionally tough decisions will have to be made. The need for education must overcome the passion for sport.

Know your Plan B.
Colm Flynn

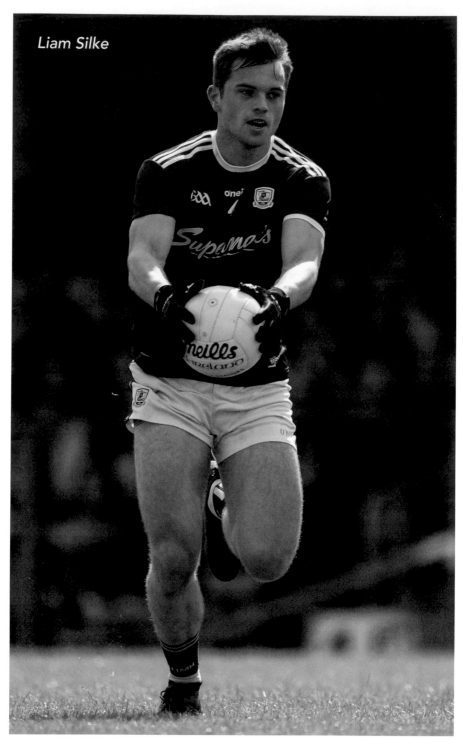

Liam Silke

Liam Silke

Liam Silke is a highly decorated Galway and Corofin Gaelic Footballer. With his spring and summer months largely taken up by inter-county commitments, and the autumn and winter months being given to club and college football, the demands on his time and energy have been unrelenting. His sporting achievements include: four All-Ireland Senior Club Titles, seven Galway Club Senior Titles, one Connacht Inter-County Title, one Division 2 National League Title, one U21 Inter-County All-Ireland Title, one Sigerson Cup with UCD as well as Club Footballer of the Year 2017/18. These has been achieved against the backdrop of an academic career that has included an Academic Scholarship in NUIG from 2012-2016 where he graduated with a Science Degree majoring in Pharmacology. Liam is currently studying Medicine in UCD, 2017-2021. Below, he gives an insight into how he has learned to balance and indeed excel in both sport and study.

Combining sport and study can be testing and time consuming but I feel there is a considerable overlap of the characteristics required to excel in both. Self-belief, determination, planning and the ability to apply yourself to the task at hand, are some of the fundamentals.

The main roadblock for most people is, time. 168 hours in a week, 56 of which should be spent sleeping, a few hours a day commuting and eating, there isn't that many hours left to achieve your goals.

Over the years I have found that prioritising time at different periods of your life is the best way to manage this. When you have exams, for example the Leaving Cert is coming up, study is where your focus must be and where you must put most of your effort. This is a period you may have to sacrifice a gym or training session because you will reap more from putting your effort into study at that point in time. Similarly, when you have an important game coming up, this is the time to focus on the sport side of things. It sounds simple, but a lot of people have tunnel vision where sport is all that matters and believe you cannot miss any training session. I've felt like this on many occasions, but I have had to prioritise what it is most important at the time in question and communicate it clearly and promptly to my coaches and educators.

As with most things in life, there is an element of balance needed. After a gruelling day in the library or working hard all day in school, sport is a channel to blow off some steam and is the perfect respite from the books. I feel when I get the balance correct it actually complements my study.

Unfortunately, prioritising hasn't always been possible throughout my sporting and academic life. Occasionally it has been a complicated juggling act. In May 2015, I was set to make my championship debut for the Galway senior football team in New York. This was to be one of my biggest days yet as a footballer. The problem was I was in the middle of my 3rd year science exams which accounted for 30% of my degree. Both were very important to me and I couldn't pick one over the other. I had a 2 hour written exam on a Friday morning and departed straight from the exam for the airport. The team had flown over on Thursday and got some sightseeing in, which I missed. I brought my laptop with me as I still had more exams to do when I returned to Ireland. I simply had to study while in New York and was fortunate that I had developed the ability to shift focus quickly which proved invaluable. We played the game on Sunday and I scored my first championship point as we ran out comfortable winners. We flew back on the Monday, arriving in Shannon airport early Tuesday morning. I had to deal with considerable jet lag while studying for another important exam the following day. This was a price I had to pay but was more than willing to do so, as I had genuine ambition in both my study and sporting domains.

Similar scenarios have unfolded with two All-Ireland club quarter finals in London with Corofin while Christmas exams have been ongoing, and last year we played London with Galway in the Connacht championship before my summer exams. These can be very stressful times but as already mentioned: self-belief, determination, preparation, planning and being able to apply yourself and shift focus quickly is how I have managed to deal with it.

Best wishes,
Liam Silke

References

Defruyt, S., P. Wylleman, N. Stambulova, S. Cecić Erpič, M. Graczyk & K. De Brandt (2019) Competencies of dual career support providers (DCSPs): A scenario-specific perspective, International Journal of Sport and Exercise Psychology.
Franck, A & Stambulova, N. (2019) The junior to senior transition: a narrative analysis of the pathways of two Swedish athletes, Qualitative Research in Sport, Exercise and Health, 11:3, 284-298,

SUMMARY POINTS - Chapter 23
- *The need for education must be balanced with the passion for sport.*
- *Further development of disciplines, habits and rituals that drive performance, hold the key to both excelling in, and balancing, education and sport.*
- *Planning and scheduling are key.*
- *The life of a student athlete requires a large degree of self-focus.*
- *Be diligent and informed when considering your future career path.*

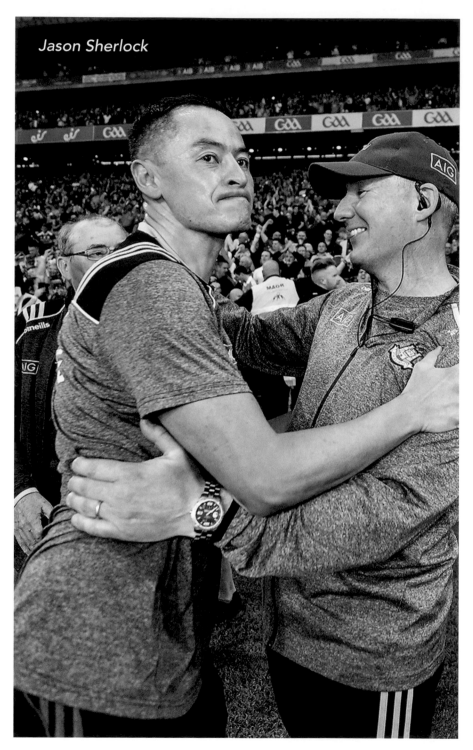

Jason Sherlock

CHAPTER 24: RACISM IN SPORT

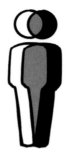

By Jason Sherlock

Jason Sherlock is a former Dublin Gaelic footballer who won an All-Ireland Senior Football Championship in his debut year at the age of 19. He went on to have a 15 year playing career with Dublin. He played professional soccer for UCD and Shamrock Rovers and made one appearance for the Republic of Ireland U-21s. He also represented Ireland in Basketball from U-15 to U-19. On retiring, Jason became involved in coaching, first managing Dublin Development Squads from U-13 to Minor before becoming part of the management team of the record breaking five-in-a-row Dublin team.

Jason is the son of an Irish mother and a father from Hong Kong. He was 'different' at a time when Ireland wasn't as multicultural as it is today. Here, he shares his insights into racism in sport and advises you, the next generation, on how to be a part of eradicating racism from sport and indeed Irish society at large.

Sport has been a huge part of my life. It has brought me many places and offered me many experiences. Most of these experiences have been positive, but some have been negative. Growing up my skin was a different colour to that of almost everyone around me. I was 'different', but back then I didn't understand that as human we are all unique; we are all different. This difference is what makes us special.

Throughout my career the colour of my skin was a source of attention for many. I experienced racist abuse and it hurt me. I am not so sure this hurt will ever leave me. I remember every situation where I was racially abused by a player, the crowd or a manager, and that never leaves you. We need education for those people that feel they can give racial abuse; they need to understand its impact. Ultimately if you've been racially abused at any time in your life, it will never leave you. It will always be part of you and it will affect your self-worth and self-esteem. As a youngster I didn't have the tools to deal with racist abuse in sport. I would get frustrated and lose focus, often ending up in confrontations that would see me booked or indeed sent off. Nowadays there is more understanding of the problem and more people there to help; that perhaps weren't there when I was young. To any youngster reading this who is experiencing racial abuse in sport, or indeed anywhere in life, I would advise the following:

- You are not the one with the problem- the racist is.
- You are not able to control the words or actions of anyone else. You can only control how you respond to those words and actions. Two wrongs don't make a right. You are educated enough to know what is happening is wrong and take solace in this.
- Empower yourself to say what has happened to you is wrong and communicate it clearly with the referee, your coach or team captain.
- Sometimes the punishment isn't what it should be, but, again, this is out of your control.
- Understand you are there to play and put your focus on this.
- Appreciate that those who are abused are often the ones that are playing the best.

In recent times I have been impressed by the stands taken by Irish athletes such as Aaron Cunningham and Lee Chin. They know what is right and wrong in terms of what has been said to them on playing fields and they have stood up to this in a strong and dignified manner. I commend them and encourage athletes throughout Ireland to continue to do likewise.

Sport is about passion and we should never seek to take this away, but at the same time, there are comments made in sport that are unacceptable. Race is a line that shouldn't be crossed. In the heat of the moment things are often said in a bid to gain the upper hand psychologically; 'verbals' it is sometimes called. Race is something that can never be used here; again, race is a line that must never be crossed. We cannot do anything about the colour of our skin and sports men and women must have an acceptance of each other.

I would now like to speak to you- the youth of Ireland at large. You, our next generation, are the ones with the power to create positive change. On a sporting front we should be looking to get as many as possible *involved in sport. Sport is good for society. It is our responsibility as athletes to welcome as many as possible into our games. Sport should welcome everyone therefore it is our responsibility to have neither an active or passive part in racism.*

Racism must be eradicated and it starts with you. Respect, responsibility and representation are all crucial elements of sport. It is the athletes challenge to leave the jersey in a better place. This is all encompassing. When you go out to play you are representing a place, a club, a group. With this comes great responsibility. Can you represent and present with genuine goodness and class? Can you improve yourself, your team, indeed your sport? It is imperative that you provide what impact you can. In sport, we are given the opportunity to improve our community by how we represent them.

> *"The only thing necessary for the triumph of evil is for good men to do nothing".*
> *Edmund Burke*

Now is the time to get this right in our society and youth sport can be the place it starts. I would call on you to be actively anti-racist in sport. Don't accept it from a teammate to an opponent or indeed a coach or fan to an opponent. Never be a bystander. Stand with your teammate if they are being wronged.

If this short piece can positively influence one youth and make things better for them, it has been worthwhile. However, the power of sport can be much greater and has the potential to change society. Sport is for everyone, and as athletes it is becoming of us to make everyone welcome. Being the best you can be in sport involves so much more than performing well come game time. Never underestimate the power of your influence to change and improve yourself, your team, your community and your sport. Racism has no place in sport and by extension, life. My challenge to you is to part of stamping it out.

Yours in sport,
Jason Sherlock

SUMMARY POINTS - Chapter 24

- *Racism is wrong and must be eradicated.*
- *If you experience racial abuse, know that you are not the one with the problem.*
- *Sport has the potential to change society.*
- *Sport should welcome everyone, therefore it is our responsibility to have neither an active or passive part in racism.*
- *Never be a bystander to racism or racist behaviour in sport.*
- *Stand up against racism.*

CHAPTER 25: WOMEN IN SPORT

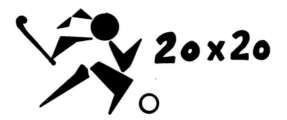

By Sarah Colgan of 20x20

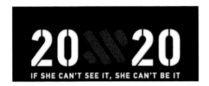

Sarah Colgan is Co-Founder of the 20x20 movement which she conceptualised and delivered with Heather Thornton under their company Along Came a Spider. For more information, see www.20x20.ie

In 2018, my family gathered round the television to watch Ireland's women play the Netherlands in hockey's World Cup Final. My children had never experienced anything quite like this – where we were all together watching a major women's sporting event live on TV.

My daughter, then aged seven, turned to me with a look on her face of both incredulity and joy and asked, "Is it really girls playing on the telly?" I felt I was witnessing a moment in slow motion, and as I sat there, looking at her being transfixed, it reinforced strongly to me what we mean by 'if she can't see it, she can't be it'. The message is more than a slogan, it is actually laying down a challenge to a culture which has marginalised the involvement of women in sport throughout history.

At the end of 2018 we founded the 20x20 movement, so called as it aims to achieve 20 percent more attendance, participation and media coverage for women in sport by the end of 2020. Our mission was to spearhead a shift in society's perception, to challenge a non-malicious but deeply ingrained subliminal bias so that women's sport can become part of our cultural DNA in the way that men's sport is.

What results from a shift in mindset is a new norm whereas many girls as boys participate, our sportswomen are valued, making our society more equal as well as healthier and happier, and giving a nation of sport-lovers more sport to follow.

On that summer's day in 2018, my mind raced back to the message for my daughter, that the games you saw your grandparents, uncles, aunts gather together for were only men's games. Our relations didn't come around and cheer for women playing on the TV.

Thankfully, that is changing for the next generation. But there remains a long road to travel.

Having interviewed scores of men, women and teenagers since 20x20 launched we keep hearing common threads in their stories: Dads who have daughters recognising unconscious comments from people commiserating with them for not having a son to create sporting memories with, as though these memories cannot be created with girls. Women who gave up sport as kids who are now regretting what they have missed, not only the health benefits but the leadership skills, the sense of being needed and part of a team. And teenage girls who felt uncomfortable simply because the culture wasn't there for them to be valued as athletes in the same way as it was for boys. It was only the ones with an unusual grit or talent who broke through.

But the zeitgeist, and a shift in mindset, means many green shoots are emanating. We've also heard of young boys collecting football cards and not seeing a difference between the male or female players; and of men in pubs analysing Katie Taylor's technical ability rather than the previous well-worn patronising commentary around female athletes. When the Irish women's rugby team asked that pundits analyse their performances with exactly the same tone and language as they would the men's team, they helped to start a shift in the public consciousness about how all women's sporting events should be viewed.

In 20x20's two year run, there have been some seismic events in Irish sport which will undoubtedly leave a legacy. For instance, Ireland broke six attendance records across our biggest women's fixtures in 2019, and the GAA gave centre stage to women at an All-Ireland men's semi-final in front of a sell-out Croke Park crowd – asking everyone in attendance to show their stripes for 20x20 and women in sport. This would not have happened five years ago and the message of men's sport supporting women's sport is a welcome one.

There is no doubt there is a massive commercial gap between men's and women's sport but we can never set about correcting that gap if first we don't invest in women culturally and show their sport the respect it deserves. Women in sport needs to be part of our societal norm and then, like with anything else, the demand and the ability to generate revenue will follow. But it needs a shot in the arm now, an element of positive discrimination, in order to rebalance the investment in Irish sport over so many years.

If you push yourself to explore the implications of failing to make it, it paints a bleak picture. A lost opportunity for Ireland, for us all. I hope today's young athletes never stop playing. That they keep backing themselves. And that none of us forget to champion the women in sport around us.

Sarah Colgan

SUMMARY POINTS - Chapter 25

- *'If she can't see it, she can't be it'.*
- *In 20x20's two year run, there have been some seismic events in Irish sport which will undoubtedly leave a legacy.*
- *Never stop playing.*
- *Champion the girls and women in sport around you.*

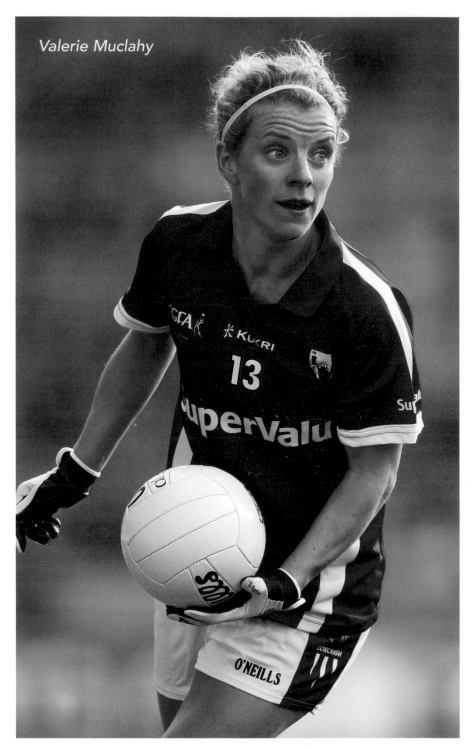

Valerie Muclahy

CHAPTER 26: SIMPLY BE

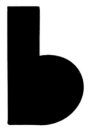

By Valerie Mulcahy

Valerie Mulcahy is a former Cork Ladies' Gaelic footballer. Throughout her career she won ten All-Ireland titles, nine National Football League titles, and was an All-Star on six occasions. She also played soccer for Cork Women's FC and Cork City in the Women's National League, as well as representing Ireland in the sport. In January 2015, Valerie publicly came out as gay. She subsequently campaigned in favour of marriage equality in the Republic of Ireland during the 2015 Referendum and has been an advocate for the LGBT community since.

Sport has always been a happy place for me. It has afforded me many great experiences and I have made great friends through my involvement with many teams. Sport is part of my identity. Another part of my identity is my sexuality. It is a part of who I am, but only one of many parts. It does not define me.

We are all unique. Our differences makes us who we are. The challenge for us all is to embrace who we are and be the best we can be, play the deck of cards we were dealt- so to speak. 'Be yourself, everyone else is already taken', is one of life's great truths from Oscar Wilde. Our challenge is to embrace all the elements of what makes us unique.

For some people, part of their uniqueness is their sexuality. Sexual orientation can be a difficult thing to figure out. Some find it easier to navigate than others. For some it may be more complex and challenging- often worried about what others will think, more than feeling uncomfortable themselves with it- at least that's what it felt like for me. My first piece of advice to any youngster exploring their feelings or untangling their sexuality would be to take your time. There is no need to rush to a 'conclusion'. This is only part of who you are. It is not something that has to consume you. I let it occupy my mind far too much, and made a bigger deal about it in my head than it needed to be. Looking back now, I would have approached things differently. I would suggest you find a trusted peer or adult to discuss any areas that are concerning you. They say talk is cheap, but talk is also valuable. It is good to talk, good to share feelings and good to seek insight and guidance. You don't need to have all the answers straight away. Follow your feelings, rather than your thoughts!

Although it may now be easy for me to say, but there really is no need to carry so much fear around this topic. Sometimes we can get preoccupied with things and thoughts, and make them out to be bigger than they need to be. Again, your sexual orientation is only a part of you. If you find yourself struggling with it, take comfort in the fact that many have gone before you. Every human encounters various challenges on their journey. I found that exploring my sexuality gave me a greater insight into me as a person and my character. I essentially saw it as something that made me stronger as a person and a personal challenge that I overcame.

Irish sport and society are now more open, understanding and inclusive than ever before. There is a greater awareness of diversity; the visibility is growing. For example, the GAA walked in the Dublin Pride Parade last year. For GAA people in the LGBT community, this was a landmark day. The work that has been done on behalf of our community is starting to become evident in obvious, tangible ways. This good work continues and the awareness and understanding that we all belong, continues to grow. As a country, we are starting to welcome and appreciate diversity. We all belong. We are all valued.

In any team environment, there are many different types of people who come from so many different backgrounds and walks of life. This diversity is often what makes a team successful. At its highest level, sports teaches us how to care for, and work with, one another. Good teammates want their peers to be happy and as a result perform better on the field of play. Good teammates are aware of the language they use. They are considerate and compassionate. Their actions speak for them. Their humanity makes those around them feel valued and empowered. Throughout my sporting career I was fortunate to be surrounded by great teammates. They were understanding and accepting of my differences and provided me with a strong support network which emboldened me to be the best and most honest version of myself. The influence of the teammate is indeed far reaching, and one we must all appreciate.

'Treat people the way we would like to be treated ourselves', is another of life's great truths. Occasionally you find people in sport, and life, who say mean and nasty things and react in a negative manner. What I like to remember is that a person's reaction is a reflection of them and not a reflection of you. Being indifferent to others' small minded opinions is one of life's great freedoms, and often this comes with age and experience.

If you are a person who is currently figuring things out with regards to their sexuality you can take comfort from the fact that I, and many more, was once that person. Looking back, if you told me as a youngster that I would be talking openly about my sexuality, or an active advocate for change, I wouldn't have believed you for a second. But honesty, courage, strength and the support of good people has led me to a place where I can be totally open and happy in myself. I have found that being myself and owning my sexuality has been empowering for me and others around me. Know that the courage and strength required is inside you and support is there for you. Simply be you.

I wish you well,
Valerie Mulcahy

SUMMARY POINTS - Chapter 26

- We are all unique. For some people, part of their uniqueness is their sexuality.
- Your sexuality is only part of who you are. It is not something that has to consume you.
- Find a trusted peer or adult to discuss any areas that are concerning you.
- Follow your feelings, rather than your thoughts.
- Irish sport and society are now more open, understanding and inclusive than ever before.
- Good teammates are aware of the language they use. They are considerate and compassionate. Their actions speak for them.
- Know that the courage and strength required to simply 'be you' is inside you, and support is there for you.

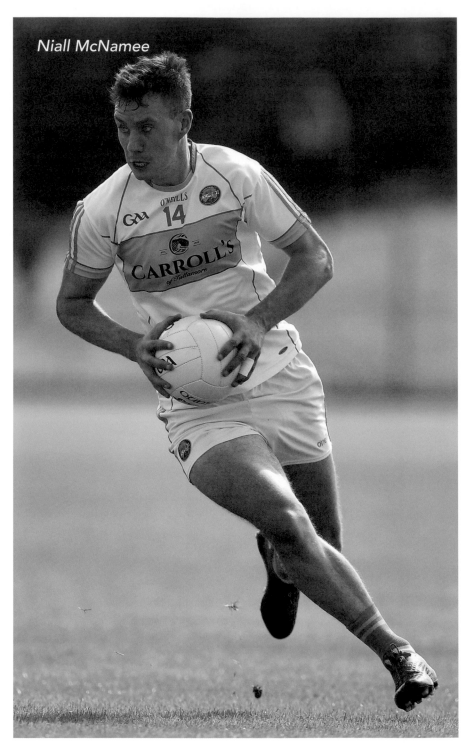

Niall McNamee

CHAPTER 27 : TOUGH TIMES

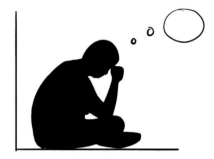

For me, this is a really important chapter in the book. This world we live in can be challenging to navigate. Some of us narrowly avoid certain pitfalls and traps; others are not so fortunate. Addiction and depression are all too common in today's world. The stories below are stories of hard times, but also stories of hope and recovery.

Niall McNamee

Niall McNamee made his senior intercounty football debut for Offaly in 2003 at the age of 17. He continues to play for Offaly and has won 10 Offaly Senior Football Championships with his club, Rhode, as well as a Dublin Senior Football Championship with UCD in 2006. He has also played for Leinster and represented Ireland in International Rules. He started gambling in his mid-teens and it became progressively worse over a short number of years. There was a period in time where he had no control over it. Today, he helps young athletes in trouble with addiction and works with the Gaelic Players Association in this area.

Competitiveness is in all of us. It's a positive trait, but can also bring us to places that cause us more harm than good. I have always loved the idea of competing since I was very young. Sport has the magical ingredient of bringing all the challenges of life into a 70 minute match or a 100m sprint. The thrill of winning; the devastation of losing. Unfortunately some of us can be defined by those events. People begin to see us as being..... just that moment in time, that sporting moment that defines the person. Sometimes the player begins to believe it too; they are just this, a sportsperson on a never ending search to find those moments of joy through the winning of a championship or personal awards.

Without this validation, some sports people find it difficult to exist in the world. They have this endless struggle of not knowing who the person is behind the sport. The days in between competition can seem meaningless. It is a wishful spiral of time passing until that first whistle blows and you are away from the troubles, and back to doing what makes you feel alive.

So how can a person feel alive in those lonely midweek days? For me it was simple; go to the bookies and pass the time. Feel that same adrenaline rush that you feel just before the dressing room door opens. In the bookies though, it is different. You can feel that adrenaline rush every couple of minutes. As each horse race begins I'm repeating the dose until it becomes something that I must have. And what happens if the game at the weekend didn't go our way? Well what better place to hide away, not only from the world and its people, but from the disappointment and sadness and anger.

Sport in itself can be addictive. It's that obsession to be the best that can often have a detrimental effect on other aspects of life. Playing an amateur sport can mean that career goals can often be put on hold in pursuit of sporting dreams. While this can be a noble pursuit, and sport can teach us all the wonderful skills and behaviours that it takes to be a valuable member of a work team and indeed society, it can also leave us blinded to the fact that bills need to be paid. As a result, for me anyway, gambling was a sure fire way to win money, in a very short period of time, without much work. This I thought, would allow me to pursue my sporting dreams uninterrupted.

There is a massive downside however. Trying to be a good teammate and indeed human being is challenging at the best of times. My experience has shown me that gambling compulsively brings out the absolute worst traits in a person. Anger, impatience, aggression, arrogance and greed are but a few. The person in the middle of this type of merry-go-round of emotions and behaviours doesn't know how they got there and also how to get off. One minute you're up, life is good and all the problems before you walked in the door, or placed that bet online, are gone. Then however, there are the downs: the chasing, the borrowing, the checking under the seat of the car for change. But we never talk about the stuff that isn't glamorous. It is only the winning stories that make it into the public domain.

The strength however lies in the broken stories, in the ones of loss and feeling like you have no control. Once you cross that line of knowing gambling is destroying your life, there is no going back. You may gamble on and place bet after bet, but deep down you know it isn't *the answer. All the while sport will continue. You will have those special performances and for a few days all will be well with the world. When the dust settles though, where are you? Are you comfortable with the person that is living this life? Can you endure another few weeks, months, perhaps even years before that special sporting tale comes true again? Or are you going to make a decision that you need help? Will you finally realise that the reason you are having that bet, taking that drink, trying that drug is because actually..... you aren't happy. You have found something that has filled the void but it ultimately will kill the best parts of you.*

There is a way out though. There are a lot of support services available for people who may be experiencing what I have just mentioned. The biggest challenge is to admit that there is a problem. A lot of the time it feels as though nobody will be able to help. The burden is too great to carry so why should we inflict that on somebody else. The fact is, and I know this from experience, once you share that big part of you that you have been keeping secret for so long a whole new world will open up for you. Who you choose to tell is entirely up to you, but there are many options. Bear in mind also that the person you tell may not have all the answers. The beautiful thing is that they don't have to. One or two phone calls later and they will have found a person who will be able to empathise with you and help you. That could range from a counsellor, a therapist, a gambler's anonymous member to a treatment centre. The support structure already exists, it's just a world you haven't been shown yet.

Best of luck,
Niall McNamee

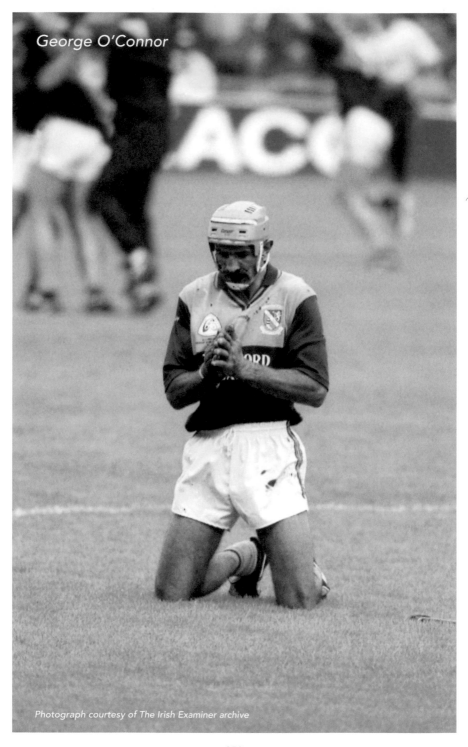

George O'Connor

Photograph courtesy of The Irish Examiner archive

George O'Connor

George O'Connor is a retired Wexford hurler. After seventeen years playing senior hurling he won his first All-Ireland Hurling medal in 1996 at 37 years old. It was his last game for Wexford and his second last game of hurling ever. He played one more game for his club and left it at that. He had given his all.

After he retired he devoted his time and energy into building coaching structures in Wexford and beyond. George ran into tough times and experienced severe depression but came out the other side a stronger and wiser man. Today he is happy and healthy, and likes to help people who are suffering and struggling with their inner demons.

It is ironic that I sit here on a beautiful first of May evening at the beginning of summer. All I can think of is getting out to the land and experiencing its beauty. Nature has its great properties of healings and searching the body and soul. It is calling me. I sit with my unconscious hat on and feel the flow. I am afforded this opportunity by Paul to give what I feel is an honest and truthful account of my experiences to date.

Today I was with a great friend of mine, a man of depth and resilience. A man that has lived to date, four lives in one, and continues to surprise me with his knowledge. We spoke for what I thought was an hour. In fact, it was closer to three. He spoke of his deep understanding for young people. "Ah sure," he said, "we protect them, feed them, care for them and most important of all, give them the great gift of time." Music to my ears. So simple, yet it sounds idyllic. "So George," he continued, "we give the children time, not presents, not money, nothing extravagant, just time" he said.

Life feels great for me now, however there were times when this wasn't the case. There have been times when I have suffered. Times when I have felt little hope for the future: anxious, stressed, depressed, devoid of life… an empty vessel, only hanging on. I have reached some highs in my life, but have also reached many lows. I have needed help and I have sought help. In a dark period of my life I have had a number of false dawns where I thought I was better and fully recharged, only to run flat again. I have been forced to learn about myself and the inner workings of my mind, my body, my spirit and my soul. I have learned to love myself. It has been a journey of self-discovery.

I am writing this short piece for young people who may experience tough times. Times in their life when the mood is very low and they feel alone and down. Times when there is little or no light. The batteries feel like they are dying. I know how it feels. Life can be tough. It can be busy and unrelenting, leaving no time to recharge the batteries and reinvigorate the spirit. The never ending demands on a person- go, go, go! The batteries get worn down, a wave hits us and we become susceptible to viruses of the mind. The spirit seems broken and the soul is darkened. Sadness comes over us. A way out of it is unclear. Help is needed and we must ask for it. We must learn how to cope, learn how to survive and then, go and learn how to thrive.

How do we understand stress, anxiety, and depression? Can one fully understand themselves first under the headings of physical, emotional, mental and spiritual? This must be in our toolkit if we are to succeed in bringing the colours back into our lives. No doubt some of the tools in this book can help. For me it always helps to reconnect with nature. Look, a blackberry! There, a wild strawberry! See the trees connect to one another. Hear a thrush bird sing. See the swallows arrive and wonder how they know when to leave? Engage and spend time in Mother Nature. Observe myself in it, and through it, gain the strength and composure to thrive in the hustle and bustle of this modern world. For me, we have to 'listen to ourselves' and 'learn ourselves', learn how to spend our time in ways that will open our mind and soul, and strengthen our spirit. Time well spent is a healer. Time is precious. Learn to spend it wisely.

We are all wired differently. Some of us are gentler souls than others. Some of us go through hardships in our lives that affect us deeply and if not healed properly these wounds are always there, ready to reopen. We all have our demons. We all have parts of ourselves that we don't like to acknowledge, but we see lurking inside. These can cause some of us to do irrational and selfish things, not out of love for ourselves, but out of fear for ourselves. When times are bad you must ask for help. There are people that can help you understand this life and the struggles it can bring. You must also learn what works for you and what is the best way to spend time that can nourish your mind, body, spirit and soul. I wish you well on the great journey of life.

God bless,
George O'Connor.

Conor Whelan

Conor Whelan is a current Galway Senior Hurler. He was part of the 2017 Galway team, that ended the 29 year wait for the Liam McCarthy Cup. He ended that season, winning an All-Star and being named Young Hurler of the Year. Conor is a supporter of Jigsaw, a mental health charity for young people. Below he tells his story of what led him to become involved with Jigsaw and of his passion to help spread the word and contribute positively in the area of youth mental health.

I have been hurling for as long as I can remember. Hurling has always been a source of enjoyment for me; somewhere I can just be myself, in my own little world. Hurling has always given me an outlet. The pitch in Kinvara has often been a source of inspiration, even on the darkest of days. I am rather fortunate that I have somewhere I can go, somewhere to escape the world to find utter peace. Unfortunately, not everyone has such an outlet. Some people find it difficult to switch off, to escape their worries on a daily basis, regardless of what they do.

My first cousin, Niall Donoghue, was one such person who struggled to deal with certain aspects of life. Niall was a happy-go-lucky, kind-hearted person. Hurling for the Galway senior team, he had it all going for him. However, he found himself worrying and anxious about things which in hindsight didn't really matter. His mental health spiralled and he came to the point of no return. Surrounded in darkness, with no light at the end of the tunnel, just emptiness. He was only 22 years old and had played in the All-Ireland Final (and replay) for Galway the previous year. Niall was fantastic that summer and was nominated for an All-Star. Just over a year later, he was gone.

As it turned out, this was the first time I had ever heard the word 'suicide'. I was 17 years old and found myself googling the term; what does this mean and why is it relevant to Niall's death? I came to understand that suicide could be the most severe consequences of a mental health illness known as depression. This was all new to me and a lot to digest as a teenager. Niall's death raised the topic of suicide and depression in his hometown and the surrounding areas of south Galway. As a direct consequence of Niall's death I feel that a lot of people, old and young, came to realise they had been experiencing the same feelings as Niall had. His death was immensely sad; such a talented and bright young man gone. It is still very raw, really hard to take, but I like to think Niall is looking down knowing he has helped to impact others for the better.

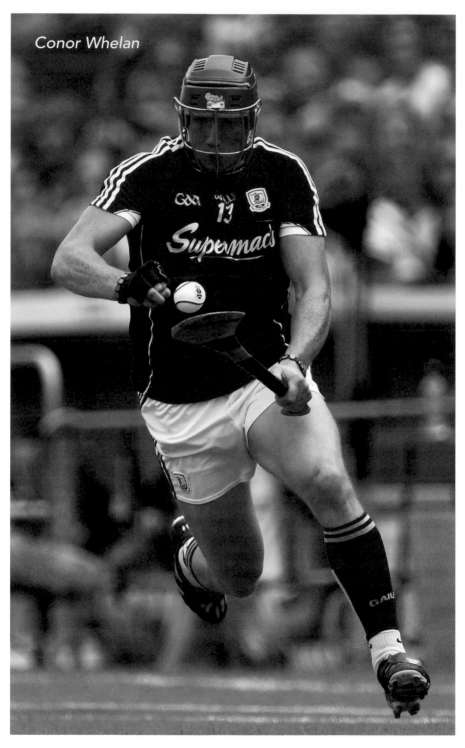

Conor Whelan

In the months after Niall's death I wondered how I had been through primary education, and then onto secondary education and had never heard anything related to mental health. As a result, I felt it became part of my identity to set about helping to change this. Breaking the silence around mental health is my goal. As an intercounty GAA player, I am in a privileged position in Irish society. As part of this role, I feel it is important to give back to society in any way I possibly can.

I am hugely passionate about the topic of mental health, the importance of looking after our mental health and most importantly the main message – talking to someone and reaching out for help. This passion has brought me on my journey with Jigsaw Ireland, a non-profit organisation which provides vital support in the area of mental health for young people from the ages of 12 to 25. To see first-hand the work that these people do, the lengths they go to in order to help people and unfortunately the struggle to help finance this work, made me feel compelled to contribute in any way possible. In truth, I feel we all have a responsibility to raise awareness around mental health in any way we can.

As a supporter of Jigsaw, I try to reiterate the key messages they share. Your mental health and your physical health are interlinked, if you don't maintain one aspect of your health, the other will suffer as a result. For me, exercise was never an issue. I always found sport an outlet. Exercise positively impacts the brain and is proven to improve your brain function. I feel it is the best cure to any problem; but that's just me. We are all different.

You must grow to understand and appreciate the importance of 'minding your mind' and work to develop the appropriate skills and tools to stay both mentally and physically strong. From time to time, I believe everyone experiences ups and downs. Sometimes these downs become longer, more sustained. I cannot overstate the importance of speaking about your emotions and what is getting you down. A problem shared is a problem halved. This is a message we are thankfully getting across in schools. I have seen first-hand, the wonderful work that is being done in my own school, Coláiste Mhuire, Ballygar, among others. We need to further emphasise this message and continue to educate our teenagers and young adults on the importance of looking after your wellbeing.

Life didn't come with any instructions or user manual; just the gift of life. We are all extremely fortunate to have this wonderful gift. Sometimes this gift can become blurred, and we can get lost in the journey. We should never lose perspective of what really matters in our lives. There will be challenges, and lots of them, however these challenges should not define us. They should simply mold us into stronger characters on the journey to our destiny.

Best wishes,
Conor Whelan.

JIGSAW
Young people's
health in mind

To see how Jigsaw can support you visit www.jigsaw.ie

SUMMARY POINTS - Chapter 27

- This world we live in can, at times, be very challenging to navigate.
- Understand and appreciate the importance of 'minding your mind' and work to develop the appropriate skills and tools to stay strong in mind, body, spirit and soul.
- Never lose perspective of what really matters in your life.
- Seek help from trusted people.
- There are a lot of support services available for those who may be experiencing tough times.

CHAPTER 28: THE OBSTACLE IS THE WAY

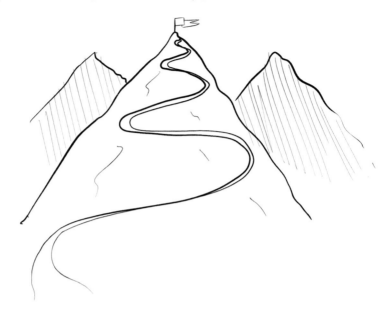

One of the core messages of this book is that sport is for everyone and if harnessed and utilised to its full potential it can and should be the cornerstone of a healthy and happy society. With this said, it cannot be denied that the opportunities to engage in and with sport appear more obvious for some than others. For some, there appear to be more obstacles to overcome and indeed some of these obstacles can appear insurmountable.

I have borrowed the title of this chapter from the book, 'The Obstacle is the Way' by Ryan Holiday. In the book Holiday explains how to apply the principles of Stoicism to overcoming challenges. He uses the example of the Roman Emperor Marcus Aurelius who ruled the Roman Empire for 19 years and articulated the Stoic approach to overcoming obstacles with the quote:

> "The impediment to action advances action.
> What stands in the way becomes the way".
> Marcus Aurelius

The stories below may help you think differently and reframe your challenges. Sport is for everyone. The obstacle is the way.

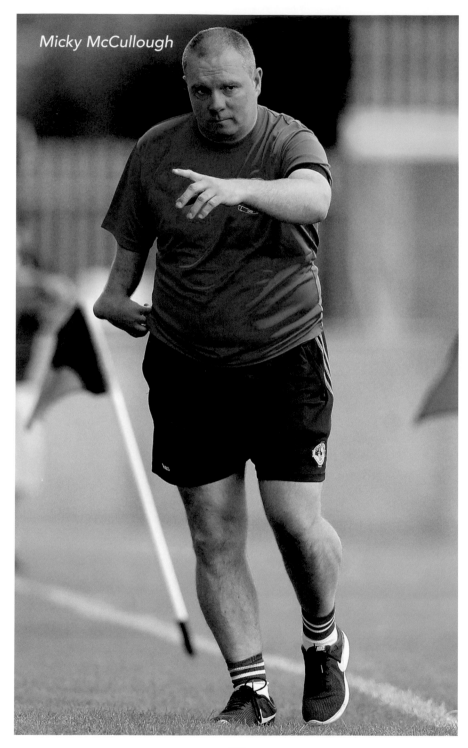

Micky McCullough

Micky McCullough

Micky McCullough was born with what he loosely terms a 'deformed' arm. He has no radius or thumb in his right hand and no movement in his fingers except his baby fingers. Despite this he enjoyed a long and distinguished hurling career winning eight Ulster colleges' titles, one Ulster Colleges All-Star, an Antrim and Ulster Senior Hurling Championship with his club Rossa, two Ulster Minor and three Ulster U21 Championships with Antrim as well as three nominations for The Belfast Telegraph Sports Awards. This is what he learned along the way.

I honestly never knew I was different until I reached secondary school. Looking back, to begin I played for the friendship because I definitely lacked the skills. I couldn't strike the ball out of my hands. My options were simple; go join in, get on with it or run around the streets on my own.

I was always game. I never hid from a tackle, whether I could protect myself or not, and I always had a decent awareness for the game. I learned to adapt, I learned to think and see things differently. I was a rogue but in my defence, I had to be. I knew my limitations.

By the age of fourteen, I still couldn't play the game to any level. If I'm honest, I didn't even enjoy it most of the time. But I stayed going, partly for the social element and partly because I wasn't a quitter.

I still remember the two milestone moments when my hurling career changed forever. The first one was as a 15 year old at Rossa Summer Scheme. It was the first time I ever felt the sweet- spot strike; the first time I struck it out of hands correctly. I felt that snap on the hurl, heard that crack off the boss and watched the ball fly 40 metres to the target. I was hooked. After nearly eight years of not being able to, now I could. If I could do this, then surely I could do anything. So, along with my sense of belonging and my inability to quit, I now added the confidence that I could do it!

The second milestone moment was while playing for my school, St Mary's. Tony and Eddie were the coaches in school and they would have pushed us very hard. They helped me add an ability to work hard, to my list of qualities. We were thought to fear no one but respect everyone. I had definitely noticed an improvement in my game by sixteen. I was now coming more and more into the reckoning to start and getting more game time. I developed a great hunger to see how good I could be at this game.

In 1997 we were preparing for the colleges All Ireland semi-final and the school took us on a training camp to Wexford. While there, we played a challenge game against St Peters. I started on the bench but was mad to get out on the pitch. Fifteen minutes in, the call came, 'Micky strip off'. I was only on the pitch 30 seconds when a ball was fired into my corner. I was out in front as usual, but normally my first touch was terrible. For some reason, this time I went with the hand; the ball was low to ground but bouncing. Next thing I knew I had the ball in hand on the half turn and was gone. My confidence shot through the roof, I wanted every ball, and I wanted scores. Why had I wasted 10 years trying to control a ball with my stick when it was just easier to use my hand? I think I finished that day with about 1-6 and from that point I never looked back. I had hunger, I had camaraderie, I never quit, I could work hard and now I could really play. It took time, it took patience, but now I had it. The years of perseverance began to bear fruit.

From that moment on I went on to play county, to be an automatic starter and a key player in teams, to win a college All-Star, to win senior championships. Seven years later my club, Rossa, won the Antrim Senior Hurling Championship, the only Belfast team that has won the Antrim championship in over 30 years at the time of writing. I contributed 5 points to the win and would go on to win Ulster and lose out in the All-Ireland semi-final stage to an excellent James Stephens from Kilkenny. On Antrim championship final day I received a ball late in the first half with two players making a run off my left side. I was able to flick the 'behind the back hand pass', long before Joe Canning became famous for it. This was in no way a show boat or arrogance, it was necessity. I simply wasn't physically able to hand pass off my right so I had to adapt. If I was asked to sum up the key lessons from my playing career it would be to work harder, think better than everyone else and adapt. I played county in both hurling and football and believe it or not was actually a very useful handball player.

I owe a lot to my coaches and mentors. My grandfather would never have accepted an "I can't" attitude from me. Joe Quinn was the same.

Eddie and Tony too, and in later years Aiden Hamill showed great faith in me as a senior hurler. I also must thank Micky McCollum as county minor manager that also took the chance on me. It was only years later it hit me how hard it must have been for these men to not only put me out there, but also to trust me to do a job. Let's call a spade a spade, hurling isn't easy, but here was some idiot at county level trying to do it with one arm. Is it comparable to trying to play premiership soccer with one leg? As Aiden Hamill stood on the line in a county final, steeped in Rossa tradition, did he think it would be the man with one arm that would play a role in bringing the Volunteer Cup back to Belfast. For all my resilience and determination I needed the lucky breaks and people that trusted me.

I could have walked away a million times, I could have just played seconds or thirds, and no one would have said a thing. Just 'having a go' was never going to be me. My Granda wouldn't have allowed that. But up until those two incidents that's all I did; I had a go, messed about. Looking back, it takes resilience to keep coming back, to face failure, dust yourself off and go again. My rewards for sticking at it were greater than all those years of failure.

I now work as a coach and I like to think I have learned from everyone I have encountered. Work hard, show respect and fear no one are still my core principles that Eddie and Tony instilled in my St Mary's days. Hone your skills, as Joe Quinn taught us. Take your time, as every player will develop at a different rate. Micky McCollum taught me to take chances, embrace risk and never give up because it's always darkest before the dawn. I'd like to think I have Aiden Hamill's sheer desire to win mixed in there too.

Remember, everyone in every team is the best at something. How can you judge if someone has the best skills? Well, you can see them. How can you judge if someone is the fittest or the strongest? Their gym results will tell you. I would imagine I was the most resilient on any team I played on. How? Because I just was never going to quit, I was never going to accept defeat and those are the traits I learned without realising in those days, weeks, months, years before I ever learned to hurl properly.

Thanks,
Micky McCullough.

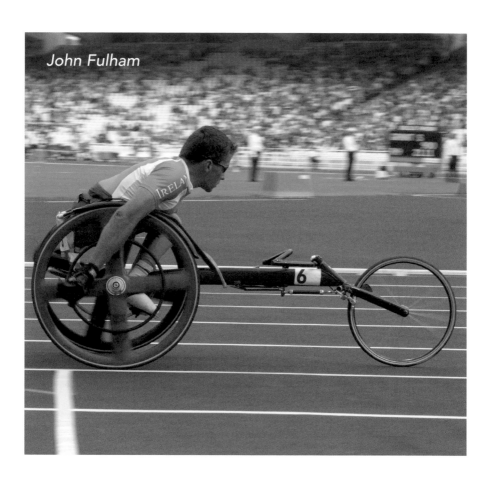

John Fulham

John Fulham

John Fulham is a four-time Paralympian wheelchair racer over 100m and 200m, winning European and National Titles. He won the Dublin Marathon three times and played on the Irish Wheelchair Basketball Team for 14 years. He is currently President of Paralympics Ireland. John was born with Spina Bifida, a congenital defect in the spine. Here he tells his story of a great life in sport.

Expectations weren't high. "Hard Luck Gerry" my Dad was told as he played golf with his friends after I was born. "We don't know how long Johnny is for this world, so we won't operate," my mother was told as she waited for me to have surgery that would help me along. Such were the levels of expectation that people had for me back in 1971, it's any wonder I managed to achieve anything at all, let alone be successful in sport.

Thankfully, I had a mother who allowed me to go headfirst down the slides, climb trees, go to 'normal school' alongside my friends and adventure wherever they adventured. I had a family who entertained my fantasies that I too could be a Jedi Knight like Luke Skywalker. My family encouraged my childhood innocence, allowing me to understand that I was unique, and that world was my oyster. I might do things a bit differently, but that world was still my oyster, full of my own anticipation and expectation. This was a belief that would form the foundation I would call on for when I wanted to achieve; for when sport and life came my way and brought challenges along with them.

What would I say to my 15-year-old self if we crossed paths now? If I knew then what I know now? Alas, there would be too much to say and not enough time to say it. Also, it would be unfair to deny my young self that education which we call experience. The reason we go through experience is because we need to learn as we go, it makes us who and what we are. So, what would I say?

I did not get involved in sport until I was fifteen. My childhood innocence took a few knocks as I grew older and picked up on the perceptions of the world around me. I started to believe their expectations that sport was not for me as there was only Football, Golf, Rugby and GAA. In school PE teachers tried in vain to include me, but just did not know how. Sport for people with disabilities was only developing; the Paralympic Movement was not what it is today. I did not see any people like me taking part. However, eventually I was spotted by some people with disabilities and discovered amazing role models like Harry Pierce and Sean O'Grady, who showed me that there was a way, even if I could not then see how.

I tried everything from table tennis to athletics and found my love, track racing. I borrowed, shared and tried all types of track chairs. I raced, crashed, stripped skin off my fingers as I learned my racing trade. Through it all, I wondered about what worked for others which did not seem to work for me. Thankfully, the role model (the aforementioned Harry Pierce) I found or more accurately, found me, took me under his wing and showed me so much. He built me a one-off unique chair for me. In those moments of trial and error as we created the chair which would be my stepping stone to an international career, I discovered that what worked for others, may not be right for me but could contribute to what was, the how. That lesson gently imparted by a wise and patient man to an arrogantly impetuous messer stood by me in years to come. I came to realise it always had been and would remain my mantra, there is always a way, it's just the matter of 'how'!

When a gym had no hand crank to help me warm up for the early morning weights sessions, I sat on the ground and used the pedals of a stationary bike. Unusual for people to see, but necessary for me. When I moved from Limerick to Dublin to work and train, I lived in a two-storey house for many years. A wheelchair upstairs and a wheelchair downstairs, crawling up the stairs to get from one to the other sorted me out. Not ideal, but it worked for me. Whether during the extreme devastation after my first international competition where I was truly trounced or in the 'call room' before the European Championships where the inevitable pre-race nerves could have stopped me winning that day, that lesson about believing in my own expectations and remembering there is always a way was often the reserve I called on.

I look at my three-year-old son now and marvel at his belief that 'I can do anything'. Even when climbing or playing football, as he says, "Come on Dad keep on trying". A reminder to me to keep pushing on those expectations.

So that is what I would say. Surround yourself with people who believe in you, you will need them and remember other people's expectations of you should never matter. What you expect of yourself will be what counts and when faced with a challenge, there is always a way, it is simply a matter of figuring out your own 'how'. Sport is truly for everyone.
Yours in Sport,
John Fulham.

Dylan McLoughlin

Dylan McLoughlin is a young man who was born with Spina bifida. He is a lover of sport and enjoys a busy and varied sporting life. Here he shares his story of getting out there, getting involved and seeing where sport can take him.

My sporting journey began as an eight-year-old when a stranger approached my mother and me in Smyth's Toy Shop. That stranger, who we would later learn to be Joe Coughlan, was a basketball coach in Titans Basketball Club in Galway. He asked would I be interested in joining a wheelchair basketball team they were in the process of setting up. I said 'Yes' and so began my sporting adventure.
I have been playing competitive wheelchair basketball for 14 years and am now part of the senior team. We train once a week with about 12 on the panel and as we are the only Galway team in the league, we travel all over Ireland to compete. The highlight of my basketball career so far has been winning the Senior Cup against Fr Matthews of Cork in 2017. I love basketball and have made many new friends through the game.

I began Karate when I was 13 years old. I stepped into the unknown with it. I could have limited myself to just basketball, but I wanted a deeper involvement in sport and liked the individual nature of the challenge. Since then I have competed in all competitions; Connachts, All Irelands and The Worlds. The highlight of my Karate career has been winning Gold in the 2017 World Championships in Cork. It is something I am extremely proud of.

Hurling is the game I love the most. The skill and speed of it excites and thrills me. I started going to matches with my Dad from an early age. I followed Galway and my local club Carnmore. When I was 15 years old Tom Cogley, the manager of the Carnmore U15 team, asked me would I help out doing 'stats'. I was delighted to be involved. Back then it was very primitive- a pen and paper approach. Soon after, I was asked by Kevin Shaughnessy to help out with 'stats' for the senior team. The more I did it, the better I became at it and the more value I could add to the team. 2019 was a big year for me. Carl Donlon, the Intermediate Camogie Manager asked me to get involved; again, helping out with the stats. The girls went onto win the county final and gained promotion to senior for the first time. I was thrilled for them and was happy to be there on the sideline contributing in my own way. The same year Enda Flaherty (RIP) was the club minor hurling manager, and he asked me to help out with the team. I was more deeply involved with this team and attended

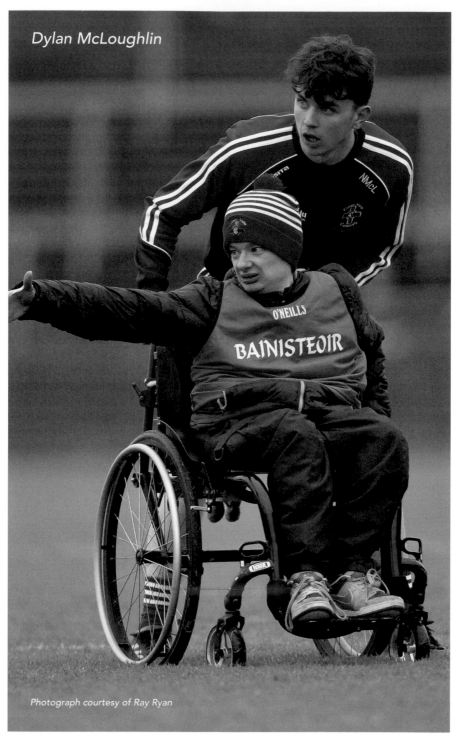

Dylan McLoughlin

Photograph courtesy of Ray Ryan

all training sessions. My role included: keeping attendance, monitoring RPEs (rate of perceived exertion) in training, collating and sending on stats which would help players get a better insight into their performance, and encouraging players to help with their confidence. Often, players would confide in me and this allowed me to give the team management insights into them. Enda was a really kind and thoughtful man, and he made me joint- manager for the semi- final and final. The team went on to be the first Carnmore team to win a County Minor A Championship, and that was my best day to date on a sporting field- to be involved was brilliant.

Today I am still involved with the club minor team and the senior camogie team. I like to think I make a meaningful contribution. My stats work is evolving with new metrics all the time. My dad has started recording the games, and this adds an extra dimension to what we do. I have also been the Club PRO for the past three years. This involves updating the club social media platforms with fixtures, results and match reports. I try to attend all games from underage to adult and I like to write up match reports afterwards. I feel this is useful for people who can't attend the games and also nice for the players.

There are opportunities for everyone in sport. My message is to get involved and put yourself out there. Don't let anyone tell you that you're not able to do this, that or the other- everyone is equal. I am gone almost every evening with sport and this enriches my life greatly. In the future, I hope to stay involved in both playing and management. I love it all... it energises me. I am excited every day to know there's training and games coming up. I think everyone should have excitement in their life and that is why I feel sport is for everyone.

Yours in sport,
Dylan McLoughlin

SUMMARY POINTS - Chapter 28

- Sport is for everyone.
- Some people may have more obstacles to overcome than others.
- There are multiple avenues to involvement in sport in both a playing and coaching/ administration capacity.

CHAPTER 29 : THE END IS THE BEGINNING

"Genius is 1% inspiration and 99% perspiration".
Thomas Edison

Congratulations, you have reached the end. Remember, the final mile is the one that gets walked the least, so very well done for persevering with this book. However, as with almost everything in life, the end is always the beginning and my wish is that you will return to this book in the months and years ahead. I sincerely hope that you have enjoyed the book and found it thought provoking, challenging, useful and inspirational. I hope it has either reinforced your thinking or perhaps ushered in the dawn of a new beginning in your sporting life and beyond. I hope it has helped you look at both sport and yourself from a different perspective and that this new perspective will lead to improvement. I hope it has given you some of the skills and tools to develop in sport, and, indeed, all domains.

Be patient and have faith in yourself. You are enough. Change doesn't happen in a moment, it comes with a series of moments. The road to real achievement takes time and has plenty of bumps on the way, but persevere. Remember, things work out best for those who make the best of the way things work out. If you search yourself hard enough, I am confident you will find a champion. Find a sport or sports you love and stick with them. Appreciate that desire to achieve something only comes when your goal is aligned with your passion and purpose.

Believe things will turn out as they should, provided you purposefully and consistently do as you should. Consciously learn as you go. Invest in yourself and develop as both an athlete and a person. Go to bed an improved version of the person that woke up. Embrace the fact that there are so many potential futures available to you.

I have a fundamental belief in the power of sport for the betterment of the individual and of society and, my wish is that you can now fully appreciate what it has to offer you as you move forward in life. The challenges it will present you, are the opportunities you will need in order to learn and grow. Remember, you don't stop playing because you grow old, you grow old because you stop playing. Work through any fears, setbacks and disappointments that you may encounter along the way.

You can do this; at times you will doubt yourself but don't fall into the trap of selling yourself short. Love your sport, enjoy the friendships it offers you, have fun performing, cherish your victories but don't rest on your laurels. Learn as you go and use those learnings inside, and outside of, sport. Learning is the essence of everything we do. Sport is for life.

TO CONCLUDE I WOULD LIKE YOU TO IMAGINE THAT YOU HAVE RETIRED FROM COMPETITIVE SPORT.

WHAT WOULD YOU LIKE TO BE ABLE TO SAY OF YOUR SPORTING CAREER?

_____

_____

Be the best you can be,
Paul Kilgannon

APPENDIX

SAMPLE DAILY JOURNAL ENTRY

1. What Relationships did I improve/ not improve (+/-) today and why?

+ (Plus)

- George - I gave him a call to catch up
- Anthony - I gave him more time than I normally would at training.
- Damien - we had a good laugh together at school. We are becoming closer.
- Mr Loughlin - I thanked him and acknowledged his good work today when leaving class. I think he really appreciated it.
- Coach Cathal - I asked him for feedback after training and we had a nice chat.

- (Minus)

- Gary - I should have stopped and listened to him when he was trying to talk to me. I can chat to him tomorrow and make up for this.
- Barry - we had words at training and I didn't get to chat to him after. Text him now...
- Joe - Told him I'd call to see him today and I didn't. Call him tomorrow and apologise.
- Kim - didn't return his missed call. Call him tomorrow and apologise.

2. What did I learn/relearn today?

- In hurling my skills are vital. The more I master my skills the more I can simplify the game. I must continue to commit to my individual deliberate practice.

- Scheduling is a powerful tool to plan my day and make the most of my time.

3. 3 good things about today.
- I concentrated and applied myself really well at training.
- We had a lovely dinner this evening with the whole family present.
- I feel I am maturing in my approach to my school work.

4. Did I live by my values (kindness, truth, effort and joy) today?
- By and large I did. I feel I am making progress in how I interact with others and present myself.

5. Did I take care of my priorities/goals?
- 10 minutes individual deliberate hurling skills practice daily - YES.
- Quality time with my family - YES
- Building and Improving relationships - YES.

Visualisation Script

(You may find it useful to adapt this script to fit your sporting context and record it onto your phone so you can listen to it).

- *I want you to take 4-5 deep breaths inhaling all the way in, through the nose for 4 seconds, holding for 2 seconds, and exhaling out for 6 seconds. Releasing any tension, negativity and doubt on each exhalation.*
- *I want you to take yourself forward in time to your next match. I want you to see the crowd, as you enter the stadium, hear and feel the __noise, energy and excitement__ in people's voices as you enter the dressing room.*
- *See yourself taking your seat in the dressing room and notice how __calm__ and __confident__ you feel as you prepare to tog out. Feel the cotton of your socks and shorts on your skin as you get ready. Notice how much __stronger, fitter and healthier__ you are in quite some time. You are __focused yet relaxed__.*
- *Feel __the energy__ in the team huddle before you go out and hear the __powerful communication__ and __encouragement__ from your teammates and management.*
- *See yourself running down the tunnel and soaking in the __energy__ and atmosphere from the crowd. Feel the grass underneath your feet as you bounce onto the pitch in a __powerful manner.__*
- *See yourself going through your warm-up, notice how __sharp__ your touch is as you __strike__ the ball effortlessly. __Feel__ that ball in your hand as you make each catch, on each skill you execute feel the __confidence surge__ through your body as you remind yourself... __'This is my arena – I love the big days. I am powerful- I am prepared'.__ See yourself controlling the ball, catching and passing the ball to your teammate. Hear their communication. Feel the speed and power in your legs as you accelerate.*
- *As you stand for the national anthem, see and feel how __powerful__ your body language is as you stick your chest out and prepare for battle. __'I can overcome any opponent, on any team, under any conditions'.__ Hear the crowd and your teammates sing the anthem. Notice how __focused__ and __confident__ you are.*
- *Now see yourself getting into position and the ref throwing in the ball. See yourself reacting __aggressively__ and __tenaciously__ and winning the ball in front of your man. Feel the surge of __adrenaline__ and __confidence__ as you win it and play it to your teammate.*
- *I want you to see yourself in 8-10 challenges now responding with __huge reactions, and great speed and strength__. See yourself doing all the basics well and winning each outcome.*
- *See yourself winning high ball above your opponent – feel the power and confidence surge through your body on every catch. See yourself: striking that ball with great accuracy and conviction to your teammate, winning the ball with a sharp pick-up, spinning out of the tackle and delivering a fast hand pass to your teammate, chasing down and dispossessing your opponent. See a high ball coming down and see the ball breaking and yourself reacting like a tiger to the breaking ball.*

- *What does that **feel like** when you win these challenges and come out on top with your man?*
- *Now imagine yourself making a mistake or an opponent beating you on that next play. Saying to yourself '**It is not what happened that matters, it's my response.** I am 100% in control of my response. I can't change the past'. Breathe in, reset your body language – head up, shoulders back and chest out. **What's important now? WIN the next play and win the moment now.***

- ***I let nothing upset me, I reset quickly** after every play and focus on winning the next ball.*
- *I am **relentless** and I have a **ravenous hunger** to win every ball.*
- *I am **confident, tenacious and tigerish**.*
- *I am **committed and decisive** on every ball I go for.*
- *I am **dominant and aggressive** on every high ball.*
- *I love hitting the ball well my striking feels **effortless** and as I hit my target.*
- *I am **alert and vigilant** on the breaking ball.*
- *I am **calm and relaxed** .Nothing disturbs my **attitude and focus**.*
- *I have an advantage due to my mental and physical preparation.*
- *I can overcome any challenge- **my mind adapts** to any obstacles. **I work hard, I am clever, and I make good decisions on the ball.***

- *I want you to now see a player you really admire in front of you. Notice how confident they look and the qualities they bring every time they play.*
- *I want you to take on some of their characteristics by stepping into his/her boots and absorbing **the confidence, the strength, the character** that they possess and adding it to the qualities that you already **possess**.*
- *What does it feel like to perform even **more confidently** on every ball? See yourself beating your opponent and finding a teammate with a great pass. Feel the **energy and confidence** in your body as you run back into position.*
- *Now every time you practice your visualisation you get **even more confident**, feel more **focused**, feel more **emotions**.*
- ***I am a warrior. I am a champion of my mind. I am relentless. I have an exceptional attitude and I understand what those words mean.***
- *Now each time listen to this audio, I will feel more **belief, more confident** in where I am going, a real sense of having a plan and implementing it.*
- *I am going to count from 1 to 5 and on each exhalation, you will feel even more confident, refreshed and relaxed.*
- *1 – feeling loose, limp and relaxed*
- *2 – from head to toe feeling calm and refreshed*
- *3 – a real sense of confidence and readiness*
- *4 – begin to open your eyes*
- *And 5 feeling fantastic in every way.*

Affirmation Scripts

SKILL PERFECTION

*I pride myself for investing quality practice in **MY SKILLS** game **EVERYDAY**. I love to practice passing, shooting, catching and tackling.*
I practice this when I am fresh but also when I am mentally tired as I know this will give me an advantage over my opponents, because I recognize the short games importance.
*This is what makes me a **GREAT PLAYER**.*
*Practicing short grip shots regularly with quality and focus is a key to the quest and a critical part of the process. I am dedicated to seeing how **GREAT I CAN BE** at my sport.*

RELENTLESS WILL TO WIN

*I love the last fifteen minutes of a Game. Regardless of score this is a time for complete concentration and focus on the process. I can best **IMPACT THE GAME** when I **CONTROL** what I have control of, that is my mind.*
*In the last 15 minutes I play **EVERY SINGLE MOMENT**. In **THIS ZONE** nothing distracts me or upsets me. I see other players tiring and making mistakes. I get stronger and my concentration gives me this edge.*
*Being in this Zone is why I play. It's a testing Time and I am **AGGRESSIVE** and **FOCUSED**. I keep a clear mind on **EVERY BALL**. I live in the present moment. Any time I even begin to get ahead and think about winning or losing, I catch that thought and throw it away. I get back to my next ball. I never care about scoreboards or what others are doing because **I TRUST MY OWN ABILITY**.*

CHALLENGE AND ADVERSITY

I TAKE GREAT PRIDE IN MY MENTAL STRENGTH. I THRIVE BY TURNING ADVERSITY INTO EVEN MORE STRENGTH.
*When the Game gets tough, **I WILL ALWAYS STAND TALL AND TAKE CONTROL**. It is my strength in the face of challenge that makes me **GREAT**.*
*I know I will be challenged along the way, I know the opposition and challenge will be strong but **I DEMAND OF MYSELF THAT I WILL BE STRONGER**.*
*If I make a mistake I know it's **TEMPORARY**. By Resetting and **FOCUSING ON THE PRESENT** is how I respond to the situation. I Believe in my skill, believe in my desire and **RESET**.*
I CAN'T CHANGE THE PAST BUT I CAN CHANGE THE FUTURE
It is not about where I have been. It is about where I am going. It is not about how I have been playing. It is about how I am going to play

---

I AM A GREAT PLAYER

I never let how I am playing affect how I feel about my ability to win the ball. I love it when I am hitting it well and I love it when the ball isn't always coming the way I wanted it to come.

*I take it as a personal challenge and a real source of **pride** to win when I'm not on top of my game in spite of being diligent and dedicated in practice.*

*These days test my patience but **I AM STRONG INSIDE**. I keep fighting for the ball until I run out of time. I see other players who start making excuses to justify playing poorly when they are not playing the way they'd like.*

I ACCEPT THIS CHALLENGE AND WILL RELENTLESSLY ATTACK THE GAME AND BE BRAVE AND UNFORGIVING IN MY ATTEMPTS TO WIN.

*I stay on my mission **AND ENJOY** the challenge of beating my man.*

I believe it is days like these that keep me in the championship. It is days like these that separate me from others who give into despair. It is my chance to separate myself from others.

I will trust myself and honour my commitment to my talent and myself. I love being strong and patient when others cave in or give in to self-pity. I am focused.

I never waver in my attitude when playing competitively

Emotional Maturity

*I pride myself in being a **CONSISTENT** and **CONTROLLED** in GAMES. **Nothing distracts me.***

I AM LIKE GRANITE, I AM SOLID.

RESILIENCE** is my middle name. I always **DELIVER IN ADVERSITY**. I stay patient, look for the next ball. I have the heart of a lion and the mind of a champion. I never let myself get frustrated, try to force things or try to make anything happen. **I FOCUS ON MY OWN GAME** always in control of my mind and emotions, **NOTHING FAZES ME

*I take **GREAT PRIDE** in this emotional maturity and patience because no one gave me this attitude. I developed it. I gave it to myself. I earned it. It is now one of my most valued strengths.*

THESE CAN BE READ DAILY AND RECORDED AND LISTENED TO AFFIRM AND ENFORCE POSITIVE PERFORMANCE BEHAVIOURS

Reasons for a Shorter or Longer than average Menstrual Cycle *(list is not exhaustive).*

	Shorter cycle	Longer cycle
Biological	Endocrine pathology: • Thyroid problems	Endocrine pathology: • Thyroid problems • Diabetes mellitus
	Uterine pathology: Endometriosis (condition whereby the tissue that normally forms the inside of the uterus grows elsewhere in the body)	Uterine pathology: • Uterine fibroids (muscle and fibrous tissue growth) • Endometriosis
	Pelvic inflammatory disease	Ovarian pathology: • Polycystic ovarian syndrome (PCOS; cysts in the ovaries) • Ovarian fibroids (muscle and fibrous tissue growth) • Ovarian cysts (fluid filled sacs)
	Anovulation (lack of ovulation)	Medications – anti-inflammatories, hormonal contraception, anti-epileptics (to treat epilepsy)
	Age (cycle generally gets shorter with increasing age above 40)	Puberty – for the first few years a prolonged menstrual cycle can be normal.
	Illness	Early pregnancy
Psychological	Stress	Stress
	Eating disorders	Eating disorders
Social	Birth control	Birth control
	Weight loss or weight gain	Weight loss or weight gain
		Excessive exercise

QR CODES

1. Double-Leg
Squat

2. Hip Hinge

3. Split Lunge

4a. Squat
(Single-Leg)

4b. Single Leg
Skater Squat

5. Trunk
Stability Drill

6. Hip Lock

7. Lower Limb
Stability Drill

8. Hop and
Stick

9. Deadlift
Comparison

10. Wall Drill
Posture Holds

11. Wall Drill
Acceleration

12. Band
Marches

13. Band
Skips

14. Tall
and Fall

15. Two-
Point Starts

16. Gareth
Bale

17. Christen
Press

18. Ankling

19. A Skip

20. B Skip

21. Dribbles /
Bleeds

22. Wickets

23. Ronaldo

24. Declaration

MOVEMENT EFFICIENCY

Exercise 1: Double-Leg Squat

Technique

The entry level squat exercise is the Body-Weight Squat. Set up with your feet approximately hip-width apart and your hands folded across your chest. Ensure the sole of your foot has FULL contact with the ground and that both feet are facing directly forwards (in some cases the anatomical constraints of the individual will not allow this and it is best point the toes out a little). Slowly lower yourself towards the floor by bending at the hips, knees and ankles. Keep Trunk Upright and Hip/Knee/Ankle aligned throughout.

Target: Achieve Position of Thigh Parallel to Floor without loss of Trunk alignment or Hip/Knee/Ankle alignment

Common Faults

Movement errors that we want to eliminate during the double-leg squat include:

i) Excessive Rib Flare: where the rib cage pokes through the front of the shirt, most commonly during the lowering portion of the squat movement. This is usually a sign that you have lost control of your Upper Trunk position.

ii) Increased Forward Tilt of the Pelvis: This is often visualised by an exaggerated "arch" in the lower back, usually seen again during the lowering part of the exercise. This is a sign that you may have lost control of Pelvic positioning.

iii) Excessive Forward Trunk Lean: This is demonstrated by the trunk moving too far forward relative to the position of the feet. This may reflect an inability to control the Lower Trunk appropriately during the squat movement.

iv) Inward Knee Drift: Loss of Hip/Knee/Ankle alignment most commonly occurs by the knee drifting too far inwards during the lowering movement of the squat. Whilst this is not a massive problem when performing a bodyweight movement, it can be a problem once weight is added to the exercise. This movement fault is usually a sign that you have lost control of Hip alignment during the squat.

Training Cues

The key to performing a quality squat is to ensure good control of the trunk and pelvis while coordinating movement well through the hips, knees and ankles. As mentioned earlier, proper weight transfer through the hips is often a missing link; this results in excessive stress being placed on other regions, such as the spine, groin and knee.

If this is the case, try reaching forwards with both hands as you begin the lowering movement. This helps to counter-balance your weight so that you can "sit back" through your hips to initiate the squat movement. In addition, placing a small loop of resistance band around knees, can further assist in engaging the gluteal muscles at the back of the hip to assist this movement.

Dosage

Repetition range will vary depending on the focus of the exercise but you should be able to complete 12 bodyweight reps maintaining perfect form throughout.

Exercise 2: Hip Hinge/Deadlift

Technique

The entry-level exercise to train the hip hinge is the Waiter's Bow. Stand with feet hip-width apart and arms folded across the chest. Keep both knees on a slight degree of bend and consciously press your feet into the floor, exaggerating pressure through the middle part of your foot (area between arch of foot and ball of big toe).

From here, bend from your hips by "sitting back" into the movement. Ensure you maintain a neutral spine as your shoulders move forward; also, ensure the slight angle of bend at your knee does NOT change throughout the movement. If you are performing the exercise correctly, a stretch should be felt in both hamstrings reasonably early in the movement. Once you've reached this point, return slowly to the starting position, again making sure that all movement is taking place at the hips.

Common Faults

This is generally a more difficult exercise to master than the squat, so it is crucial that you pay attention to technique throughout. Some of the movement errors to look out for include:

i) Increased Forward Tilt of Pelvis: As mentioned earlier, this may be demonstrated by excessive arching of the lower back and is usually a sign that control of the Lower Back and Pelvis region is not sufficient. This may also be a sign that your ability to recruit your Gluteal muscles to extend your hips during this movement is not efficient.

ii) Insufficient Backwards Weight Shift of the Hips: This is a common fault that needs to be identified and corrected early. As the trunk lowers, the hips should simultaneously shift backwards to ensure a true hip hinge. Compensations that occur if this fails to happen include excessive bending of the lower back +/- collapse at the knees.

Training Cues

The 3 main things to remember when performing this exercise are:
-Tall Hips
-Soft Knees
-Neutral Spine

Your foot connection with the floor also needs to be maintained throughout. As you shift your hips backwards, your toes may want to lift off the ground as the weight shifts onto your heels. Avoid this by consciously keeping them pushed into the floor.

If you are struggling to execute the exercise as detailed, make it a little easier to begin with by holding onto a chair or pushing your hands into a wall. This will provide extra trunk support that should help in performing a proper hip hinge movement.

Dosage

Repetition range will vary depending on the focus of the exercise but you should be able to complete 12 bodyweight reps maintaining perfect form throughout.

Exercise 3: Split Lunge

Technique

Set up in a split kneeling position, with your front leg flat on the floor and your back leg extended so that you're pushing through your big toe. Both knees should make 90degree angles and your trunk should be in a neutral position. The shoulder, hip and knee of your back limb should form a straight line.

With your hands placed on your hips, lift yourself slowly into a standing position to push through the Midfoot of your front leg, while concurrently pushing through the big toe of the back leg. Slowly return to the kneeling position without losing control of the trunk and pelvis (See Fig 3b).

The 3 main things we are looking for during this exercise are:

-Vertical Thigh Position of BACK LEG

-Vertical Shin Position of FRONT LEG

-VERTICAL Trunk Position

Common Faults

i) Excessive Forward Movement: This will be manifested by changes in the positions of the Back Thigh and Front Shin-Bones where they lose the aforementioned vertical alignment that we are looking for. This reduces the activity of the hip and trunk muscles that we are looking to train in this exercise.

ii) Excessive Anterior Pelvic Tilt: As per the previous exercises, this may be seen by increased arching in the lower back region and associated prominence of your ribcage through the front of your shirt.

iii) Excessive Forward Trunk Lean: As per the squat earlier, this is seen by the trunk moving too far forwards in relation to the position of the feet. This movement pattern can result in excessive strain being placed on structures of the front of the hip and groin.

Training Cues

The main training point here is that we adhere to the 3 rules above, i.e. Vertical Back Thigh, Vertical Front Shin, Vertical Trunk throughout. To assist with maintaining this position, engage the core at the start of each repetition by subtly pulling the lower rib cage towards your belly button and keeping this tension in your core for the duration of each rep.

Dosage

Repetition range will vary depending on the focus of the exercise but you should be able to complete 12 bodyweight reps on each side, maintaining perfect form throughout.

Exercise 4: Squat (Single-Leg)

Technique

Stand on one leg with a bench or chair placed behind you. The height of the bench may need to be adjusted depending on your height and ability to perform the exercise correctly.

With hands reaching in front, slowly lower yourself to the chair by bending at the hip, knee and ankle, until your buttock touches the bench. As per the previous exercises, ensure that your trunk stays vertical throughout and maintain appropriate hip/knee/ankle alignment for each repetition. Sole of the foot should remain flat on the floor throughout.

Common Faults

i) Excessive Inward Drift of the Knee: This is where the knee visibly tracks substantially inside the big toe, usually during the lowering part of the squat movement. It may reflect reduced muscular control at the hip joint, particularly of the gluteal muscle group, and will generally place undue stress on other lower body tissues, such as the groin, knee and ankle if it is not corrected early.

ii) Excessive Lateral Trunk Sway: This movement compensation will usually be seen in combination to the excessive inward knee drift as outlined above. It occurs when the athlete shifts weight excessively onto the standing leg while performing the single-leg squat movement. This places extra workload on other body tissues, especially the groin.

iii) Pelvic Drop: This occurs where the pelvis of the opposite/free side drops while the athlete performs the single-leg squat. It is usually a sign that the stabilising muscles of the standing hip, in particularly the outer gluteal region, are not working optimally and may need to be trained. Persistence of this movement pattern over time may cause overstress of structures such the groin, hip or knee.

iv) Toe-Out Foot Alignment: This is where the foot turns outwards during the squatting movement. More often than not, this occurs in reaction to the knee moving inwards as mentioned earlier and is a compensation to assist the hip muscles to create stability around the hip. However, it is not an efficient movement strategy and can overload other lower limb structures if it occurs during higher intensity sporting movements such as landing, decelerating and changing direction.

Training Cues

If you're finding it difficult to perform the single-leg squat as per the guidelines above, you can again use the stability of a wall or chair to hold onto for support. Another option is to reach the opposite leg behind while reaching in front with the hand on that side. This helps to create a counter-balance effect to promote better weight transfer through the hip and trunk stability, in turn leading to a more efficient movement pattern.

Dosage

Repetition range will vary depending on the focus of the exercise but you should be able to complete 8 bodyweight reps on each side, maintaining perfect form throughout.

Exercise 5: Trunk Stability Test

Technique

Lie on your back, with your legs off the floor so that you are making right angles at your hips, knees and ankles. Hands should be placed across your chest, with your chin tucked slightly to ensure your neck is in a neutral position.

From here, activate your abdominal muscles by consciously pulling your lower ribs in the direction of your pelvis. As you do this you should feel your lower back flattens into the floor. SLOWLY drop both legs to the floor, keeping your back pressed into the floor throughout. Once you feel you can no longer keep your lower back in FULL contact with the floor, or if your lower ribs start to lift up, stop the leg lowering movement and let your legs drop to the floor. The longer you can control the leg lowering movement WITHOUT your lower back losing contact with the floor indicates a better score of lower abdominal capacity.

Common Faults

i) Loss of Lower Back Alignment: This is seen by the lower back lifting off the floor at any stage during the exercise. It reflects an inability to maintain stability and control of the lower trunk and means the level of difficulty of the exercise needs to be reduced so that it can be trained properly.

ii) Loss of Neck Alignment: This reflects loss of control of the upper trunk and again means you need to regress the difficulty to train effectively.

iii) Change in Tempo: The slower the leg lowering movement is performed, the better. Making the movement faster indicates that some of your "mover" muscles, in particular the hip flexor and groin, are assisting. This means we are not getting a true reflection of the function of the abdominals. Therefore, the slower the better when you're performing this drill.

Training Cues

This is a deceptively difficult movement to execute properly. Thus, it is better to start at a level where all parts of the system can be controlled. Holding both ends of a resistance band in your hands, helps pull the lower ribs down to engage the abdominals effectively. To ensure you are keeping this position throughout each repetition, place a bottle of water on the upper abdominal region. Your aim is to prevent the bottle from falling throughout the course of the exercise.

Dosage

Aim to perform 4-6 repetitions without taking a break, ensuring you keep perfect form throughout. If you struggle with the movement, make it easier by only dropping ONE leg at a time.

Exercise 6: Hip Lock

Technique

Stand with your back at a wall with both arms extended fully overhead to make yourself as tall as possible. Lift one leg off the floor and place in a position where the hip, knee and ankle joints are all positioned at 90 degree angles. Keeping stability on your standing leg, aim to close the distance between the shoulder and pelvis on your UNSUPPORTED side by hitching the pelvis upwards. This movement may be accompanied by slight outward rotation of the foot on that side, which is perfectly fine. At the same time, reach the fingers of the STANDING side hand as high as possible towards the sky. The net effect of these movements is that you should feel a strong muscle contraction of the gluteal/outer hip muscles of the STANDING leg. Aim to hold this position for 3-5 seconds before switching to the opposite leg.

Common Faults

i) Excessive Knee Lift: On the unsupported/free leg, the aim is to elevate the Pelvis, not the Knee. If the knee is lifting above knee height, it usually means the hip flexor muscles on the unsupported leg are assisting the movement due to reduced activity of the gluteal/outer hip muscles of the standing leg. If this is the case, you should regress to an easier version of the drill, as explained in the Exercise Progression section later.

ii) Excessive Lateral Trunk Flexion: Again, weakness of the standing gluteal/ lateral hip muscles of the standing leg may manifest in you leaning or rotating the trunk towards that side when trying to perform the hip lock movement. This is also a sign that the exercise should be regressed to meet your ability so that the appropriate movement pattern can be achieved. You can work through the progressions of the exercise once you are able to demonstrate proper form at each level of difficulty. As with all of the drills described, the quality of how you coordinate each repetition is of primary importance. Therefore, start at entry level with each exercise and only progress once you have nailed the technique appropriately.

Training Cues
In addition to the instructions above, one simple cue to remember when performing the hip lock is to "finish tall" and really reach the stance-side hand as high as possible without any compensations taking place in the trunk. As your ability improves, aim to challenge the movement by lifting the standing heel an inch off the floor (think of just enough space to fit 2 credit cards between your heel and floor). This will reduce your support and add a greater demand in executing the hip lock properly. Finally, aim to "fight" to stay in the lock position for at least 3 seconds for each repetition as mentioned earlier. The ability to hold the hip lock reflects good capacity of the target muscles to support this position during the crucial mid-stance phase of running.

Dosage
Aim to perform 4 repetitions each leg, fighting to hold the hip lock position for at least 3 seconds per rep, as mentioned earlier.

Exercise 7: Lower Limb Stability Drill
Technique
For the lower limb stability exercise, set yourself up in a split-stance position. There should only be 3-4 inches separating your feet; this is to ensure you keep a narrow base of support that will provide a stability challenge during the exercise.

From here, the aim is to get 90% of your body weight onto your front leg. To achieve this, shift your weight forward onto that limb by bending your knee and pushing your kneecap as far as possible over your toes, to the point where your heel wants to lift. Once you've established this knee position, consciously push into the floor through the midfoot (part of your foot between arch and ball of big toe). Finally, shift your pelvis and trunk forward over that side until it feels like you're just about to lose your balance. At this point, you should feel a strong muscular contraction through the entire leg. Hold the position for 10 seconds without allowing any movement of the ankle, knee or hip joints.

Once you've established this position, you need to challenge your ability to hold it by adding movement of your trunk. Start by reaching towards the floor to touch your big toe. When performing this action, take a gentle inhale through your NOSE, then EXHALE FULLY THROUGH YOUR MOUTH as you bend forwards. You need to make sure that the positions of the hip, knee and ankle of the front leg DO NOT CHANGE during this reaching movement, i.e. you should be bending from your BACK. The ability to hold these positions fixed reflects the ability of your muscle system to produce adequate force to keep those joints stable, which is what we're ultimately aiming to train.

Common Faults

i) Not Bending from Back: The hardest part of this drill for most athletes is "letting go" of the back. We're generally told that bending our back is bad for us, which is untrue, especially as it applies to this exercise. Therefore, in order to train the lower body joints to be stable, we want to let all the movement occur through our spine.

ii) Hip Sinking or Lowering: Inability to keep proper stability around the hip may be seen by the hip "sinking" towards the floor as you perform the forward bend. Again, this is not the desired outcome so really focus on holding the hip high throughout each repetition of the exercise.

iii) Loss of Knee Angle: It is important that you hold the "knee-over-toes" position for the entirety of the exercise. Your knee may want to straighten at the point where you start to return to the upright position, as your quads try to kick in. However, the aim instead is to keep the knee in a position of slight bent by using the hamstring and calf muscles.

Training Cues

Think from the ground up as follows:

-Think of bursting a balloon under the midfoot; hold this pressure for the entirety of the drill

-Keep knee forward so that you cannot seen your toes if you look down from above

-Shift hip and pelvis forward until you feel 90% of your bodyweight is on the front leg (Heel should be nearly coming off the floor)

-Exhale Slowly and Fully as you bend forwards, think of blowing up a balloon. Reach with your fingers to make your arms as long as possible. Hip stays high throughout.

Dosage

Aim to perform 4-6 repetitions each leg. Start with a small range of movement and build that as you get more comfortable and confident in doing the exercise.

Exercise 8: Hop and Stick

Exercise Technique

Set up in the exact same start position as Exercise 7: Lower Limb Stability Drill. Once you've achieved the appropriate joint positioning of your front leg, take the back leg off the ground so that all your body weight is now on your front leg. In this position, consciously tighten every muscle from the ground up through your leg to build as strong a contraction as possible. Using this muscle force, push the ground away to jump forwards, MAKING SURE YOU

LAND IN EXACTLY THE SAME LEG POSITION. Reset your start position for each repetition to ensure you are in the desired alignment.

Common Faults

i) Loss of Joint Position on Landing: As with the last drill, the ability to execute the proper angles is crucial. If you're finding this difficult to achieve, particularly as you land, then make the exercise easier by practicing hopping from one leg to another first so that you can develop the appropriate landing technique. Also, do not worry about jump distance in the beginning. The priority with this exercise is the ability to absorb force, or decelerate, your body efficiently. You can focus on force production, or acceleration, at a later stage once your landing mechanics have reached a satisfactory level of competence.

ii) Bouncing or Sinking: When you land or stick from your hop, we want your leg to be in the most stable position possible. If there is movement or "bouncing", in particular at your knee when landing, it is a sign that you have not established sufficient muscle control of the limb. If this is the case, you should regress the exercise so that you are able to execute landing with sufficient control.

Training Cues

Focus on the exact same cues as the last exercise in order to achieve optimal joint positioning for each repetition.

Look to really challenge your starting position by shifting enough weight onto your stance leg that it almost feels like you're about to lose balance and stumble forwards.

Dosage

Aim to perform 4-5 repetitions each leg. As you get more comfortable and confident with the exercise, progress the difficulty by increasing the distance of each hop. Progress further, by increasing the height of each hop.

Types of Injuries

Site	Acute Injury	Overuse/Chronic Injury
Bone	Fracture Periosteal contusion	Stress fracture Stress reaction Osteitis Periosteitis Apophysitis
Articular cartilage	Osteochondral/chondral fracture Minor osteochondral injury	Chondropathy
Joint	Dislocation Subluxation	Synovitis Osteoarthritis
Ligament	Sprain/tear (Grade I - III)	Inflammation
Muscle	Strain/tear (Grade I - III) Contusion Cramp Acute compartment syndrome	Chronic compartment syndrome Delayed onset muscle soreness Focal tissue thickening
Tendon	Tear (complete or partial)	Tendinopathy - Paratenonitis - Tenosynovitis - Tendinosis - Tendinitis
Bursa	Traumatic bursitis	Bursitis
Nerve	Neuropraxia	Entrapment Minor nerve injury/irritation Altered neuromechanical sensitivity
Skin	Laceration Abrasion Puncture wound	Blister Callus

Reproduced from Clinical Sports Medicine Fourth Edition

Sample Recipes

Porridge Bread
Makes 6-8 slices

- 3 cups porridge
- 2 Eggs
- 2 tablespoons honey
- 2 bananas
- 1 cup of walnuts and flaked almonds mixed
- 1 cup of mixed frozen berries
- Flaked coconuts

Preparation
- In a large mixing bowl mash bananas and eggs together
- Mix porridge, berries and nuts with the banana and egg mix in a large mixing bowl
- In a baking tray lined with non-stick baking paper, add mix and spread evenly
- Place in oven @ 220 for 45-50 minutes

Homemade Pizza
Makes 4 Pizzas

- 4 Wholemeal wraps
- 1 can of chopped tomatoes
- 1 can of drained chickpeas
- 1 can of drained kidney beans
- Sliced Ham/chicken
- Baby Spinach

Preparation
- In a large mixing bowl mix chopped tomatoes, chickpeas and kidney beans to make pizza base
- On each wrap, transfer the mix to the top of the wraps and evenly spread.
- Add as much spinach and meat as you wish
- When placing pizza on tray, spray oil on tray so to allow for easy removal when cooked
- Place in oven @ 200 degrees until the edges of the wraps begin to crisp.

About The Author

Paul Kilgannon is an Author, Sports Coach and Coaching Consultant. He is the creator of the CARVER Coaching Framework, which is used internationally by coaches across multiple sports.

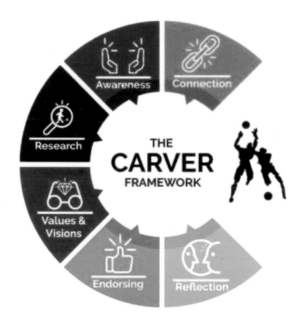

Paul's services include:
Coach Mentoring.
Coaching Seminars & Workshops.
Club Consultancy.
Team Workshops.
Team Management Consultancy.
Athlete Mentoring.
Athlete Development Workshops.

Contact Paul on www.carvercoachingframework.com
Follow Paul @carver_coaching on Twitter, Instagram & TikTok and at
Carver Coaching on Facebook.